Triangle Pose: Yoga's Happy Pose; Modified Triang

Anyone can do yoga's Triangle pose (*trikonasana*), known as the happy pose because it opens your Venus *chakra* (the energy center located behind your heart) and allows joy to fill your body and radiate within you and from you. Triangle tones your spine and waist, stimulates your bowels and intestines, strengthens your legs and ankles, improves your circulation, develops your chest, and strengthens your breath.

Modified Triangle is a perfectly correct form of Triangle for beginners. Reach for your knee. As your torso and shoulders become more flexible, you'll be able to reach farther.

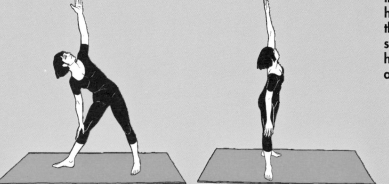

In Triangle, hand to knee, the hips, pelvis, shoulders, and heart are all aligned.

How Many Triangles in Triangle?

The triangle is used as a spiritual symbol in many different cultures: Pagan goddess traditions used the triangle to symbolize the virgin, mother, and crone. In Egypt, the triangle represented the female principle, motherhood, and the moon. In Arabia, the triangle symbolized the three lunar Goddesses. The Celtic shamrock was a three-way design originally representing the three mothers. The double triangle symbolizes creation in the Tantric tradition. The downward-pointing triangle is the *yoni yantra* or symbolic representation of feminine sexuality and the Mother Goddess, while the upward-pointing triangle symbolizes the Mother Goddess's son and spouse to whom she gave birth repeatedly and who was her mirror image. And while Brahma, Vishnu, and Shiva later took the title of the Hindu trinity, it was originally a Goddess trinity. Mindbodyspirit is a triangular relationship, as is mother, father, and child, or even "me, myself, and I." You can find triangles and three-way figures and concepts all over your life if you look. Think about that as you bend into Triangle.

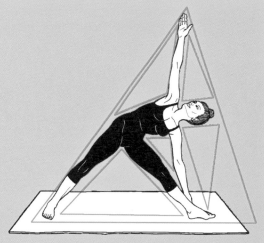

Downward Facing Dog: Another Triangle

Downward Facing Dog pose (*adho mukha shvanasana*) brings heat to your body, strengthens and stretches your spine, and restores your heart by stimulating *kundalini* energy in your Venus *chakra*. In Kundalini Yoga, Downward Dog pose is often called Triangle pose. *Kundalini* energy moves through the *chakra* centers along the spine, leading to awakenings of enlightenment.

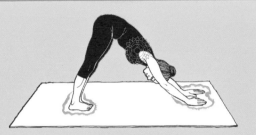

Namaste: Yoga Calm and Center

Namaste means "I salute the divine light within you."

Whether standing in Mountain pose (*tadasana*) or sitting in a meditation pose, practice yoga breathing—full, deep breaths. Yoga helps maintain balance and posture, which leads to internal balance and good health. *Namaste*, the prayer *mudra*, honors each one of us as the divine beings we *are!*

Inhale and lift your arms.

Exhale and return to *namaste*, prayer pose.

Yoga's Guidelines for Living

Incorporating these yoga guidelines for living into your yoga practice will enhance your success—in yoga and in life!

Yoga Don'ts: *Yamas*

Do no harm (*Ahimsa*)

Tell no lies (*Satya*)

Do not steal (*Asteya*)

Cool it, Casanova (*Brahmacharya*)

Don't be greedy (*Aparigraha*)

Yoga Do's: *Niyamas*

Be pure (*Saucha*)

Be content (*Santosha*)

Be disciplined (*Tapas*)

Be studious (*Svadhyaya*)

Be devoted (*Ishvara-Pranidhana*)

A
A L P H A

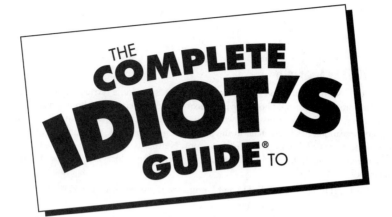

Yoga

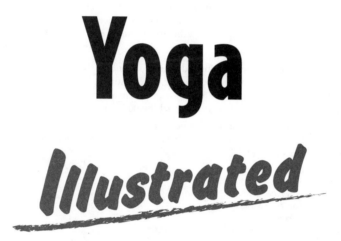

Third Edition

by *Joan Budilovsky and Eve Adamson*

ALPHA

Publisher: *Marie Butler-Knight*
Product Manager: *Phil Kitchel*
Senior Managing Editor: *Jennifer Chisholm*
Senior Acquisitions Editor: *Mike Sanders*
Book Producer: *Lee Ann Chearney/Amaranth*
Development/Senior Production/Copy Editor: *Christy Wagner*
Cartoonist: *Chris Eliopoulos*
Illustrator: *Wendy Frost*
Photographer: *Saeid Lahouti*
Cover/Book Designer: *Trina Wurst*
Indexer: *Angie Bess*
Layout/Proofreading: *Angela Calvert, John Etchison, Trina Wurst*
Graphics: *Tammy Graham, Dennis Sheehan*

Joan Budilovsky, yogi and co-author of this book, demonstrates the yoga poses depicted in the photographs.

Contents at a Glance

Contents

Foreword

The world-famous violinist Sir Yehudi Menuhin said about yoga that it is "a technique ideally suited to prevent physical and mental illness and to protect the body generally, developing an inevitable sense of self-reliance and assurance." Yoga did not make him a musical genius, but gave him energy, balance, and a sense of well-being for the last half of his life, allowing him full expression of his great talent.

Yoga can do the same for anyone. Old or young. Male or female. Busy or super busy. In fact, yoga in one form or another is practiced by several million people today. It has been part of the kaleidoscope of our Western culture for more than a century now and has proven incredibly effective in the maintenance of a sound body and mind and even the restoration of one's health. This is why several progressive insurance companies are now including yoga in their alternative therapies coverage.

Yoga is a tradition that looks back upon at least 5,000 years of experience and experimentation. Although it was created in India in a different cultural environment, the basic insights and laws on which it is based are valid anywhere in the world. Of course, there is much more to yoga than its potency as a system of health care. But this is for you to discover.

In this book, you will be gently but persuasively guided into the beginnings of yoga practice. The authors serve as knowledgeable and cheerful friends, motivating you all the way. Within these pages you will find no lack of encouragement, and everything is explained step by step. So please, take the leap into what you will discover to be a rewarding and healing experience.

Georg Feuerstein, Ph.D., M. Litt.

Georg Feuerstein, Ph.D., M. Litt., is director of the Yoga Research Center; author of *Shambhala Encyclopedia of Yoga* and *Shambhala Guide to Yoga*; and a contributing editor of *Yoga Journal.*

Introduction

Imagine waking up one morning to find that all stresses in your life have been replaced with total joy. Yes, joy—the kind of pure joy you felt as a child when it was summer and the sun was shining and you had nothing to do but explore the whole world. Now, imagine possessing a strong, flexible body over which you have complete control. To top that off (literally!), imagine a mind free of chaotic thought, confusion, and uncertainty. Imagine pure health, pure consciousness, and pure bliss. This is the realm of the yogi.

And that yogi is you! Even if this realm seems far away now, you will soon be on an amazing journey. We have each traveled down our own yoga paths a little way. We've looked ahead, peeked over the horizon of the next few hills, and now we'd like to give you some hints about how to make the most of what's in store for you on your journey into yourself. Yoga is a process of self-discovery, and everyone's discoveries will be different, but we hope to steer you toward the potential "you," the perfect "you," the "you" waiting to be set free.

It won't be difficult. Yoga is beautifully simple. In fact, we think you're gonna love it!

How to Use This Book

This book is divided into seven parts, each bringing yoga into your life in a different way.

Part 1, "Yoga Union and You," eases you into the concepts of yoga. We talk about why this ancient Eastern system of health has become such a hit with modern Westerners and how yoga can improve all aspects of your fitness, including your performance in other sports. We introduce you to your body, yoga-style, and reveal what yoga can do to improve your mental state as well as your physical condition.

Part 2, "Getting Spiritual with Yoga," includes a little history, just to put yoga in context, then explains the various types of yoga. Next, we talk about the "rules" (yoga's guidelines for living), and the finer points of Hatha Yoga, the most popular form of yoga in the West.

Part 3, "Starting Your Yoga Practice," will help you do just that. We offer advice on how to find a yoga class and teacher, how to practice yoga at home, what to wear, how to overcome any mental stumbling blocks, when to practice, how to squeeze yoga into a busy day, and how to craft your own, personalized practice. This part of the book will help you make yoga your own.

Part 4, "Strength: Postures to Build Endurance," is the first part of exercises. We show you outstanding standing postures, beautiful backbends, terrific twists, and inversions, including the famous headstand posture.

Part 5, "Calm: Postures to Quiet the Body and Mind," is the part of calming and centering postures, including sitting and meditative poses, breathing exercises, forward bends, *chakras* (energy centers in the body), *mudras* (meditation hand positions), *mantras* (centering chants), and *mandalas* (circular art designed to focus the mind), and a detailed discussion of *shavasana*, or Corpse pose. You'll learn how to let go of your mind, and you'll discover how great stress management can feel.

Part 6, "Yoga Sessions: Energy Flow," will bring you sequences of yoga postures you can use in your practice. We'll start with *vinyasanas*, dynamic combinations of postures that will have you breaking a sweat. Then we'll give you some 5-minute yoga sessions and 15-minute yoga sessions for when you only have a little time, and a sample 30-minute and 60-minute yoga session for when you've got more time to spend.

Part 7, "Living Your Yoga," is all about the yoga lifestyle. We'll show you how to practice yoga with a partner, whether a friend, your life partner, or your child. You can even practice yoga with your whole family! You'll learn why yoga is great for all the stages in a woman's life, from PMS to menopause, then we'll go on to explain the yoga philosophy of food, how to eat for a healthier yoga practice, and at last, how yoga can optimize your body's healing capacity, whether you suffer from minor headaches or a more serious chronic condition.

Yoga Jewels

Throughout this book, we've added four types of extra information in boxes, for your enlightenment:

 Know Your Sanskrit _____
These boxes give you definitions for Sanskrit (the classical language of India) terms and correct pronunciations, too, so you can talk the talk.

 A Yoga Minute _____
These boxes are full of fun anecdotes and trivia about the fascinating world of yoga.

 Wise Yogi Tells Us _____
These special boxes offer you tips and advice for living your yoga.

Ouch! _____
These cautionary boxes contain information about how to avoid potential problems.

Acknowledgments

Far more people than can ever be mentioned here have, directly or indirectly, helped to make this book what it is. We'll name a few, but we send sincere and grateful energy out to all of you: Joan's dear friend and webmaster Kathie Huddleston, who convinced Joan that she needed a yoga website, and who consequently created the most beautiful Yoyoga! website (www.yoyoga.com). All Joan's students, who have taught and continue to teach her so much, and to all her many inspiring teachers along the way who encourage her to flex her mind and her muscles. Swami Kriyananda and Katie Lahiff, of the Temple of Kriya Yoga in Chicago, who stand out brilliantly as Joan's teachers during this edition. Eve's children, Angus and Emmett, who are even more accomplished yogis than they were when this book first came out. Joan's foster children, who, however briefly hold the key to her home, will forever hold the key to her heart. Eve's dog, Sally, who was her constant under-the-desk companion throughout the writing of all three editions of this book. Joan's feline companions, Mufasa and Simba, who regularly volley for laptime with Joan as she writes—helping to extend her flexibility in reaching and writing. Dr. Georg Feuerstein, for his invaluable advice and counsel. Saeid Lahouti, the photographer for this book, who has shared at least a few lifetimes with Joan (the photos for this book alone took several!). Wendy Frost, for her beautiful illustrations that have magnificently expanded with each edition of this book. Lee Ann Chearney at Amaranth, our book producer, for always giving us "all the best," and always promising "More soon!" We amore you, LAC! Witty and charming Gary Krebs, for finding Joan on the Internet. The whole team at Alpha: Marie Butler-Knight, Mike Sanders, Jen Chisholm, and the ever-fabulous Christy Wagner. William Hunt, for walking his talk, for consistently being one of Joan's most inspiring teachers, and for his high-caliber tech review. Bruce Symonds, for bringing perspective and laughter into the teachings. Bob Rumba, for so eloquently modeling with Joan in the water yoga pictures of this book. Fr. Frank Stroud of Fordham University for increasing Joan's awareness in the awakened deMello way. Katrina Ryan for being such a fantabulous example of yoga. Eve's two favorite yoga teachers in Iowa City, Joyce and Kelli, and her yoga buddy (and buddy otherwise), Lois, who comes along despite her wrists. Joan's friend Chuck Reiter, whose simultaneous nostril breathing and continual encouragement are each appreciated in their own way. Joan's beautiful twin sister, Jane, who since birth has been the deeply felt "THA!" in Joan's "HA!" The many wonderful bookstores (the people in them, really) who have encouraged both of us as writers. Joan's parents, John and Leona, and Eve's parents, Richard and Penny. Joan wishes to thank Eve, and Eve wishes to thank Joan, and both of us wish to thank our families and friends who have been there or are there to lend an ear, a hand, a good thought, the right words, or whatever it takes—offering yet another view of the "many limbs" of yoga.

Special Thanks to the Technical Reviewer

The Complete Idiot's Guide to Yoga Illustrated, Third Edition, was reviewed by an expert who checked the technical accuracy of what you'll learn here, to help us ensure that this book gives you everything you need to know about yoga. Special thanks are extended to William Hunt.

William Hunt is a certified yoga instructor, ordained priest, and the director of the Hatha Yoga teacher's training program at the Temple of Kriya Yoga in Chicago. He also co-teaches with Dr. Bruno Cortis, cardiologist, in wellness seminars.

Special Thanks to the Book Producer

This book would not have been possible without the expert vision and editorial guidance of Lee Ann Chearney of Amaranth. The team at Alpha is immeasurably grateful to her for her hard work and diligence. Thanks, Lee Ann!

Trademarks

All terms mentioned in this book that are known to be or are suspected of being trademarks or service marks have been appropriately capitalized. Alpha Books and Penguin Putnam Inc. cannot attest to the accuracy of this information. Use of a term in this book should not be regarded as affecting the validity of any trademark or service mark.

In This Part

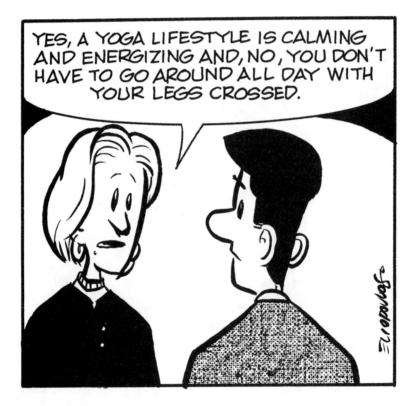

Yoga Union and You

Part 1 is an introduction and more, filling you in on why the ancient and venerable system of living called yoga is not only relevant but extremely popular today. If you want to get in better physical, mental, emotional, and spiritual shape, yoga is the key. No matter what your fitness level, no matter what your personal philosophy, no matter what your religion or lack thereof, yoga can make a positive impact on your life.

We go on to help you get more familiar with your body and on better terms with the body you call your own. We also show you what yoga can do for your body's strength, flexibility, balance, grace, and muscle tone. Do you know whether you are an ectomorph, an endomorph, or a mesomorph, and what each of those terms means? You'll find out in Part 1. You'll also learn how yoga can make your mind as toned, strong, sharp, and effective as it makes your body strong and supple. Learn what yoga's true and original purpose has always been and how this ultimate objective can lift you to a new level of personal achievement. Best of all, learn how yoga can set you free to feel and enjoy pure, unfettered bliss.

In This Chapter

- ◆ What yoga is

- ◆ How yoga helps alleviate stress

- ◆ Using yoga to promote strength, balance, and flexibility

- ◆ Using yoga as preventive medicine

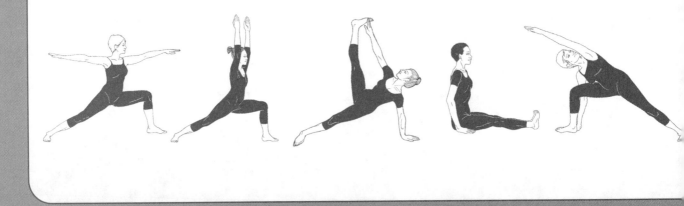

Chapter 1

Everybody's into Yoga

When it comes to yoga, idiots just don't exist. Banish the thought that yoga is something you'll never be able to do. These days, yoga classes are everywhere, and yoga students are so varied, they have become impossible to stereotype. Yoga is neither too esoteric to understand, too mystical, nor on the fringe. Not anymore! The Western world has embraced yoga and, in our usual way, we have adapted it, searched out "new" ancient forms of it, renamed it, recast it, cast aside trends that don't work in favor of new trends that work better, loved it, fought with it, made peace with it, and in general, made yoga our own.

Yet yoga is still the ancient and venerable tradition it once was. It's simply now wonderfully and irrevocably accessible to anyone and everyone. Just about every city and most small towns have someone teaching a yoga class, and often, the choices are amazingly varied. Where once there was nothing resembling "yoga" in the "Y" section of the Yellow Pages, today you might find classes in beginning yoga, advanced yoga, Iyengar Yoga, Bikram Yoga, Ashtanga Yoga, Hatha Yoga, or such Westernized hybrids as power yoga, relaxation yoga, fitness yoga, yoga for seniors, yoga for pregnancy, and yoga for kids. You can find yoga classes at traditional yoga studios, high-tech health and fitness clubs, in city recreation centers, community colleges, and even in people's homes. Yoga is mainstream.

So you can forget about the notion that yoga is only for double-jointed people who've been able to fold themselves into a suitcase since birth or for perpetual 1960's flower children who sit around and chant all day. Yoga is user-friendly. Anyone—at any fitness level, and with a wide range of personal and fitness goals—can benefit from beginning a yoga practice—even you.

Maybe you want to try yoga because you've never been able to touch your toes and you'd like to do it before you retire. Maybe you're seeking a quiet place to center yourself, to meditate by taking your mind somewhere far away from the house, the kids, the office, and the million nagging details of everyday life. Maybe you're an athlete who wants to learn yoga breathing for the advantage gained by stronger lungs and better circulation, not to mention the strength, balance, and agility you can gain from a regular yoga practice. Or maybe you've heard that yoga is great for migraine headaches, relief from chronic lower back pain, or good physical therapy after an injury or during an illness. It's all true.

The ancient and venerable art of yoga is neither a sport nor a religion; it's a journey of the body and mind. When you do yoga, you nurture the movement of *prana*—life force. You'll read a lot of Sanskrit words in this book because yoga terminology originated thousands of years ago in this ancient language. But there's nothing ancient about the concept of *prana: Prana* is the life "force." May the force be with you as you begin your yoga practice.

What Is Yoga?

Yoga is a system of techniques that reflects real and proven scientific concepts. Many things Western scientists understand about the body have actually been known by yoga practitioners for centuries. Yoga sees the body from a different perspective than traditional Western medicine, but the basic principles are the same. What we Westerners call *nerve plexus*, yoga calls *chakras* (although these terms don't coincide precisely—*chakras* include psychospiritual energy). What we Westerners call *spinal alignment*, yoga accomplishes through various poses or exercises designed to do what some of us

pay chiropractors to do. The human body is in a constant state of flux, continually adjusting internally to the influence of a changing external environment. Western medicine calls this process *homeostasis*. Yoga's *five sheaths of existence*—in essence, the body, the breath, the emotions, the intellect, and happiness—reflect the same need for balance between internal and external forces. The terminology may be different, but the concepts are universal.

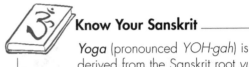

Know Your Sanskrit

Yoga (pronounced *YOH-gah*) is derived from the Sanskrit root *yuj*, meaning "to yoke or join together." *Prana* (*PRAH-nah*) is a form of energy in the universe that animates all physical matter, including the human body. *Prana* is the soul of the universe. Doing yoga maximizes your body's flow of the universal life force, giving you better health and increased vitality. *Chakras* (*CHAH-krahs*) are centers of energy located between the base of your spinal column and the crown of your head. Each *chakra* has a corresponding color, sound, perception, and biological function. Note that the actual spelling of *chakra* is *cakra*, but this spelling isn't commonly used.

Yoga is a fun activity that can produce powerful results. Yoga will wake up your body, sharpen your mind, and clarify your spirit. Yoga doesn't hurt, is only as difficult as you make it, and allows you to proceed at an individualized pace. Yoga can be a tiny part of your life, or you can incorporate its theories, rituals, postures, diet, and philosophy into every aspect of your life. You control how deeply yoga touches you. But if you begin a steady practice, be assured that yoga will transform the way you look, feel, move, breathe, and interact with friends, family, and co-workers.

Yoga Is Occident Insurance

Life in the West (the Occident, as opposed to the Orient) is no picnic. Sure, it's exciting, even exhilarating, but after all the pressures, stresses, responsibilities, frustrations, resentments, choices, temptations, and obsessions the average Westerner has faced by the end of a typical working day, it's no wonder we are a culture eagerly searching for ways to simplify our lives.

So how can yoga help? In the face of a daily existence that is so vibrant it almost vibrates us apart, yoga is an oasis. Yoga teaches the frantic mind to settle and find peace, and it helps the ravaged body heal itself by optimizing our natural ability to heal and by building physical confidence as well as emotional well-being. Yoga removes scattered energy, replaces depleted energy, and keeps your body—including all its internal systems—toned and in good working order.

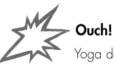

Ouch!

Yoga doesn't hurt and isn't about unnatural contortion. Sure, accomplished yogis might be able to move into seemingly impossible positions, but these postures are for people who have progressed to a level where such positions are possible and helpful. Some bodies are born more flexible than others. Each person has to find his or her own edge—the point just before discomfort occurs—and grow into it at a comfortable pace. We're all working the same edge, just in different places!

So what are we getting at here, you ask? Yoga is the best life insurance policy there is. It helps you slow down, center yourself, and get the most out of your life so every day is precious. By holding the body in a series of yoga postures that stretch and strengthen your muscles, loosen your joints, focus your breathing, and tone your internal organs, you'll find a new friend in your body. While you continue to hold each posture, your mind will learn how to tune out the distractions of life and hone in on how things are for you in this moment of living. Doing yoga makes you *listen* to how you feel—physically and mentally. This newfound power of concentration will carry over into every aspect of your life. Signals you once ignored—that crick in your neck or your obsessive worrying over a detail that keeps you from seeing the forest for the trees—are instantly acknowledged and seen for what they are: warning signs that you are heading down the wrong path. Yoga can help you regain your sense of self-fulfillment and joy, ensuring a more satisfying, not to mention fitter, existence.

Yoga Is a Great Stressbuster

Stress is a simple fact of life on earth in the twenty-first century. Stress is so common that countries all over the globe are incorporating the English word *stress* into their own languages: "*¿Que stress? ¡Me siento agobiada/o!*" (translation from Spanish: "What stress? I am totally overwhelmed!"). If you've never been under stress, we'd like to know your secret. (It's probably yoga!)

Yoga tackles stress on many levels. The postures, or *asanas*, help you control your wayward body, making it stronger, more flexible, better functioning, and, consequently, more resistant to disease and other physical problems. Practicing the *asanas* trains your body to do exactly what you tell it to do. Your doctor knows that moderate exercise, deep breathing, and relaxation are all great ways to relieve stress—yoga accomplishes all three. Yoga's breathing exercises, or *pranayama*, consciously channel the flow of the life force, *prana*, into and out of the body. Physiologically, deep, regular breathing sends a signal to each cell of your body to relax. Yoga meditation calms your racing thoughts and exercises your ability to master your own mind rather than let your mind master you.

Know Your Sanskrit

Asanas (pronounced *AH-sah-nahs*) are the postures, or exercises, of yoga designed to help you master control of your body. *Asanas* are also meant to facilitate meditation. *Pranayama* (*PRAH-nah-YAH-mah*) are breathing exercises designed to help you master control of your breath.

Yoga is a physical, mental, and spiritual way of life that puts reality into perspective. Yoga doesn't change your stressful circumstances, but it does teach you how to react to them without neglecting or injuring yourself.

Yoga Promotes Whole-Body Fitness

Maybe you're an accomplished athlete, or maybe you're a couch potato. To you, exercise might mean breezing through a five-mile run in the morning and a requisite visit to the gym three times a week or it might mean getting up to look for the remote control. Either way, yoga is perfect for you!

Because yoga combines so many different fitness elements and is so easily tailored to the individual, it can be practiced with great benefit at the beginner level as well as at the most advanced level. Whether you're a beginning or advanced practitioner, yoga will slowly, gently, and easily open up your body. You'll feel taller, breathe easier, and move about more comfortably.

Nonathletes might also be attracted to the idea that yoga isn't competitive. In fact, a sense of competitiveness is in direct opposition to the yoga frame of mind. Your yoga practice is personal and has nothing to do with anybody else. Plus, yoga will give you so much energy and such an improved self-image that you might find exercise isn't as bad as you thought.

A Yoga Minute

According to the National Heart, Lung, and Blood Institute, heart disease is almost twice as likely to develop in physically inactive people.

Yoga is designed to work all your muscles, not just a few isolated major muscle groups. Many of the postures, such as the twists and inversions, stimulate particular internal organs or release energy from stress-prone areas such as the lower back or neck. Yoga's fine-tuning exercises are the ultimate full-body workout. Other exercise programs tend to develop only one part of you—cardiovascular fitness, leg strength, or fat burning, for example. Yoga does it all.

Although many types of yoga exist, *Hatha Yoga* is the branch of yoga that concentrates on the body and is the form of yoga most emphasized in this book and practiced by Westerners. Many of the well-known forms of yoga, such as Iyengar and Bikram, are Hatha Yoga as practiced by particular yoga teachers, such as, in these cases, B.K.S. Iyengar, who popularized a form of Hatha Yoga that concentrates on proper alignment (sometimes using props to assist) and strength building, or Bikram Choudhury, who developed a set of 26 yoga postures practiced in order, often in a heated room. There are many other examples of yogis who developed and named their own systems of yoga, but most of them have something in common: They are all based on Hatha Yoga, and they all have the goal of harnessing or yoking the body to make it stronger, more flexible, and healthier.

Know Your Sanskrit

Hatha Yoga (pronounced *HAT-ha YOH-gah*, not *HATH-ah YOH-gah*, as it is frequently mispronounced) is the type of yoga most commonly practiced in Western culture. *Ha* means "sun," and *tha* means "moon," so *Hatha* is a combining of complementary forces. Hatha Yoga is the branch of yoga that transforms the human body via physical strengthening and purification to make the body a worthy vehicle of self-realization.

Hatha Yoga is an excellent fitness program, but it's also more. Hatha Yoga is based on the idea that gaining supreme control over your body is the key to control of your mind and freedom of your spirit. Through postures (*asanas*), breathing exercises (*pranayama*), and meditation, Hatha Yoga exercises, tones, and strengthens the whole person—body, mind, and spirit. Even if you start with the physical exercises alone, Hatha Yoga will quickly begin to work its magic.

Fitness today means more than a healthy body. Our culture is experiencing a growing trend toward things spiritual. With a growing passion for holistic health alternatives, we are a society looking for balance in a world that is out of balance. Holistic fitness is quickly becoming a mainstream concept, and yoga fits comfortably into this trend. Yoga is the answer to the spiritual seeker's *and* the athlete's search for physical excellence because it's the best all-purpose, all-person, whole-self, individualized fitness program—time-tested over centuries.

Yoga Is Healing Power

Yoga is a boon to the healthy body, but it can also be of supreme benefit to the body in need of healing. Of course, the best route for a healthy person to take is one of prevention. Healthy habits, maintenance of the body, peacefulness of mind, and calmness of spirit will go a long way toward protecting you from compromised health. Yoga is great preventive medicine, because it keeps all of you—body, mind, attitude, outlook, immune system—in top form.

Your spine, the "Grand Central Station" of your body, is stretched, loosened, and aligned by yoga—postures are designed to allow energy to flow freely through your spine and entire body. Many holistic health practitioners and even traditional practitioners argue that if the spine is aligned, the entire body works better, feels better, and fights disease more effectively.

In addition, yoga aids each of the following:

◆ Circulation

◆ Digestion

◆ Respiration

◆ Reproduction

Yoga also …

◆ Tones your organs.

◆ Improves your posture.

◆ Frees your breathing.

◆ Is cleansing.

Yoga helps your body purge itself of toxins that can negatively affect your health, both by releasing negative energy and, more directly, removing obstacles to the proper stimulation of the body's *lymphatic system.* The lymphatic system, the centerpiece of the immune system, protects and maintains the body's internal fluid environment, both filtering toxins and transporting nutrients to the blood. Lymph is pumped through the body by movement—when we breathe, contract or release our muscles, or even with the motion of our beating hearts or our digestive systems as we process food we've eaten. Yoga helps our bodies go with their natural flow. Even if you're not very mobile, you can practice yoga with eye exercises, simple stretches, and conscious rhythmic movements. Take your fitness personally and craft a yoga fitness plan that is all your own.

If you're sick, injured, or bothered by nagging health complaints, yoga can be a therapeutic addition to your physician's treatment plan. Of course, yoga should *never* be used in place of competent medical care. Ask your doctor or physical therapist about how yoga can be helpful in alleviating your specific health problems or concerns.

> **A Yoga Minute**
>
> According to the World Health Organization, an estimated 691 million people worldwide suffer from high blood pressure.

My Yogi, Myself

Once you've created your yoga plan and have begun to practice, guess what you are? Healthier? Sure. In better shape? Of course. But you're something else, too—you're a *yogi!* (A female *yogi* is actually called a *yogini,* pronounced *YOH-gee-nee,* but let's be contemporary and say we're all yogis.) Anyone who practices yoga is a yogi—that's what yogi means. You needn't be wise, you don't have to wear a loincloth, and you certainly don't need to practice for 10 hours every day. Even if you start with just a little yoga, you're a yogi. Of course, the more yoga you practice, the more you'll gain, and the wiser a yogi you'll become.

Yoga is practiced to varying degrees around the world, but some exuberant practitioners who have devoted their lives to the practice of yoga have achieved amazing control over their bodies. Although, according to yoga, such feats aren't important to the goal of spiritual enlightenment (self-realization), yogis have been known to …

◆ Stop their own hearts (then start them again, of course).

◆ Live to be well over 100 years old.

- Suspend their breath for an hour or more a day.
- Stand on one foot for several years (don't ask us why).
- Lie comfortably on a bed of nails.
- Eat razor blades without harm (we prefer a nice salad).

Here are a few more incredible feats that border on the supernatural, but these we'd have to see to believe:

- Become invisible at will.
- Remain suspended in mid-air (handy when all the chairs are taken).
- Move through space at the speed of light (saves on gasoline).

It doesn't matter why you approach yoga—whether for fitness, stress relief, enlightenment, or healing. It doesn't matter how advanced you are, whether you are out of shape and inflexible or an athlete extraordinaire. It certainly doesn't matter how much you already know about yoga. If you let yoga help you, it will help you in whatever way you require.

If you're intrigued but still need just a little more convincing before you're ready to perform pretzel-like contortions or begin *dhyana* (your daily meditation), read on for 10 great reasons to practice yoga:

- Yoga will tone your muscles and trim excess weight. It might even change your attitude about your body for the better.
- Anyone can do yoga. It's just a matter of starting at the appropriate level and remembering that you aren't competing with anyone.

> **Know Your Sanskrit**
>
> *Dhyana* (pronounced *dee-YAH-nah*) means "meditation"—the process of quieting the mind to free yourself from preconceptions and illusions. The result is a clearer vision of the truth about yourself, your life, and the world. For more on meditation in its many forms, read *The Complete Idiot's Guide to Meditation, Second Edition*, by the authors of this book.

- Yoga doesn't hurt. You go at your own pace, do what feels good, and stop before you feel pain. What could be better?
- Yoga will give you the gift of boundless energy.
- The increased energy and vitality you receive from regular yoga practice will make you feel as if hours have been added to your day.
- Yoga lets you dare to be different. People who tease you about doing yoga don't understand what you're doing—explain it to them!
- You can do as much or as little yoga as you like. Start with the postures, and you might find that your interest in breathing, chanting, and meditation develops later—or not at all, which is fine, too. It's all up to you.
- Yoga is definitely not about guilt! You can benefit the most from regular yoga practice, but practicing the postures whenever you have time is still beneficial and certainly better than no yoga at all.

◆ Contrary to popular belief, yoga isn't a religion. It's a method for life that can complement and enhance any religious system of beliefs, or it can be practiced completely apart from religion.

◆ Yoga will help ease your aches, pains, and stiffness. You'll feel like a kid again.

But don't take being a yogi lightly just because you've become one without too much effort. Your body, your mind, and your happiness are *your* responsibility. Your yoga program is a great start, but you need to have the right yoga plan. Learn as much as you can about yoga and consider taking a yoga class. The best way to learn yoga is with a teacher who can help you with the finer points of the postures, answer your individual questions, and guide you in finding a sequence of postures that best suit your needs and personality.

Wise Yogi Tells Us

If you are overweight or have a problem with overeating, yoga is the perfect exercise for you; it's gentle on the out-of-shape body, stiff joints, and heart. You'll feel better about your body as you begin to lose weight, and you can achieve an inner peace and confidence that will help you avoid compulsive overeating.

Even before you find a teacher, though, reading and learning about yoga can start you on your way. The more you know about yoga, the more you can focus on how it can help you. This book is a great start in your search for the perfectly personalized program. Apply everything you learn to your own journey. How can each new piece of information improve the personal program you are creating for yourself? Think about what you've learned already. Are you beginning to see how yoga might fit into your life? Yes? Then you are wiser already.

Yoga Sets You Free

Perhaps you're flirting with the idea of yoga because you imagine it's an interesting fitness plan, but perhaps you're looking for something more. People have been practicing yoga for thousands of years, not because they want to be "in shape" (a fringe benefit), but because they are seeking meaning in life. Yoga can be a fitness program, but it can also be a path to greater self-knowledge and, ultimately, self-actualization. Yoga helps you reach the fullness of your human potential. You will be more confident, stronger, healthier, and more at peace with who you are. You will make better decisions, set and achieve worthwhile goals, and become the person you want to be.

The ultimate goal of the yogi is to achieve the experience of truth, which might mean different things to different people, but which is, to some degree, a consistent experience for all—a clarity of vision, supreme focus, and a feeling of oneness with the earth, even the universe. This ideal state is called *samadhi* and involves consciousness to such a heightened degree that individual ego falls away and oneness with the universal force of love and goodness, or *brahman*, is achieved. It is the state of pure bliss.

 Know Your Sanskrit

Samadhi (pronounced *sah-MAH-dee*) is the goal of yoga. It's when the yogi finally becomes aware of nothing but *brahman* (*BRAH-mahn*)—the all-pervading Supreme Self, or God—everywhere. It's a state of absolute bliss and might be transitory or, ideally, perpetual.

A few rare and diligent yogis have been able to maintain this state for extended periods, but for most of us, *samadhi* is an elusive experience. We might get occasional glimpses of it, or sudden rushes of bliss that fall away but become imprinted in our memories. After all, we do have to live in the world, which is often a less-than-blissful place. On the other hand, you and your world are what you make them, and yoga can help you optimize yourself, your experience, and your all-important perception of the world around you. Yoga is fitness plus peace and fitness plus joy.

The Least You Need to Know

- ◆ Yoga has become mainstream. Yoga classes are available everywhere and people of all types enjoy yoga.
- ◆ Yoga reduces stress and improves concentration.
- ◆ Yoga is a great workout at any fitness level.
- ◆ Yoga helps prevent illness and keeps the systems of the body in order. It increases energy and vitality, promoting well-being.
- ◆ Anyone who practices yoga is a yogi!

In This Chapter

◆ A self-test for the yoga-challenged

◆ Understanding how your body works

◆ Using yoga to learn to trust your body

Chapter 2

How Comfortable Are You in Your Body?

You know the types of people who are comfortable in their bodies. You've seen them gliding through life looking ready for anything. They don't slouch or slump or hunch over. They don't have flawless bodies. (Nobody does.) But they don't seem to mind! They look like they feel great in their own skin, no matter what shape or size they happen to be.

Are you comfortable in *your* body? Are standing, sitting, and lying down easy, or do you feel your clothes binding, your stomach sagging, your back aching, and your knees cracking? Can you spring up from a sitting position on the floor like a child, or is hoisting yourself to a stand always accompanied by grunts, long sighs, and various strange popping noises from assorted joints?

The truth of the matter is that most of us aren't comfortable in our bodies. Why? Two reasons: We don't maintain them as well as we might, and we are convinced, for any number of reasons, that we *should* look and feel different than we do. Fitness expert Jack LaLanne once said that if more people treated their bodies with the same care and upkeep they give to their most precious possessions (their houses and their cars), everyone would be fitter and healthier. Isn't a little maintenance worth the effort?

And what about maintenance on your body image? That could probably use a little ratcheting, too.

A Self-Test for the Yoga-Challenged

Are you yoga-challenged? In other words, are you so far out of touch with your body that yoga seems like an impossibility? Take this test to find out how in tune you are with your body. Choose the one best answer for each question.

1. The longest amount of time I can sit on the floor without feeling some sort of pain and discomfort is …
   a. Thirty minutes or longer.
   b. Fifteen minutes, max.
   c. Maybe two minutes.
   d. Why the heck would I want to sit on the floor? That's why they invented the couch.

2. My back …
   a. Never hurts.
   b. Hurts 24 hours a day.
   c. Hurts after I've been sitting for too long.
   d. Hurts when I don't exercise regularly.

3. My coccyx is …
   a. The vertebrae at the base of my neck.
   b. My kneecap.
   c. A small, triangular bone at the base of my spine.
   d. I'm quite sure I don't have a coccyx!

4. I get sick (cold, flu, gastroenteritis, etc.) or injured (sprained ankle, twisted knee, back goes out, etc.) at least …
   a. Once a year.
   b. Once every few months.
   c. Once every few weeks.
   d. I hardly ever get sick or injured.

5. My vision is …
   a. Excellent (20/20 or better).
   b. Pretty good. I have glasses or contacts, but my prescription isn't a very strong one.
   c. Terrible. I can't see well at all without my glasses or contacts.
   d. I'm sorry, I couldn't quite make out the question. It's too blurry.

6. Whenever I feel a cold coming on, the first thing I do is …
   a. Push fluids, get more sleep, go in late to work, and drag myself through the day.
   b. Try to talk myself out of it or ignore it. I don't have time to get sick!
   c. Go to work, but whine and complain that I'm getting sick while sneezing and coughing all over my co-workers.
   d. Rest, bundle up on the couch with some herbal tea with lemon and honey, increase my vitamin C intake, and stay home so I can get better.

7. The difference between tendons and ligaments is …
   a. Tendons connect muscles to bones; ligaments connect bones to bones or hold organs in place.
   b. Tendons connect bones to bones or hold organs in place; ligaments connect muscles to bones.
   c. Tendons and ligaments are those things I'm always pulling and tearing, after which my doctor says, "There's nothing I can do."
   d. Huh?

8. The way I feel about my body can best be described as follows …

    a. I dislike certain parts of my body, but other parts are pleasing. I'm good at disguising my faults with my clothing.

    b. My body is okay, but I don't pay much attention to it.

    c. I love my body. I think it's beautiful, and it feels good to be in it. I take good care of it so it will stay that way.

    d. I practically have a heart attack every time I look in the mirror, so I just don't look in the mirror.

9. I can …

    a. Bend down and touch my toes easily.

    b. Bend down and touch my knees easily.

    c. Fold completely in half, bending forward, hugging my calves with my arms, and resting my head and entire upper body against my legs.

    d. Look down and almost see my feet.

10. My muscles are visible …

    a. In a lot of places if I flex. I can see the line of my calf muscle if I stand on my toes, and I can see my biceps and triceps if I flex my arm.

    b. All the time. I can see my thigh muscles, calf muscles, biceps, triceps, deltoids, and abdominal muscles, even without flexing them. I am truly buff!

    c. Possibly on an x-ray—that is, if x-rays showed muscles.

    d. Every now and then. Especially when I'm at a lower weight, I can see something that looks a little bit like muscle, but mostly I just see smooth, rounded surfaces with some bumpy cellulite here and there.

Now score your test by giving yourself the correct number of points for each answer. For example, for each question you answered with an a, give yourself three points. For each b, you get two points. Add up your points, then check the following section to see what your score means.

a. 3

b. 2

c. 1

d. 0

Your score: _____

What Your Body Is Telling You, and Whether It's Good News

So how did you do on the quiz?

If you scored 25 to 30 points: Are you already a yogi and just reading this book for fun? You have a wonderful awareness of your body. If you aren't doing yoga, you'll probably love it.

If you scored 16 to 24 points: There are a few things you don't like about your body, but at least you pay attention to it. As you work through yoga's exercises and meditations, your bad habits will eventually disappear on their own. You won't need will power, because treating your body well will feel so good!

If you scored 8 to 15 points: Yoga can help you become more aware of your body and improve your self-image. You'll discover feelings, muscles, positions, and energy you never imagined you had. If you don't pay attention to your body, it will break down faster, and you don't want that!

If you scored 0 to 7 points: Talk about somebody who needs yoga! You're barely aware of your body at all, either because you ignore it or because you dislike it so much that you want nothing to do with it. Yoga can gently coax you into a new relationship with your body—one based on respect and appreciation.

Most of us have many illusions about our bodies. Unfortunately, these illusions affect not only our feelings about our physical appearance, but also our self-esteem and our relations with others. Be aware that the following italicized statements about your body are *not true*:

◆ *Your body is without consciousness, and your mind is separate from your body.* **Not so.** Many of your organs and tissues have properties similar to your brain, sending out messages, receiving information, reacting accordingly, and letting you know when you're being abusive or kind to your body. Your entire body is awake, alive, and aware.

◆ *You can't change your body.* **Of course you can!** Not only can you change your body profoundly through your actions and thoughts, but your body continuously changes itself: All your cells are replaced every five years. Your body is supremely mutable.

◆ *Your body is solid.* **It only looks that way.** Actually, at the atomic level, your body consists of vibrating atoms with lots of space in between. You are more energy than matter!

◆ *Bodies are a curse.* **Not at all!** Bodies are an opportunity and a tool through which the inner soul can be discovered.

◆ *I am a victim of genetics.* **You don't have to be a victim.** Genetics only reveal the make and model of your body. What you do with that body and that mind and how you care for them can be as powerful as your genes.

◆ *People judge you by your body, first and foremost.* **No they don't, even when they think they do.** Your self-concept is a powerful force that emanates from you and influences others more than you might think.

Ouch!

Stop punishing yourself! Hating your body is unnatural; why not give yoga a try? The postures will improve your health, and yoga's meditation will help your mind feel more benevolent toward your body. Life is too short to ignore or berate the primary mechanism that houses your soul.

The Shape You're In

To know your body is to love your body, with all its unique characteristics. Whether you tend to be muscular, curvy, slim, or some combination, look around and you'll see others with many of the same qualities—and different physical characteristics of all kinds, too.

But knowing your body type can do more than make you feel satisfied that there are plenty of other people who have a similar shape. Your body type can give you clues to what types of yoga poses will come more easily to you and what types of poses might be more challenging and balancing for your body type.

(Keep in mind as you read the descriptions for each of the body types that any body type can belong to either men or women.)

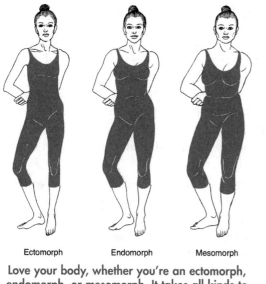

Ectomorph   Endomorph   Mesomorph

Love your body, whether you're an ectomorph, endomorph, or mesomorph. It takes all kinds to make a world!

The Slim Ectomorph

The ectomorph body type tends to be tall and slender with narrow shoulders and hips, long limbs, relatively low body fat, and underdeveloped muscles. Although the stereotypical ectomorph is slender because of a tendency to have a lower muscle mass, ectomorphs can develop a high fat-to-muscle ratio if they don't get enough exercise.

Luckily, exercise is easy for ectomorphs, who tend to be highly energetic and who, when in shape, can bounce effortlessly through a high-impact aerobics class followed by a three-mile run. Good luck keeping up with an ectomorph's pace. Unless you are also an ectomorph, it won't be easy.

Aerobic activity, however, while healthy in moderation, isn't as important for ectomorphs as developing those muscles. Everyone needs cardiovascular exercise, but ectomorphs might tend to overdo this type of activity because it comes so easily. Not so easy for ectomorphs is weight training.

Yoga is great for ectomorphs because it can help slow that frantic pace they tend to maintain. Yoga is also a weight-bearing activity, so it is the perfect, gentle way to introduce ectomorphs to their own muscles. Because many yoga poses lift, hold, and/or balance the body's own weight, yoga provides ectomorphs with the muscle-developing and strength-building exercise their body type requires to maintain a physical fitness equilibrium.

Your ectomorph summary:

- Narrow shoulders and hips
- Long limbs
- Low body-fat-to-muscle-mass ratio
- High energy
- Benefits from yoga poses that are calming and that develop muscle strength

The Curvaceous Endomorph

The endomorph is the classic Rubenesque figure: all curves and rounded surfaces. Endomorphs aren't automatically overweight, but they do tend to have a higher fat-to-muscle ratio than the other body types, accumulating fat on the abdomen, buttocks, hips, and thighs. They tend to be pear-shaped, with narrower shoulders and wider hips than ectomorphs.

Endomorphs have slower metabolisms and might seem more languid or serene than the energetic and active ectomorph. This natural tendency, when not countered with regular activity, might result in a sedentary lifestyle—something that isn't healthy for anyone. Endomorphs burn fat more slowly, and it takes more steady, low-intensity aerobic exercise for them to burn fat than it would for an ectomorph, making exercise crucial to maintaining a healthy weight.

Yoga is perfect for endomorphs, too. Many yoga exercises are low-intensity aerobic exercises that burn fat. Endomorphs might want to pay particular attention to *vinyasanas*, such as the sun salutation (see Chapter 19), groups of yoga poses strung together with coordinated breathing patterns. These pose series are just what the endomorph needs to burn off any extra fat that develops and impart the energy some endomorphs have difficulty generating.

 Know Your Sanskrit

Vinyasana is a steady flow of connected yoga *asanas* linked with breathwork in a continuous movement. It is a dynamic form of yoga.

Endomorphs also tend to have a naturally strong lower body, but the endomorph's upper body often needs development. Many yoga exercises involve lifting and holding body weight with the upper body. These poses will help the endomorph develop a more balanced body.

Your endomorph summary:

◆ Narrow shoulders and wide hips

◆ High body-fat-to-muscle-mass ratio

◆ Strong lower body

◆ A relaxed disposition, sometimes bordering on inactive

◆ Benefits from an aerobic series of yoga poses like the sun salutation and poses that build upper body strength

The Muscular Mesomorph

The mesomorph develops muscle mass easily and has a high muscle-mass-to-body-fat ratio. Mesomorphs tend to accumulate fat around the waist, triceps, and back, but mesomorphs who get physical activity have well-developed muscles. It doesn't take much for a mesomorph to sport washboard abs, cut triceps, or an impressively muscled back.

Strength is the mesomorph's forte, so the weight-bearing aspect of yoga makes the mesomorph feel right at home. Too much weight-bearing exercise can actually bulk up a mesomorph too much.

 A Yoga Minute

The classic muscle-bound weight-lifter tends to be a mesomorph. Mesomorphs who don't want to look too bulky should limit weight-bearing activities to those that use lighter weights and more repetitions.

Mesomorphs tend to be more easily motivated than endomorphs and might feel right at home with the weight-bearing yoga poses, but stretching is another matter. Those tight mesomorph muscles don't tend to be particularly flexible.

Yoga to the rescue! Yoga is perhaps *the* best exercise for developing long, strong, flexible muscles. The aerobic aspect of yoga is also helpful for mesomorphs, because their tendency to develop fat around the middle might put them at greater risk for heart disease.

Your mesomorph summary:

◆ Muscular upper and lower body

◆ High muscle-mass-to-body-fat ratio

◆ Accumulates fat around the middle

◆ An easily motivated disposition

◆ Benefits from moderately aerobic yoga poses and poses that lengthen and increase the flexibility of muscles

Your Body and Yoga 101

Yoga can help you optimize the particular physical body you've been given, but your physical makeup isn't the whole picture. You are also animated by energy. Your cultural background determines the way you see or understand your body in all its layers and complexities, and your own personal level of confidence and trust in your own body can teach you even more about the complex package otherwise known as you.

Where Do You Stand?

To see how aware you are in your body right now, stand up, with your feet together, and lift your toes up from the floor. See if you can feel your arches slightly rise as you do this. If you can feel this, try to maintain the lift of the arches as you lower your toes. If you don't feel much of anything, don't fret. A regular practice of yoga will make you more aware of subtle areas of your beautiful body—areas you might have been ignoring or have not even aware of yet!

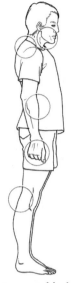

Poor posture can block the flow of energy through your body.

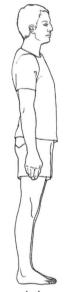

Yoga practice can help you align your body for increased energy and vitality.

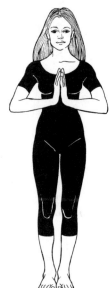

Yoga's Prayer pose centers, restores, and renews. Inhale and lift your heart. Exhale and lower your shoulders.

Your Personal Energy Cycle

No matter how in or out of touch you are with your body, everyone has energy cycles. You know, even without consciously knowing, when your energy levels fluctuate. Sometimes your energy peaks; sometimes it lags. Sometimes you wake up ready to go-go-go; sometimes you can barely pull yourself out of bed. Energy cycles can be affected by increased activity, over- or undereating, or too little sleep. Your monthly cycles, the weather, lunar cycles, your health, your diet, and your regular level of exercise can all have an effect, too.

Just as people have different body types, they also have different energy patterns. Maybe you tend to wake up ready to take on the world, but by nighttime, you can't wait to crawl into bed. Or maybe you don't want to see another human face before 10 A.M., but at midnight, you are ready to rock. Although individual energy fluctuations can be a matter of habit (you can accustom yourself to working the night shift, for example), working with your natural energy flow will make yoga easier and more enjoyable, and a regular yoga practice will smooth out your natural energy flow.

A Yoga Minute

Are you a night owl or a lark? Night owls typically enjoy energy peaks about two hours later in the day than larks, who are the classic "morning people." Typical larks enjoy the morning and a good breakfast, feel most alert and creative early in the day, and prefer to retire early. Night owls often dislike eating breakfast, enjoy their peak later in the day, and prefer to stay up late and sleep in.

When energy shoots up or plummets too suddenly, you are left feeling exhausted, out of balance, and even confused. That sudden five-story drop on the roller coaster might be thrilling for a few seconds, but those nice, smooth hills and valleys are a lot less jarring on your system. Yoga helps your energy cycles flow smoothly. Instead of super highs and abysmal lows, you can enjoy a steady stream of energy, like an exhalation of air you control by the size of the opening of your lips and the force of your exhalation.

With the regular practice of yoga, energy lows blend into energy highs, and the highs flow easily into the lows. Yoga helps you get in touch with and pay closer attention to these cycles as it softens the transitions between them, making you feel more even and balanced all day and all night.

The Muscle and Bone Connection

Yoga postures make more sense if you know a little bit about how your bones and muscles make your body work. Your particular physical challenges will also become more specific to you if you understand your anatomy.

Your skeleton is your frame. It contains 206 bones and supports your muscles and organs. Connecting the muscles to the bones are tendons. Muscles help you bend your joints and perform all sorts of tasks. Strong muscles go a long way toward supporting your frame, making it easier to achieve good posture. Think about how effortlessly infants curl up and raise their toes to their mouth. Your back and spine are completely loose before you learn to walk. Once walking begins, the spine tightens and flexibility diminishes and diminishes and diminishes. Yoga is the caretaker of the spine, lengthening and extending it to release the energy that runs through this neural superhighway.

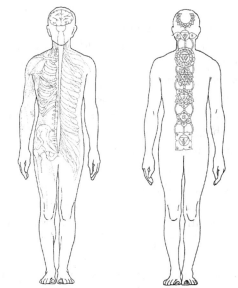

The Western anatomical model of the human body's musculoskeletal and nervous systems (left) is complemented by yoga's seven energy centers, called *chakras* (right), which store and release *prana*, the life force.

Eastern Body, Western Body

Is your body different than the body of someone from a different part of the world? Of course not, but different cultures have different theories about the body. The concept that the body and the mind are one is an easy concept for the Easterner. The physical body is merely one of several "bodies." It's a temple to house the spirit but should be well tended and rigorously cared for because of the importance of what it holds. The *astral* body is the vehicle of the spirit and is maintained through breathing, meditation, and concentration. The *causal* body is the place where the spirit works. The ego is absent from the causal body, and the spirit can know its true potential here. Ideally, the spirit transcends all bodies and becomes pure consciousness, an individual expression of the divine. To the traditional Easterner, the mind-body is sacred, not to be abused, but to be used as a vehicle for the spirit's expression, which results, finally, in enlightenment.

On the other side of the spectrum is the Westerner. Traditionally, the Westerner sees one part of the self at a time. The body is the body. Healthy food keeps it running, and exercise keeps it strong. End of story. Then there is the mind. The mind is the source of intelligence and thought. Activities that stimulate the mind, from philosophical conversations to crossword puzzles, keep the mind active. End of story. Then there is the spirit. The spirit might be nurtured and maintained by going to church or by a personal philosophy or spirituality. In many, the spirit is ignored. End of story.

Wise Yogi Tells Us

Moderation is the wisest, most peace-inspiring course. Nothing should be so important that it must be had in excess, and nothing should be so unimportant that it must be utterly denied.

Westerners have certainly survived—and thrived. So why should we change a system that works? Because it keeps us off-balance. Westerners are movers and shakers, yet many of us exist on the edge of health and sanity, surviving on caffeine, nicotine, and sugar, wracked by stress and saddled with materialism, ego, desire, and greed. We need something to even us out, calm us down, and get us in touch with ourselves again. Don't believe that this will slow you down or make you less effective. Integrating mind, body, and spirit can only make you a better, more effective, and productive person—Westerner or Easterner.

Do You Trust Your Body?

Maybe you've never thought of your body in terms of something you should or shouldn't trust, but you do have an intimate relationship with your body. It's your vehicle for communicating with the world. Do you trust your body? How many of the following statements do you agree with?

◆ "When I get a craving, I can't control my eating. I'll eat an entire quart of ice cream, a huge steak, a pound of chocolate, candy, a whole pizza, and a pie. I can't stop myself."

◆ "I'm accident-prone, especially when I play sports or exercise. I always twist an ankle, jam a thumb, or injure myself in some other way."

◆ "I always get sick just when an important event is about to happen. My body betrays me when I need it most!"

◆ "I don't know what to think about myself, because what I see in the mirror is totally different than how other people describe me."

◆ "I'm uncomfortable in most of my clothes."

If you agreed with any of these statements, you have problems trusting your body. Your body is not your enemy, and it's not a stranger. Although you might need professional help to cure an eating disorder, chronic illness, or negative self-image (you'll want to enlist the aid of a licensed health-care professional as well as a yoga instructor!), the wonderful thing about yoga is that it reacquaints you with your physical self. You'll get to know your body like never before, and you'll even learn to make peace with your body, enjoy your body, and even *like* your body.

Your body will begin to respond the way you intend it to. You'll know what your body is going to do. You'll be paying attention. You'll have more control over your physical being and mental state, so you'll be injured less, more sure about what you think, in better control of what you do, and more self-confident.

The Least You Need to Know

◆ Yoga helps you feel better in your body.

◆ Body awareness, including posture, is an important part of practicing yoga.

◆ The ectomorph body type tends to be tall, thin, and energetic; the endomorph body type tends to be curvy with wide hips and a more relaxed temperament; the mesomorph body type tends to be strong with well-developed muscles and an even temperament.

◆ The more you pay attention to and learn your own personal anatomy, energy cycles, and body image issues, the more you will integrate your mind and body for greater confidence and self-control.

◆ Yoga can help you learn to trust your body.

In This Chapter

- ◆ Yoga as a bodymind workout
- ◆ Yoga as your ultimate fitness power source
- ◆ Cross-train with yoga
- ◆ Yoga enhances your sports performance

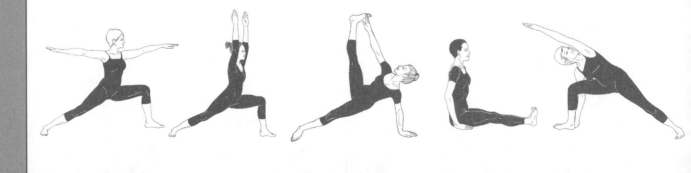

Yoga Body Power: Fitness Beyond Stretching

So you thought yoga was about getting flexible? It is indeed, but it is also much more than stretching. Yoga is a fantastic strength-builder because many yoga poses involve the manipulation and holding of your own bodyweight. Yoga is an incredible endurance builder as you learn to hold challenging poses for longer and longer, and as you try *vinyasana*, or moving sequences of yoga poses, that challenge and increase your aerobic capacity and improve cardiopulmonary function.

Yoga also increases your ability to balance, fine-tunes your coordination, tones your digestive system and other internal organs, ratchets up your immune system, and helps you pay closer attention to the movements and nuances of your body, both obvious and subtle. In other words, yoga makes you more fit, more athletic, and more physically aware than ever before. If you're looking to yoga for bodymind fitness power, you've come to the right place.

Yoga Means Connection

Yoga taps into your inner power, connecting your body with your mind. It's easy to fall into a pattern of associating fitness with the body alone. We run, go to step aerobics or kickboxing class, bicycle, and perform sit-ups and pushups—all for our bodies.

But the yogi will soon see the absurdity of the notion that the body is separate from the mind. Body and mind are one, and although they can become isolated and dissociated from each other, yoga brings them back together where they belong. Everything works better when all the circuits are connected. Your mind can boost your physical performance to new heights, and control over your body is training for control over your mind. Can you say "super athlete"?

Are You Off-Balance?

Perhaps you've been feeling "scattered" lately. Do you lose things easily? Forget appointments or information? Are you overwhelmed by the buzz of activity in your life? Maybe you think you don't have time to slow down and get "centered," but you must know this: You don't have time *not* to get centered. If you're feeling out of balance, you're wasting your days, your energy, and your power. You're like a house with the heat on and all the windows open. Yoga can help you close the windows (or turn off the heat) and center on making the most of each precious moment of your day.

Sometimes stress is a good thing. It can give you the power to escape from a dangerous situation. It can help you succeed in life, both in your physical pursuits (say, running a marathon) and in your intellectual challenges (say, passing a test). Too much stress, however, wreaks havoc on the body. When experiencing stress, the brain stimulates the adrenal glands, resulting in certain telltale symptoms:

- Your heart rate speeds up.
- Your blood pressure rises.
- Your breathing quickens and becomes more shallow.

- Your pupils dilate.
- Your muscles tense.
- You sweat.
- Your senses become heightened.
- Blood flows to your muscles and brain.

Too much of this kind of activity will wear out anyone's system. Yoga's bodymind fitness power can channel stress more efficiently, helping you instead of hurting you.

Mind Meet Body, Body Meet Mind

Beginning to practice yoga is like introducing your body and your mind for the first time. Sure, they have resided in close proximity your entire life, but do they really know each other? If you want to be truly fit, you must introduce your body to your mind and your mind to your body. Even though they are inextricably combined, they might still be living as strangers.

Hatha Yoga, the yoga that concentrates on strengthening and purifying the physical body while simultaneously strengthening and purifying the mind, is the perfect introduction. As we begin to work body and mind separately, in time we recognize that they are really one and the same. Through the practice of Hatha Yoga, we can come to this realization.

Practicing Hatha Yoga means finding the balance in the union of your bodymindspirit. Hatha Yoga is truly a holistic exercise (bodymindspirit = holistic), because it involves the activation, control, and mastery of every part of your body. Fitness is the inevitable result—so is restful sleep, improved health, and tranquility of mind. Hatha Yoga gives voice to what the body knows: All its parts are one.

Coming Back to Center

Just like any other sport, yoga requires a warmup period. Haphazardly practicing might build your strength to a small degree, but you won't get the benefits of yoga's bodymind discipline. Centering is a mental warmup to go along with your physical warmup. As you practice your beginning poses, consciously focus your mind on your body. Notice how your body feels and what it's doing. Commit to your yoga practice for the next 10, 15, 30, or however many minutes you have allotted yourself. The more often you make a habit of consciously centering your mind on what your body is doing, the more you'll notice a feeling of calm, of being centered in your daily life. Your yoga fitness power is showing!

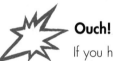 **Ouch!**

> If you have a medical condition, such as chronic back pain, yoga can be great therapy. A yoga teacher can show you which postures will benefit and strengthen your particular weak area. But be careful: The postures should feel comfortable, not painful!

Tapping Into Your Yoga Power Source

So how does all this "centering" and concentration get you in shape? Because your mind and your body are so intricately connected, a centered mind with the power of concentration works directly on the body, allowing each yoga posture to accomplish the maximum possible benefit. Don't be misled into thinking you can ignore the "mental" parts of yoga because you aren't in it for the "enlightenment." Perhaps getting in shape is priority one for you. That's great! But the key to yoga's fitness power is in the synthesis of everything you are: your body, your mind, your spirit—each part working together to make the whole stronger, healthier, and more alive. Remember, a healthy body means more than just a strong body. As any doctor will tell you, a positive attitude toward life is central to the body's natural healing powers. Yoga stimulates your bodymind power source, channeling your positive mental energy into your physical workout, and vice versa.

Bend Without Breaking

If you've always been athletic but haven't concentrated on maintaining your flexibility, you might be nervous about trying yoga. Never fear. You don't have to be able to sit in the Lotus pose for an hour or even for a minute. You don't have to do the Lotus pose at all! However, eventually, after lots of yoga practice, you might find you *want* to try it. However, just as endurance isn't necessary for the beginning runner, who attains endurance by running, yoga can help you gradually build flexibility. If you're about as flexible as a steel pole, start slowly and go only as far into a posture as you can. Every week of practice will take you farther. Before you know it, your joints will loosen, your muscles will stretch, and your body will take on a smoother, more pleasing shape.

Perhaps you've always been naturally flexible. Don't think yoga will be simple! There's always the next posture waiting for you. You can always push a little farther, a little more, working that edge until you achieve postures you never imagined were possible. And if flexibility is your forte, yoga can help you build strength, endurance, balance, and refinement.

As you accomplish postures you couldn't begin to achieve when you started, you'll understand flexibility in a new way. Who would have thought greater flexibility would make you feel more comfortable playing with your kids at the park or joining that weekend game of flag football? Who would have thought it would make your morning run easier and more comfortable? Yet it does! Plus, yoga's increased flexibility is rewarding within a yoga practice as well as throughout your everyday life. The achievement of a yoga posture you've worked on for weeks is like winning a marathon without anyone else losing—pure triumph!

Know Your Sanskrit

Lotus pose, also called *padmasana* (pronounced *PAHD-MAH-sahn-ah*) is a yoga sitting pose in which the left foot lies upturned on the right thigh and the right foot lies upturned on the left thigh. It is meant to resemble the perfect symmetry and beauty of the lotus flower.

Balancing Acts

You probably take your ability to balance for granted. You get up in the morning, walk around all day without incident, and lie back down at night. Balancing wasn't always so easy, however. In fact, during one illustrious period of your life, learning to balance took up most of your waking moments.

Through yoga, balancing once again captures your attention, and you might feel like a wobbly toddler all over again when you first try Tree pose or Warrior 3 or Crow pose or any of the other yoga balance poses we'll show you in this book. Balance is challenging. Yoga balance postures take keen muscle control and

strength, flexible joints and mental centering, and lots of practice. Once you've refined your balancing act, you'll discover that the walking you take for granted is even easier than before. Balancing is control, both in stillness and in motion.

Strength from the Gut

Everybody knows that lifting a heavy weight takes strength. But balancing takes strength, too. So does holding a posture for an extended time. Some yoga strength training is isometric (a form of exercise in which muscles are tensed in opposition to each other or to an immovable object). After assuming each yoga pose, hold it for as long as you can hold it correctly. Talk about a way to wake up muscles you never knew you had! Yoga's isometric action is easier on your muscles than the weight bearing and pounding of other sports, yet extremely effective for building strength. What's more, each yoga position in a well-structured workout includes a posture and its opposite, so your body will stay physically centered, never developing any side or particular body part out of proportion to the others.

Some yoga poses are weight bearing, too, but instead of lifting a big metal barbell over and over, in yoga, you lift and manipulate your own bodyweight in many different positions and from many different angles. After an intense yoga workout, you might feel like you've been lifting weights at the gym for an hour! Yet because the only thing you lift is *you*, yoga continually builds your self-awareness and your ability to fine-tune and adjust the movement, stillness, and position of your own body.

Yoga positions are entered and held by the body in order to find the peace within—the point where sustaining the pose is easy, natural, and feels "right." The more difficult the pose, the harder it is to find peace. Yoga postures mirror life. When things are easy, it's easy to feel good. But feeling good when things aren't going your way—whether it's a bad hair day or a serious tragedy—is a challenge. Yoga is a journey through the poses, working with each pose until you find that peace, then progressing to the next level. This progression combines the building of physical strength with the toning of the mind.

This might surprise the Western athlete even more: Strength is compounded when the body, mind, and spirit are exercised together. Strength will mean more to you once you've practiced yoga than it ever did before. It will be more than just how much you can lift, and the more you practice yoga, the more you'll know exactly what we mean.

Keeping the Faith

"But I know it will be just like that aerobics class," you may be thinking. "I'll be all excited for the first week or two, then I'll get bored and quit." In any given day, probably just as many people quit a fitness program as start one. Why should yoga be any different?

The benefits you'll soon feel from your yoga practice are so comprehensive, you might well find that you'd rather give up coffee, doughnuts, or pepperoni pizza than give up your daily yoga "therapy." Beyond the more obvious benefits of increased flexibility, balance, and strength, yoga has thousands of less-dramatic (though no less important) rewards. Yoga feels different than other fitness programs, because each posture is specifically designed to activate your body in minute ways—adjusting here, stimulating there, stretching here, strengthening there, compressing, releasing, expanding, and reaching. With all this internal maintenance, you can't help but enjoy increased health and a vibrant sense of well-being.

Wise Yogi Tells Us

Yoga is great for teenagers, who already tend to be strong, flexible, and energetic. Teenagers are frequently surprised at how challenging yoga can be. The mental focus, physical control, and spiritual development that come along with yoga are wonderful therapies for adolescents whose hormones are raging and who might feel depressed, out of control, or angry without knowing why.

Yoga vs. Other Exercise

The title of this section is a little misleading, because yoga isn't in competition with anything. It's not a wrestling match. Yet because most Western forms of exercise emphasize stress on the muscles combined with quick, harsh movements, yoga stands out as a distinctly different kind of exercise. Yoga avoids the quick and harsh, which tend to trigger lactic acid production in muscle fibers, leading to pain. Instead, yoga emphasizes breathing to deliver more oxygen to muscles, lessening the effects of lactic acid production.

However, we aren't suggesting you ditch your volleyball league or your marathon participation in favor of a yoga practice. On the contrary! Just add yoga to the program. A regular yoga practice can improve your performance in any other athletic activity. Read on to see how yoga can boost your performance in your other favorite physical pastimes.

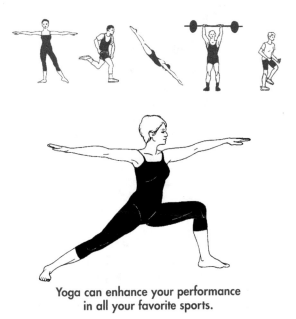

Yoga can enhance your performance
in all your favorite sports.

have more developed lower body structure. Working with the graceful shift from Downward Dog to Upward Dog strengthens upper and lower parts of your body and brings them into balance. Hold at least three long breaths in each pose before shifting to the other pose. Move back and forth with a slow, controlled movement. (We'll talk more about these poses in Chapter 19.)

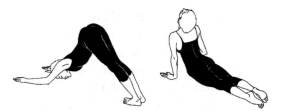

Moving from Downward Dog into Upward Dog and
back again can contribute grace, strength, and
coordination to the aerobic dancer.

Awesome Aerobics

Aerobic dance can be a lot of fun, especially for those who like music. Aerobic dancers who also do yoga are more graceful, have more fluid movements, are better able to keep up, and are more flexible. Like running, aerobic dance is primarily a cardiovascular activity; although low-impact aerobics are kinder to your body than high-impact, aerobic dancers still experience a lot of stress on their muscles and joints. Aerobics is energizing and great for people who need the motivation of a class and an instructor (something a yoga class also offers). Yoga is a great complement, because it balances aerobic dance's frenetic energy by inducing a sense of calm and inner control.

For increased aerobic dance performance, try moving from Downward Dog into Upward Dog and back again. This strengthens the body, particularly the back, legs, and upper arms. It helps build grace as the movement of the legs shift in the foot balance from the top of the foot to the toes. It balances strength of upper body with lower body. Dancers tend to

Rockin' Running

"But *I know* yoga won't give me the cardiovascular strength and endurance running gives me!" you may be protesting. Yoga doesn't challenge your cardiovascular system in the same way running does, but consider this: Runners rely on strength and balance. Flexible runners get injured less often. Runners also tend to have shallow, hard breathing patterns; they sometimes hyperventilate. Yoga's deep-breathing exercises increase your lung capacity, getting more oxygen to your brain and increasing your endurance.

Yoga is kinder to your body than running, so it makes a great alternate workout to give your body a rest from the constant pounding and joint stress runners experience. Runners frequently injure their feet, ankles, knees, and hips. You can use yoga postures to build strength in these same body parts! In fact, the New York Road Runners club promotes an official yoga program called "Power Yoga."

For increased running performance, try standing poses like Warrior 1 and Warrior 2. Warrior poses in particular help develop knee strength. Instead of the pounding effects on the knees that occur during running, Warrior poses strengthen the knees through the hold of the pose for several breaths, and both legs are active in the pose. Lift up on the quadriceps muscle as you hold these poses. Lift up on the back of the thigh on the back leg in the pose. This applies to all versions of Warrior pose.

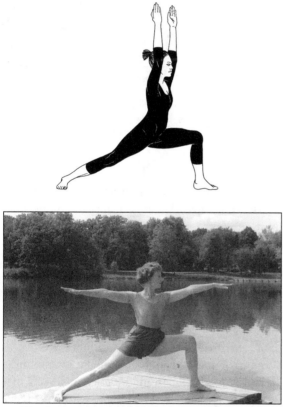

Warrior poses strengthen the knees, thighs, and calves for better running performance.

Biking and Beyond

Riding a bicycle is an excellent way to strengthen leg muscles without stress on joints, increase cardiovascular functioning, and spend time in the great outdoors. Even if you ride an exercise bicycle at home or at the gym, biking is good for you, no doubt about it. However, if the only exercise you ever do is ride on a bike, you might be courting a physical imbalance. Bicycling is great for your leg muscles, but it does very little to increase upper body strength. It improves breathing, but once your body becomes accustomed to the particular motions of cycling, it can fall into a rut to the point that cycling doesn't challenge your body the way another exercise might.

Solution? Enter yoga! Yoga is great for cyclists because it lengthens and loosens tight quadriceps and hamstrings (the muscles on the front and backs of your thighs) and keeps calf muscles limber, too. In addition, yoga can balance your physical awareness by adding upper body strengthening to your fitness routine. In addition, the balance and concentration you gain from yoga can help you be a more confident and safer cyclist.

For increased cycling performance, try Revolved Triangle pose. Revolved Triangle helps open the chest area—something cyclists might tend to keep closed as they are hunched forward on their cycles. It also gives an excellent spinal twist—something all biker's spines will appreciate. The hamstrings stretch and elongate during this pose as well, which is crucial for cyclists. It is fine to bend your knees while going into this pose, and gradually straighten the legs once in the pose. Do not overstretch, though.

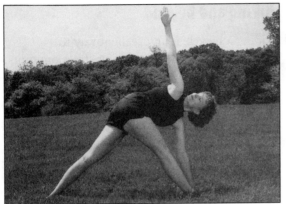

Revolved Triangle opens the chest, activates the spine, and stretches the hamstrings for stronger, more flexible, and more comfortable cycling.

Super-Charged Stretching

Most of us have had basic stretching exercises drilled into us since grade-school gym class: Bend down and touch your toes, reach to the right, reach to the left, roll your head from front to side to side. The difference between this type of stretching and yoga is that yoga stretches are specifically designed not only to lengthen your muscles, but also to stabilize your joints, stimulate your organs, balance your endocrine system, and strengthen your muscles as you hold the stretch. It's still a good idea to do basic stretches before and especially after engaging in strenuous exercise, such as running or swimming, but if you also add yoga to your fitness program, stretching will soon be a breeze. When you start to stretch, you'll feel as if your body is telling you, "Okay, yes, I know exactly what we're doing. I'm *with* you!"

For increased flexibility, particularly as a warm-up and cool-down before strenuous exercise, try Lying Down Spinal Twist pose. This pose helps create a more supple spine, ready to stretch and move in various directions. It also limbers the neck and opens the chest. After you do this pose lying down, try doing it sitting up. Straighten one leg at a time. The

toes of the straight leg are pulled back, allowing a nice hamstring stretch for each leg. Hold each twist for several breaths. Close your eyes. Internalize.

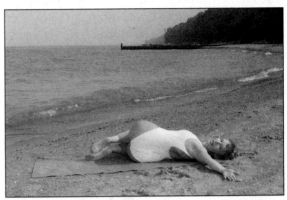

Lying Down Spinal Twist activates and gently stretches the spine, which is the core of your body and an important source of strength and flexibility. When your spine is flexible, your whole body moves more easily.

Superior Swimming

Swimming is an excellent exercise because it works your muscles and your heart without putting stress on your body. Swimming is essentially a cardiovascular exercise as well as a strength-builder. As you move through the water and increase your heart rate, you also work large and small muscles against the resistance of the water. If you're a swimmer, you'll find yoga a great addition to your fitness program, because the increased flexibility and strength gained through yoga make swimming easier. Also, the breathing practice in yoga is of exceptional benefit to swimmers, who must have good control over their breathing in the water.

For increased swimming performance, try Boat pose. Hold on to the ladder or the side of the pool. Straighten your legs and extend your back. Bring your feet close to your hands. Extend your spine, and try to elongate your spine and open your chest. Hold the pose for several breaths.

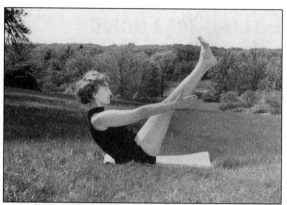

Try Boat pose in the pool holding on to a pool ladder. Modify the angle according to your comfort level. This pose helps stretch your legs, arms, and spine for easier swimming.

Uplifting Weightlifting

Lifting weights adds strength to both muscles and bone. More and more studies suggest that weightlifting is extremely beneficial, particularly for women and seniors, to fight bone loss and muscle atrophy, keep the body in good shape, and boost metabolism because the more muscle mass you have, the more fat you burn even when you are just sitting at your computer. The downside of weightlifting, however, is that weightlifting alone decreases flexibility. Although moderate weightlifting a couple times a week might not make a noticeable difference, more serious weightlifters can get "muscle-bound." Even those of us who lift weights regularly, not aiming for bulk but benefiting from the many other boons of weightlifting, might find we need to stretch more often to keep those strong muscles lengthened and flexible.

Anyone who lifts weights can benefit dramatically from yoga. Weightlifters also benefit from the breathing exercises and balance training of yoga. Also remember that yoga is really a form of weightlifting, because you lift your own bodyweight, so don't lift weights and do muscle-intensive yoga workout on the same day.

However, a relaxing, calming, stretch-oriented yoga workout incorporated into a weightlifting workout is the perfect combination of strength and stretch. After each weightlifting exercise, do a yoga pose that stretches the muscle you just worked. The more familiar you become with yoga, the more you will discover which poses work after which weightlifting exercises. We'll give you one example here.

Let's say you just did a triceps workout with dumbbells or the pulley machine (the triceps are those muscles along the backs of your upper arms). After each set, spend a minute or two in Cow pose, which specifically targets the triceps (as well as the shoulder joints and other arm muscles).

What makes yoga different than a simple triceps stretch? As you do the Cow pose, fully watch your body respond. How was the effect of the weight you just lifted? Close your eyes and notice how your body is responding to the stretch. Is it crying out in anguish or celebrating in movement? The quietness and length of breaths you hold a stretch in a yoga pose will help you center on the lessons your body is teaching you. Contracted muscles cannot breathe. They need to stretch to release lactic acid buildup. Help your body heal itself and move on to ever greater heights in physical fitness.

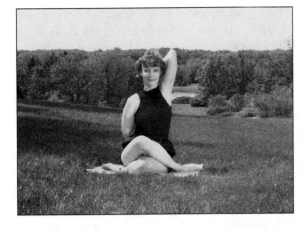

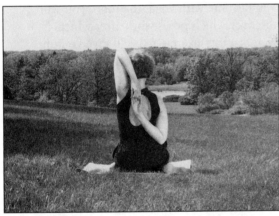

Cow pose is the perfect yoga complement to a weightlifting triceps workout. After each set, spend a minute or two in Cow pose to stretch your strengthened triceps.

A Yoga Minute

According to the National Sporting Goods Association, exercise walking was the number-one fitness activity in 2001, with 71.2 million participants over age 7. The sport that grew in popularity the most? Snowboarding!

Ecstasy: Yoga Union

The Western approach to yoga tends to be more fitness-oriented, while the Eastern approach to yoga is based on the idea that a healthy body makes it easier to progress spiritually. Either approach benefits both body and mind, however. If you're interested in yoga for its physical benefits, you can consider the spiritual "centeredness" you achieve a splendid bonus. Or if you tend more toward the Eastern way, consider fitness the icing on the cake of spiritual growth. Either way, yoga fitness power means self-confidence, self-control, and inner peace. Whatever your fitness level, let yoga challenge you.

It's All in Your Mind!

Everyone knows that a good percentage of athletic performance is mental. We've all seen our favorite team in a pressure situation get psyched out—suddenly, it can't do anything right. Think about the last time you played your favorite sport. Was there ever a time when you suddenly slipped into "the zone"? Your performance becomes flawless, and you're able to exceed your normal abilities.

Because yoga unites body and mind, it teaches you control over your mental state as it teaches you control over your body. What happens to you really is "all in your mind," so let your mind be your instrument—learn how to "play" it in the zone of peak performance.

Wise Yogi Tells Us

End every yoga session with a few minutes of complete and total relaxation. Don't move, don't think; practice sitting or lying absolutely still. Simply feel your body. This little space at the end of your yoga workout is an important part of bringing your mind and body together—grounding your awareness and allowing your body to make the most of your workout.

Maximize Your Performance

When you understand that your mind and body are one, the sense of tranquility and control you can achieve makes everything clearer and simpler. Everything you do will be affected. Do you have a big presentation at work? You are calm, confident, and empowered. Do you have a championship tennis match? You are strong, flexible, buoyant, and the ball seems to go exactly where you will it to go. Do you have a really difficult test? Your mind is so uncluttered that all your studying comes back to you effortlessly.

Of course, such power doesn't come easily. A week of sitting in the Lotus pose for five minutes a day won't be enough to send you permanently into "the zone." Yoga is a process. Your bodymind needs to learn new habits and new modes of intercommunication. But if you're persistent and follow the yoga path, you'll quickly perceive the changes blessing your life. You'll feel peace of mind, even the ecstasy of oneness with the life force. And you will be in the best shape you've ever been in, too.

So what are you waiting for?

The Least You Need to Know

◆ Yoga is about personal progress, not competition.

◆ Yoga uses mind power to build body power and, eventually, as you evolve, fuse the two into one power.

◆ Yoga's isometric action is easy on the body.

◆ Yoga makes you a better runner, cyclist, dancer, swimmer, weightlifter, and all-around great athlete!

In This Chapter

- ◆ Finding peace in a stressful world
- ◆ What meditation teaches us
- ◆ Reaching the yoga zone of flow
- ◆ Flow in an actual yoga pose

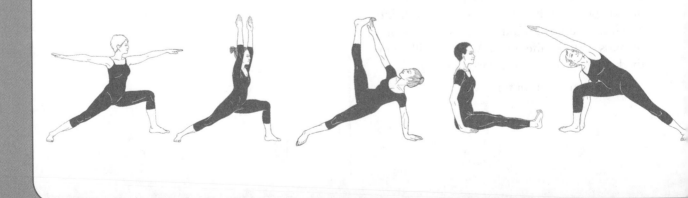

Chapter 4

Yoga Mind Power: Relax, Center, Flow

Life can be tough. Stressful, fast, overloaded, even out of control. We have so much to think about, so much to remember, so much to do, so much responsibility, and so little time. However, although it may sometimes feel like it, life is not a war, it's not a contest, and it's not a race.

Life is *being*, yet when we rush through our days with no thought to our own lives and the maintenance of our own minds and bodies, "being" might be the last thing we think about. However, incorporating a yoga practice into your day—your week … your life—can help you to stop, focus, and live consciously, even if just for a short time each day. Yoga helps you see the truth of being and helps you live each moment.

The need to name, label, evaluate, and analyze everything we come into contact with can be debilitating to the spirit. Yoga teaches you to look without classifying, to listen without judging, to feel without losing control, to learn without assuming you already know—simply, to be. Readjusting your thinking through yoga can provide you with incredible freedom— freedom from stress, from anxiety, from suffering.

Of course, everything is subjective. Realizing this will help bring peace to your busily categorizing mind and help you see the truth in difficult situations, people, and even yourself. Labels make perception seem easy, but perception isn't easy, so banish the labels and look harder and closer at yourself and the world. Let yoga show you how.

A Fight-or-Flight World

There's no doubt about it—we live in a stressful world! The human animal has a specific way to deal with stress, and it's called the *fight-or-flight response*. When confronted with a stressful situation, your adrenaline starts pumping. Your muscles tense. Your senses heighten. In essence, your body becomes primed to deal with the stress in two ways: either fight with the utmost energy and strength, or get away as fast as possible. How can fight or flight help you? It gives you energy. It gives you a quick reaction time. Your mind is sharper and clearer. If you recognize all this and work with your body, your experience of a stressful situation—say, presenting a new product line at work or teaching a class to a new group of students—will be vibrant and exciting.

The problem with the fight-or-flight response comes when it's engaged too often. Bodies can take only so much stress, and if your body and mind are forced into a constant elevated state of stimulation, muscle tension, and excess energy, you're bound to break down. Maybe you'll get sick, collapse from exhaustion, or just plain lose your ability to communicate effectively. You might forget things, you might lose things, you might feel overwhelmed and unable to concentrate.

The problem with our world is that it constantly bombards us with stressful situations. What's more, our culture rewards those who take on the most stress. Who do you admire more—your colleagues who are always taking on projects and coming up with new ideas, working late every night, and helping everyone else who gets behind? Or the colleagues who relax at their desks talking on the phone, leave at 5 P.M. with overflowing in-boxes, and never seem in a hurry to get anything done?

We want the overachievers on our team: the high-powered, assertive, I-can-do-anything types. With that kind of pressure, it's no wonder we're all under so much stress.

In a fight-or-flight world, yoga is like a daily trip to the spa. Not only will it relax you and calm your mind, it can fine-tune the fight-or-flight response. With yoga, you can learn to clear your mind and listen. You can learn to focus, concentrate, and tune in. When your muscles tense, you will become more aware of them and can direct their energy to stand straighter, move more quickly, and react more deftly. As your senses heighten and your thinking sharpens, you'll see how to clear your mind of everything but the task at hand. Answers will come to you. The perfect combination of words will flow effortlessly from your mouth. You'll be able to perceive your situation clearly—the motivations of others, your position in the circumstances, and what should be done. Panic is replaced by confidence.

We don't want to give you the impression that yoga is magic. It isn't. It doesn't turn you into someone you aren't—but yoga is the key to making the fight-or-flight response work for you, because it gives you control over your physical and mental responses to this instinct. It teaches you to focus, concentrate, and finally master your body and your mind.

Concentration, Relaxation, Meditation

Meditation is an important part of yoga. But maybe you aren't interested in meditating. That's fine—just practice the *asanas*. Chances are, however, that the more you progress through the *asanas*, the more interested you'll become in meditation. Meditation can do wonderful things for your mind and your body.

Perhaps you aren't sure what meditation is. Really, it's a simple concept. Meditation is the process of attaining total awareness through the cessation of the thought process. What? You thought your thoughts were constant, a constant part of you, the running monologue of your mind? Yoga teaches that you are not your thoughts at all. Your thoughts are a part of you, but they are not you, and they do not make you. You can turn them off the way you turn off a faucet when you aren't thirsty. Meditation gives your mind a break from the constant onslaught of thought.

But meditation isn't easy. You can't just sit down and stop thinking, much as you might wish you could. The first step is to master relaxation, which is not only crucial for stress relief and better concentration but is the lynchpin of meditation.

A beginning meditator first concentrates on relaxing. You can relax in many positions—lying down, sitting, even standing. The key is to focus your mind in a way that will help your body calm, unwind, and release its tension. Try feeling like a wave relaxing into the ocean, because that's what you are. You are a part of the universe the way a wave is part of the ocean. In fact, repetition of the *Om mantra* even sounds like waves on the shore. Soon your thought waves will decrease and become still. The wise Indian sage Patanjali said, "Yoga is the cessation of the fluctuations of the mind." We say "Still waters run deep."

A Yoga Minute

Patanjali was an Indian sage who, thousands of years ago, wrote a text called the *Yoga Sutras*, which recorded concepts that had been passed down orally for many years. This influential text, which consists of a series of aphorisms about how to practice yoga, has helped define the modern practice of yoga.

A neglected mind is one that doesn't work as well as it could. Meditation is mental maintenance. Teaching yourself how to relax your mind and release it from the stress of thought for a short period each day keeps it clear and clean. You'll think better. You'll see more accurately and with more insight. You'll be able to concentrate and focus on things like never before. You'll be able to truly relax. In fact, you'll probably be amazed at the mind power you never knew you had.

Ouch!

Even meditation can be counterproductive. Although you probably won't pull a muscle while meditating, it's possible to stay stressed, or even become more stressed, in your efforts to relax! Don't think. Don't worry that you aren't meditating correctly. Feel your body, feel your breathing, and feel who you are. Let your thoughts flow through your mind like pictures on a movie screen, flickering and passing on. Gently, lovingly, let each thought go. *Ahhhh!*

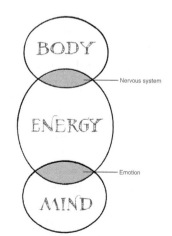

Pure energy transcends mind and body. Our emotions and nervous system are physical links to energy. Pure energy transcends the physical.

Wise Yogi Tells Us _____

If meditation sounds like something you'd like to learn more about, pick up a copy of *The Complete Idiot's Guide to Meditation,* now in its second edition (Alpha Books, 2003).

From Full Mind to Mindfulness

What is stillness? Simply a lack of movement? As you move through your daily life, stillness would probably not be an adjective you would use to describe your mental state. You are busy, you have responsibilities, and you are good at what you do. This takes a full mind, a mind always thinking about what to do next. A mind prepared to deal with conflict. A mind ready to tackle anything, whether it's a toddler's temper tantrum or capturing a multimillion-dollar account for your company. Who has time for stillness when you've got so much to *do?*

You do, because stillness will take your full mind; empty it out; give it a good, thorough cleaning; and transform it into a mindful mind. What does that mean? A mindful mind is like a mirror that is meticulously polished. It reflects what is really there and nothing else. When you become mindful, you learn to suspend everything you believe about yourself, others, and the world. Your limits, your shortcomings, your fears, what people have told you that you can and can't do—all these are put on hold. What's left is the real you, and your possibilities are limitless. Mindfulness takes courage. It can be scary to look at the real you. But if you take a good look, you'll have new power. You'll understand who you are like never before.

And as your self-concept expands, so will your concept of the world. Everything is within your grasp. Yet you aren't grasping—you're simply living, achieving, and being the best person you can possibly be. Have you heard the phrase "optimize your hard drive"? That's not just for your personal computer. Yoga optimizes the hard drive in your head! This involves extending your meditation to your daily life. Once you've made meditation a part of your life, you can gradually learn to carry its principles with you throughout your day. When negative feelings arise, gently push them away as if they are balloons. Look at them, note them, acknowledge them, then let go of the string. If people are unkind, unfair, or judgmental of you, you can learn to gently push these balloons away, too.

Ouch! _____

Do not sit awkwardly during meditation. Sitting slumped over with a crooked spine, or sitting in a position too advanced for you can cause injury to your body, as well as frustration. It's impossible to relax deeply into your meditation if your body is strained or in pain. So stay within your physical limits while meditating and concentrate instead on your mind.

Meditation in daily life means remembering the peace and stillness you've learned to achieve during regular meditation, then finding that peace and stillness throughout the day. The real you will shine through best when you're in touch with this inner peace.

Wise Yogi Tells Us _____

To help yourself meditate, think of all the definitions of yourself you know. "I am a teacher." "I am a father." "I am bad at math." "I am talented." "I am shy." "I am lazy." "I am well meaning." "I am jealous." Now pretend these definitions are untrue. Just pretend. Then look beyond. What's left is the real you, and you might be surprised at what you see. Surprised as well as pleased, as if you've met an old friend you haven't seen in years … maybe even in lifetimes!

Know Your Sanskrit _____

Avidya (pronounced _ah-VEE-dyah_) is the word for incorrect comprehension. The opposite of _avidya_ is _vidya_ (_VEE-dyah_), or correct understanding. _Avidya_ inhibits our perception in many ways—through automatic, learned responses; dependency on habits; and negative self-talk. _Avidya_ is like a cloud in front of the sun. Learning to recognize _avidya_ and dispel it is one of the goals of yoga. _Asmita_ (_ah-SMEE-tah_) is the ego, _raga_ (_RAH-gah_) is attachment, and _dvesha_ (_DVEH-shah_) is rejection. _Abhinivesha_ (_ah-bhee-nee-VEH-shah_) is the survival instinct or thirst for life. It is the desire to exist and so becomes an obstacle toward enlightenment, which is existence but beyond the personal existence to which unenlightened individuals cling.

Relax Past Your Boundaries

What are your boundaries? We all have them, and they are all branches of _avidya_, or our false perceptions of life and of ourselves. Boundaries limit us from the truth and from our potential. Some of the boundaries we impose upon ourselves are known as _asmita_, or ego; _raga_, or attachment; _dvesha_, or rejection; and _abhinivesha_, or the survival instinct.

Ego is a boundary difficult for most Westerners to avoid. Your ego is what gives you a sense of who you are to the world. To say "I am the smartest one in this class" is ego. To say "I have to win this game" is ego. To say "I am beautiful" or "I am right" or even "I am good at my job" is ego. To most Westerners, some expression of ego seems natural and even productive. Why not be proud of what you do, how you look, or what you've accomplished? You certainly should be proud of who you are. But _asmita_ means being proud of the wrong things—the things that limit you, such as material possessions, physical appearance, beating out someone, or being the best, which implies you're better than others.

Deep inside, you're a jewel. You're a beautiful soul that's part of a beautiful universe. Getting caught up in the petty and nonlasting aspects of life can only hold you back from your true potential. Maybe you still think you have to be competitive to "win," but yoga can help you to see winning in a new, more fulfilling light.

Attachment is related to ego and involves desire. Do you know what it's like to want a cookie or a piece of cake, not because you're truly hungry but just because you want the pleasure? The desire for pleasure can overcome you, and you can be fiercely single-minded until you get what you want. If you've experienced this feeling, then you know what _raga_ is. Attachment also involves material possessions—that sort of "fever" you get when you see something you really want. It can consume your entire mind—the desire for that new dress, stereo system, or hot red sports car. Attachment to any material possessions, sensual sensations, addictions, desires, or even an obsessive attachment to another person is a boundary that holds you back from truth and the true knowledge of yourself. Attachment gets in the way of who you really are.

Rejection is like the opposite of attachment and is called *dvesha*. Your spouse left you, so you refuse to get involved in a relationship again. You were thrown from a horse, so you refuse to ride again. You were in a car accident, so you vow never to drive another car. All these are *dvesha*. Rejecting experiences, people, or thoughts that have caused you pain in the past blocks you from the future. But *dvesha* needn't be so drastic, and we all experience it. You refuse to try okra because you think it will taste unpleasant. You don't go to a party because you know the social interactions will be stressful and you just don't have the energy. This isn't to say that you can't make the decision not to do certain things, but when you reject things out of a fear of discomfort, pain, or inconvenience, rather than rejecting things simply because you don't want or need them, then *dvesha* has become a stumbling block in your life.

The final obstacle is the survival instinct, or *abhinivesha*. This instinct might seem to be a positive one at first, but it is actually a stumbling block between you and enlightenment. This intense desire to remain alive is related to the fear of death (although they aren't the same). You probably want to remain you. You might fear death, but you also enjoy your life (for the most part) and, thus, fear any kind of change in your existence. Enlightenment, involving release from the material world and tangible existence, is both mysterious and scary. Does enlightenment mean that life as we know it will cease? We are animals, after all. Our instincts are for self-preservation. Moving beyond our instinctual natures into our spiritual selves isn't easy.

Wise Yogi Tells Us

"Heart breathing" is a technique that can be very renewing. Sit comfortably. Close your eyes. Notice your breathing, but don't try to control it. Feel your chest expanding and contracting. Now imagine the breath is flowing out of your heart with each exhalation and pouring into your heart with each inhalation. Don't think about anything. Just feel the breath flowing in and out of your heart. Imagine the breath is pure love. Do this for 5 to 10 minutes, then slowly open your eyes, get up, and move on. Remember the feeling throughout your day. Then do it again tomorrow!

Yoga helps dispel *abhinivesha* (the survival instinct), as well as the other aspects of *avidya* (incorrect comprehension) that cloud our perception and inhibit our growth. Sure, you'll probably always have occasional bouts of ego, attachment, rejection, and the instinct to cling to your material existence. You are only human—and not *only* human, but deeply, magnificently human. Through yoga, you can become even more deeply connected to your true humanity. You can learn to recognize your incorrect comprehension for what it is, then you can blow out the incarnations of your incorrect comprehension like matches. No more delusions!

Yoga helps you relax, think more clearly, and see the inner you that is a part of the universe and all that is good. Yoga helps reveal *avidya* for the impostor it is. And if you can perceive the stumbling blocks in your path clearly and without doubt, you can confidently step around them.

Find the Zone—and Move In!

We've already talked about the zone. The zone is that place you go when your skill is suddenly heightened, your mind is sharp, and you can do no wrong. Athletes know about the zone. When an athlete is in the zone, he or she has reached peak performance. The mind is thinking quickly, sharply, and accurately. Success is effortless.

Artists know about the zone. It's the place where nothing else exists but the task at hand. A painting seems to paint itself. The words to a novel flow effortlessly. The sculpture emerges, the actor becomes the character, and the dancer becomes one with the dance.

Students know about the zone. It's that rare time when the answers to a test are obvious to you and all the information you've studied seems immediately available. Your brain exceeds itself, the words to an essay write themselves, and the meanings to formulas suddenly become clear.

Another word for the zone in contemporary culture is *flow*. Anyone can achieve flow, but some achieve it more often than others. You have flow when you become completely absorbed in what you're doing. Time seems to stop, nothing else exists, and you become one with your work. During flow, you can accomplish things you never thought you could.

Wouldn't it be nice to achieve flow whenever you wanted—to move into the zone and live there all the time? For most, flow comes and goes, seemingly according to its own whim. But for the experienced yoga practitioner, the zone is a place to go whenever you choose. Because yoga uses control of the body to still the mind and control of the mind to manipulate the body, body and mind become integrated not only with each other, but also with the external world. If you're one with your work, your art, or your sport, you've achieved flow. You're in the zone.

Yoga is like a key to the secret door into the zone. Open it, and you'll live beyond your limits, finding new productivity, creativity, efficiency, and true delight.

Go with the Flow Right Here, Right Now

It's fine to read all about getting into the zone, but how do you actually get there? By cultivating mindful awareness and focus.

Would you like to try it? Let's take a basic yoga pose, called the Cobra pose (*Bhujangasana*, in Sanskrit), and practice getting into and out of it. Look at the following picture of the pose and read through the step-by-step instructions before you try it. Make sure you are wearing comfortable clothes that don't constrict your movement, and place a towel, blanket, or mat on the floor.

Before you jump into the pose …

1. Let's sit for a moment. Sit comfortably on the floor and breathe. Don't worry about breathing deeply. Just notice your breath. Give your breath your full attention. You can probably "hear" lots of thoughts rattling around in your mind, somewhere behind the sound of your breathing. Note them, but don't let them engage you. Back to your breath.

2. After you've been sitting for a minute or two with your mind focused on your breath, move into a lying-down position on your stomach. But don't just move thoughtlessly. As you move, really pay attention. Keep your mind centered on how you feel, on how your body moves, on which parts are going where as you come down to the floor. Your body is all that matters right now, and a great yoga pose like this deserves all your concentration. With every step of this pose, keep pulling your focus back to your body; the way the pose feels; the way you move and breathe as you get into, hold, and get out of the pose. You are practicing mindfulness. You are in flow training.

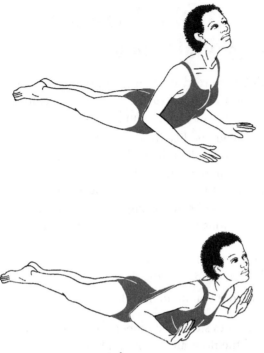

Cobra pose.

a. Lie on your stomach, flat on the floor, with your heels together and great toes next to each other. Place your hands on the floor on both sides of your chest. Your face should be resting against the floor.

b. Inhale, and lift your forehead, then chin, then shoulders, then chest off the floor. Keep your hips pressed against the floor and your elbows bent, shoulders down and away from your ears.

c. Look upward and take a few slow, deep breaths. Then try sticking out your tongue and opening your mouth wide to help release your face. Finally, slowly come back down. First your chest, then shoulders, chin, and forehead. Return to the starting position.

d. Come back up into Cobra again, and this time closely examine the current strength of your spine. Once in the pose, lift your palms off the floor, as in the lower figure in the figure See how much of your body comes down—if it's a lot, your arms are doing too much of the work. Focus on your spine instead. The emphasis of Cobra pose is to strengthen the spine.

e. Now, slowly push yourself up with your hands and sit back on your heels. Rest your forehead on the floor and relax, giving your spine a chance to stretch in the opposite direction. This position is called Child's pose.

3. Stay in this last position for a few minutes.

How was it? Did you stay focused on your body, your movements, and how the pose felt? Are you still focused on your body? As you rest in this ending position, let your body feel the aftereffects of Cobra pose. What do you notice? How does your mind feel? At any point during the process, did all those clattering thoughts in the back of your mind recede? Did they stop clattering altogether? What are your thoughts like now?

Maybe you got a little taste of flow during this exercise, and maybe you didn't. But if you practice yoga every day with this kind of attention, eventually you'll experience flow. You have it in you.

A Yoga Minute

Yoga is truly a mindbody exercise. The mind focuses on the body, and the body responds to the mind. The two are partners in the process, and your whole being becomes more fully integrated.

Practicing yoga poses is a kind of meditation itself. With this approach, you can train your mind to be flow-ready. It will happen more and more. You'll finally know what it's like to be yourself!

Release Your Inner Delight

Yoga's payoff is a big one: inner peace. The regular practice of yoga can bring calm to a harried life, comfort in grief, joy from sadness, and an inner strength and focus that can carry you through your life with assurance, confidence, and purpose. Yoga lets you live your life wide awake and aware of each moment.

Maybe you consider yourself a happy person, or maybe you suffer from depression. Maybe you had a happy childhood, or maybe you've been hurt in the past. No matter who you are and no matter what has happened to you in your life, you have the capacity for joy. Deep inside you, bliss waits for you to find it. Yoga will ferret out that joy with relentless persistence. Through yoga, you can find that joy and release it.

But make no mistake: It isn't easy to release your inner delight. A body that's undisciplined, weak, and lazy saps all your inner energy to keep it maintained. A mind fraught with chaotic thought is too absorbed on the surface level to delve deep enough to find inner joy. But with persistent yoga practice, the body becomes strong, controlled, flexible, and disciplined. The mind becomes quiet, calm, and tranquil. A restless body that at one time struggled to maintain Lotus position for an extended period and a mind that regularly wandered without purpose now both respond with focus and commitment.

Wise Yogi Tells Us

The symbolism of the lotus flower is extremely important in yoga. The lotus flower is a beautiful circle of petals that floats on a lake. The lotus's roots, however, are deep in the mud. This mud provides the nutrients to help the lotus grow and achieve its beauty. To *yogis*, the lotus represents human life. Our lives are submerged in "mud"—in the material world, in striving and grasping, in worry and pain. Yet we can use these challenges the way the lotus root absorbs nutrients from the mud—sending up a shoot that will ride to the top of the murky lake and bloom on the surface in perfect beauty.

Maybe inner joy isn't what you're looking for. Maybe you don't even believe it's something that's possible for you to find. Yoga doesn't turn you into anything you aren't. Yoga simply releases you so you can find the joy that everyone has inside. Yoga is a personal journey, and you go at your own pace. All you have to do is follow the map; that is, practice the postures. Meditate, if you feel like you're ready. Gradually, as you become prepared, the joy—the inner delight—will come.

The Least You Need to Know

◆ Yoga uses the fight-or-flight response to your benefit.

◆ Yoga teaches mindfulness.

◆ Meditation is simply relaxation for your mind.

◆ Meditation stimulates *vidya*—correct understanding—and dispels negative thoughts, feelings, and actions.

◆ Practicing yoga poses with your full attention can help you learn how to achieve flow, or total absorption and optimal skill in whatever you are doing.

In This Part

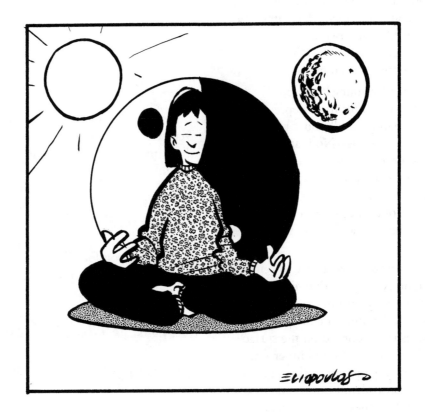

Getting Spiritual with Yoga

Part 2 begins with a mini history lesson. Yoga has been around for thousands of years, and in all that time, it has branched into various types, from studious Jnana Yoga to active Karma Yoga to mystical Kundalini Yoga. Learn about how yoga came to the West and why our culture is coming to a point in its evolution where yoga will become a powerful and pertinent tool.

Next, we introduce you to yoga's comprehensive guidelines for living. Far from hard-and-fast "commandments," yoga's *yamas* (abstinences) and *niyamas* (observances) point the way along the path that will most enhance your yoga journey. Patanjali, an ancient Indian sage who first put yoga to paper, recorded yoga's Eightfold Path (of which the abstinences and observances are the first two aspects), and we've laid it out in an easy-to-follow format, explaining the eight important facets of a yogi's life—from keeping the body fit to mastering detachment, concentration, and meditation.

Finally, we'll give you an introduction to Hatha Yoga, a system of yoga emphasizing control of the body and the most popular form of yoga in the West.

In This Chapter

- ◆ The history of yoga
- ◆ The nine types of yoga
- ◆ How yoga first came to the West
- ◆ Nonspiritual yoga: Is it possible?

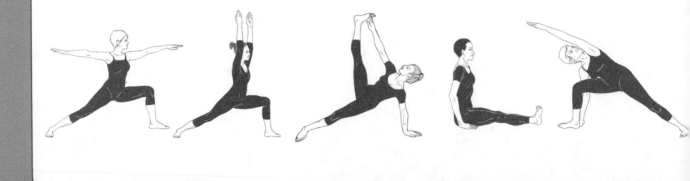

Chapter **5**

The Yoga Tradition: Many Types of Yoga

You don't have to know anything about the yoga tradition to practice yoga. After all, we're not in school, and we're not going to give you a history test. But history can be interesting, especially when there isn't a test—no pressure! Yoga's history is particularly illustrious and ancient. Understanding the deep and sagacious roots of your fitness program might help you gain a deeper appreciation of yoga's staying power and sacred origins.

People Practiced Yoga in 2500 B.C.E.

Yoga has been around for a long, long time. "How long?" you ask. The *Rig Veda* is possibly the oldest known text in the world, and it contains definite elements of yoga. Although the only remaining written versions are a few hundred years old, the earliest hymns are believed to be more than 4,000 years old. The hymns of the *Rig Veda* were passed down via an oral tradition with great accuracy. Hindu priests were trained to memorize the hymns precisely. If the *Rig Veda* is indeed thousands of years old, its existence might coincide with the existence of the Vedic people who lived along the Indus River.

But just because yoga is old doesn't mean it's old-fashioned. Yoga is timeless, transcending cultures, eras, and philosophies. It's said that you never know if something will be a classic until it has stood the test of time. Need we say more?

How Yoga Was Made

Nobody knows for sure exactly how yoga first came to be. Ayurveda, an ancient Indian system of health, includes yoga exercises designed to master the body and increase health, and yoga might have evolved from ancient ayurvedic practices. Today, ayurveda practitioners still use yoga as part of their practice. Because yoga or elements of yoga are mentioned in so many ancient texts without exact reference to their origins, however, we will probably never know for sure. However, yoga was likely an important part of the sacred rituals practiced by Indian holy men and an essential component of meditation. The poses themselves were likely handed down directly from teacher to student for centuries.

What we do know is that, several thousand years before the birth of Christ, a man named Patanjali first began recording information about yoga in writing. These were written as a collection of pithy, sometimes enigmatic aphorisms that described yoga's purpose, practice, and guidelines for living. Patanjali's "Eightfold Path" is still used today as the quintessential yoga reference. (Check out Chapter 6 for more details about Patanjali's Eightfold Path.) As for the exact details of how to do the many different yoga poses, these have evolved over thousands of years, gleaned from different texts, from word of mouth, and, as always, from teacher to student, teacher to student. Today, many traditional yoga poses continue to evolve, but many have remained in what are, as far as we know, their classic forms.

East Meets West

After all those centuries in India, how did yoga get all the way to America? Nineteenth-century America was largely unfamiliar with Eastern thought. Then, in 1893, *Swami* Vivekananda addressed the Parliament of Religions, causing quite a sensation. He quickly became a popular figure and was followed by many other gurus who came to the West and profoundly influenced their followers, such as Swami Paramahansa Yogananda, Swami Sivananda, and many more.

Know Your Sanskrit

Swami is correctly spelled "svamin," but Westerners write and pronounce it *swami*. **Svamin** is a title of respect for a spiritual person who is master of himself rather than of others. **Guru** literally means "dispeller of darkness." Gurus are self-realized adepts who initiate others into self-realization.

The 1960s rock group The Beatles became interested in Eastern thought and even visited India, befriending Maharishi Mahesh Yogi. George Harrison in particular was fascinated with Indian culture. He became enamored with the sitar (a Hindu stringed instrument that looks a little bit like a mandolin), and was one of the first to bring sitar music into rock 'n' roll. The Beatles, through songs such as "Norwegian Wood (This Bird Has Flown)" and "Within You, Without You," introduced Hindu melodies to modern music and opened Westerners' minds to different sounds and new experiences.

The Maharishi came to the West in 1959. America's "hippie generation" took to yoga in the 1960s, perhaps because traditional values were being questioned and yoga offered an alternative set of values attractive to spiritual seekers. After a few decades of excessive materialism and a world of violence, drug abuse, broken families, and the absence of any firmly held, widespread spiritual beliefs, yoga is more popular than ever before. We are seeking the spiritual with new vigor as an answer to a world we can't control—and not just the spiritual in theory. We are seeking the spiritual in *action*, in a way that can be meaningful to each of us.

Yoga Studies All Religions

So after all that history, you might be suspecting that yoga must surely be a religion. Yoga might seem like a religion. It offers guidelines for living, spirituality, study of sacred texts, and communion with the "divine." Some branches of yoga seem more religious or mystical than others, but yoga itself is certainly *not* a religion.

Yoga is open to all religions and encourages the study of all religious and spiritual texts. Yoga is not biased, prejudiced, or exclusive. You needn't be a Hindu, a Buddhist, a Muslim, a Christian, or a Jew, but you may be any of these. You can also be an agnostic or completely nonspiritual. Whatever religion you practice, yoga will help you understand your beliefs more clearly and get you in closer touch with your spiritual side. Yes, you have one, even if you don't go to church or synagogue or mosque or Zen center.

In Search of the Sacred (*Svadhyaya*)

Because yoga encourages the study of the sacred (*svadhyaya*), you might find it interesting, even helpful, to take a look at some of the world's major spiritual texts. Reading and studying any or even all of them will benefit your yoga practice as well as your mind by expanding your consciousness to possibilities you might not have considered. The more you know about the wonderfully varied and diverse world around you, the more you'll be in tune to the oneness that brings us all together.

 Know Your Sanskrit

Svadhyaya (pronounced *svahd-YAH-yah*) means "inquiring into your own nature, the nature of your beliefs, and the nature of the world's spiritual journey." Accomplished by the study of sacred texts, such as the *Bhagavad Gita* and the Bible, as well as through self-contemplation, *svadhyaya* is one of yoga's observances and one aspect of Patanjali's Eightfold Path, as described in the *Yoga Sutras* (and further explained in Chapter 6).

We aren't saying you should give up your other pursuits and devote your life to the minute study of ancient religious scriptures (unless you think that sounds like fun). However, reading the sacred texts of our world, or even just those of your own religion, can help you get in touch with the spiritual journey our species has undergone since we were first able to comprehend the concepts of spirituality, divinity, and the universe.

How about starting with the sacred texts that arose from the culture that invented yoga? Here are a few of the major sacred texts of India, but don't feel limited to these. The world is full of much, much more!

◆ The *Rig Veda,* considered the most ancient of sacred texts. Meaning "Knowledge of Praise," it's been orally passed down via sages who memorized it. Consisting of 1,028 hymns, the *Rig Veda* is now believed to be more than 4,000 years old.

◆ The *Upanishads,* the scriptures of ancient Hindu philosophy, which describe the path of Jnana Yoga, the discipline of wisdom as a path to self-realization.

◆ The *Bhagavad Gita,* perhaps the most famous Hindu text and the epic story of Arjuna, a warrior-prince who confronts moral dilemmas and is led to a better understanding of reality through the intercession of the god Krishna.

Wise Yogi Tells Us

The *Bhagavad Gita* is one of India's most beloved sacred texts. It tells the epic story of the warrior-prince Arjuna as he stands at the edge of a battlefield preparing for war. He discusses his universal moral dilemmas with the Hindu god Krishna, who is driving Arjuna's chariot. Is war justified? What if your loved ones are on the opposing side? What is right when your duties conflict? What does it mean to be born, to live, to die? The *Bhagavad Gita* is widely available and still a good read. (And it isn't even very long!) Pick up a copy and see what the fuss is all about. It's a beautiful story of inner quests and spiritual awakenings.

◆ Patanjali's *Yoga Sutras,* the source of Patanjali's Eightfold Path. Many call Patanjali the father of yoga because of this significant and influential text, but yoga was around long before Patanjali, who only made it more accessible.

◆ The *Hatha-Yoga-Pradipika,* a fourteenth-century guide to Hatha Yoga—everything you always wanted to know about Hatha Yoga but were afraid to ask!

Planting the Seeds: Yoga Branches for All Growing Personalities

Up to this point, although we've been focusing primarily on Hatha Yoga, we haven't really been distinguishing between all the different types of yoga. Yoga has a unified goal (a state of pure bliss and oneness with the universe), but each of the various methods emphasizes a different way to get to that goal. Let's go over some of the main types of yoga to see how they differ.

Hatha Yoga: Know Your Body, Know Your Mind

As we've mentioned before, Hatha Yoga works under the assumption that supreme control over the body, or the physical self, is one path to enlightenment. Hatha Yoga is a sort of spiritual fitness plan in which balance is a key. Attention to the physical is foremost in Hatha Yoga; this particular type of yoga involves cleansing rituals and breathing exercises designed to manipulate the body's energy through breath control, in addition to the postures or exercises for which Hatha Yoga is commonly known.

Wise Yogi Tells Us _____

If you're ill, whether you have a cold, chronic pain, or something more serious, Hatha Yoga postures, meditation, and the practice of mindfulness can be of great benefit. Learning to relax, physically and mentally, can comfort you and aid in healing. If you're in physical pain due to illness, however, or find yourself too distracted to even think about meditating, start slow, as little as five minutes a day. Even taking a series of full, deep breaths can be centering to body and mind.

Raja Yoga: Know Your Mind, Know the Universe

Raja Yoga, also known as *The Royal Path*, emphasizes control of the intellect to attain enlightenment. Meditation, concentration, and breath control are paramount in Raja Yoga, the yoga of the mind. Hatha and Raja Yoga work well together; Hatha Yoga is often considered a stepping stone to Raja Yoga, because after control of the body is mastered, control of the mind comes more easily.

Kriya Yoga and Karma Yoga: Act It Out!

Kriya Yoga and Karma Yoga are the yogas of action. *Kriya* means "spiritual action," and Kriya Yoga involves the practice of quieting the mind through scriptural self-study, breathing techniques, *mantras*, and meditation. Kriya Yoga understands that divine energy is stored in the lower part of the body. The study of Kriya Yoga breathing and meditation techniques helps bring this energy up the spine. As the energy builds, the yogi's body (physical and astral) is strengthened.

In *Karma* Yoga, the emphasis is selfless action. Karma Yoga transcends concerns of success or failure, egoism, and selfishness. What emerges is service to all beings. Because yoga teaches that every person is part of the divine universal spirit, Karma Yoga encourages that all beings on this earth be served with the respect deserving of a divine presence. The follower of Karma Yoga proceeds through daily life attempting to increase virtue and decrease lawlessness in the world by working for others and foregoing personal desires, resulting in greater empathy for and understanding of the world—and eventually, full understanding, or enlightenment.

Know Your Sanskrit _____

Karma is the law of cause and effect, or "what goes around comes around." Everything you do, say, or think has an immediate effect in the universe and in you. Karma is not negative. It is neither bad nor good. It is the movement toward balanced consciousness.

Bhakti Yoga: Open Your Heart

Bhakti Yoga places sincere, heartfelt devotion to the divine ahead of all else. Bhakti Yoga involves reverence, devotion, and perpetual remembrance of whatever divine presence is meaningful to you. Unsettled minds, intellectual concerns, the material world—everything falls away as love takes over and the heart is enveloped in thoughts of the divine. The heart is Bhakti Yoga's focus and is cultivated as the primary way to achieve unity with the divine.

Jnana Yoga: Sagacious You

Jnana Yoga is the path of knowledge and wisdom. Inquiring minds are what Jnana Yoga is all about, and because all knowledge is hidden within us, Jnana Yoga's goal is to inquire deeply into ourselves through questioning, meditation, and contemplation until we find that knowledge. Jnana Yoga involves a radical shift in perception. Everything you know, think, believe, or feel is questioned—temporarily. When everything you know is suddenly untrue, all that remains is you and the universe, which are the same thing. The goal is wisdom, which is far beyond the mere accumulation of information. It's direct knowledge of the divine through the elimination of all that is merely illusion.

Tantra, Mantra, and Kundalini Yoga

Tantra, Mantra, and Kundalini Yoga are grouped together here because they are all somewhat different than the other types of yoga. Although they share many practices and ideas, Tantra, Mantra, and Kundalini Yoga are more esoteric than other forms of yoga. Tantra Yoga involves the study of sacred writings and rituals. Mantra Yoga is the study of sacred sounds. Kundalini Yoga is the study of *kundalini* (energy) movement along the spine, which is released through breath and specific Hatha Yoga movements. All types of yoga are best learned under the guidance of a qualified teacher, and all require a degree of emotional, mental, and moral preparation.

Know Your Sanskrit

Tantra means "technique," and **Tantra Yoga** involves the techniques of ritual and study to eliminate obstacles to enlightenment.

Tantra Yoga has been associated with sexual rituals in popular culture, but that is an inaccurate portrayal. Tantric thought assumes that we live in a dark age (*kali yuga*) and, therefore, must use every method possible to boost our spirituality. Because Tantra Yoga emphasizes the power of ritual, it has become most famous in Western culture for its notion that sexual energy is an important store of energy that can be rechanneled to further you along your way to spiritual enlightenment. Our culture has expanded on the idea of sexual energy and sometimes perverts the concept into something it was never meant to be. Tantra isn't about the rampant search for extreme sex and the fulfillment of sexual desire. Remember, yoga is about mastering desire and refusing to let it control us. However, sexual communion as a way to generate spiritual energy can be a part of tantric ritual.

Know Your Sanskrit

Kali yuga (pronounced *KAH-lee YOO-gah*) is the fourth of four ages (*yuga* means "age") and the age in which we are now living. The shortest of all the ages, *kali yuga* is 432,000 years long. The other ages are **satya yuga,** the first age (1,728,000 years); **treta yuga,** the second age (1,296,000 years); and **dvapara yuga,** the third age (864,000 years).

Tantra is a complex, ancient, and esoteric discipline with a wide range of practices, often involving sacred rituals based on the idea that humans are reflections of divinity.

Tantra is also meant to be studied under a qualified adept, and its rituals and philosophies are kept secret from others who aren't receiving professional guidance. The idea is to prevent Tantra's precepts from being misunderstood and misused.

Mantra Yoga centers around the principle that sound can affect consciousness. *Shamanism,* yoga's probable precursor, considered sound an extremely important aspect of the search for spiritual enlightenment, and even today many religions use singing, chanting, rhythm, and recitation in their rituals. Mantra Yoga arose as a result of mystical experiences rather than philosophy. A *mantra* is a syllable or sequence of syllables designed to clear the mind and encourage spiritual awakening. Some people believe that Sanskrit syllables may even awaken reflexology points, those key spots on the hands and feet that correspond to different organs and organ systems in the body.

Once awakened, the body is energized to higher states of consciousness. *Om* is the most commonly known mantra syllable and sounds curiously (but probably not coincidentally) like "amen," the sound that punctuates so many religious hymns and prayers.

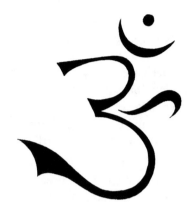

Om, written in Sanskrit.

Know Your Sanskrit

Shamanism (pronounced *SHAH-mahn-ihzm*) is the religion of certain northeast Asian peoples and is based on the philosophy that the workings of good and evil spirits can be influenced, but only by *shamans* (*SHAH-mahns*), the priests of shamanism.

Kundalini Yoga involves techniques meant to awaken energy, which is symbolized as a snake that "sleeps" at the base of the spine. When released correctly (that is, when the recipient is properly prepared), *kundalini* energy, sometimes called "serpent power," is potent and results in enlightenment. If released too soon, *kundalini* energy mixes with a person's negative emotions and can turn into intense and painful experiences.

Pure *kundalini* is a balanced and compassionate state of being. A person cannot have a negative *kundalini* experience. If someone has a negative experience, it is due to something other than *kundalini*. A *kundalini* awakening is thought to result not only in enlightenment, but also in the ability to control involuntary bodily functions such as the heartbeat.

To awaken the *kundalini*, you must go through complex mental and breathing exercises that should be practiced only under the guidance of a qualified teacher. Sometimes (though it's rare), a *kundalini* awakening will happen spontaneously, but don't be scared away.

Kundalini Yoga is, at its heart, searching for the same thing as all other types of yoga. Classes are available in this interesting branch of yoga; with proper instruction, the practice of Kundalini Yoga can be enjoyable, energizing, and ultimately enlightening.

Know Your Sanskrit

Kundalini is energy that lies curled like a snake at the base of the spine and can be awakened through various techniques and movements, after which it travels up the spine, activating the *chakras*. Kundalini Yoga is specifically designed to release this energy and channel it.

Can You Do Yoga Without Being Spiritual?

"All right, all right," you might be saying, "I'm interested in yoga, but this whole spiritual angle just isn't me." Worry not. You can do yoga without being spiritual, even though yoga is traditionally a spiritual pursuit. The postures, as we've said before, are great for fitness. Breathing exercises have wonderful physiological benefits. Even meditation needn't be spiritual—just a fitness program for the mind.

Wise Yogi Tells Us

Maharishi Mahesh Yogi was the inventor of Transcendental Meditation, or TM, a form of meditation that uses the ancient concept of *mantra* meditation and the mental repetition of a *mantra*. A *mantra* can be provided to you by your TM instructor, or you can create your own.

Yoga is so personal that it's impossible to say what it "should" be for anyone. In fact, yoga is distinctly "anti-should." It involves doing what feels right for you, what you want to do. The purpose of yoga is to maximize your potential—to help the best possible *you* emerge. Maybe the best possible you has no use for spiritual enlightenment. Whatever your potential and whatever your gifts, yoga will help you find them and make the most of them.

Why Practicing Yoga Is *So* "Right Now"

The world today is a lot different than when yoga first came to the West in the 1960s. The political climate continues to change, materialism waxes and wanes, optimism sparkles and fades and glimmers yet again. As people gradually become disillusioned by—or recover from—the hard lessons the world has taught us, many are searching for a more satisfying and fulfilling way of life than one designed around acquiring material possessions or getting ahead. As we discover that the nice car, the big house, and the fancy job title don't necessarily make us happy, we might be wondering more and more often: What really matters? Is it each other? Community? Love? Political action? Service to others?

If it isn't *stuff*, or relationships based on stuff, or a culture built around the acquisition of money, then what is it? Throughout history, priorities change and fashions come and go. The pendulum is swinging back toward spiritual priorities and self-actualization and away from more worldly concerns. This trend is apparent in the popularity of books (like this one) on subjects both spiritual and holistic. People have been disappointed, hurt, and disillusioned by the external world. As we realize we can't control what other people do, from family members to friends and work colleagues to actions in the international community, we are returning to the one place we can control. We are looking inward again.

Yoga fits easily and serenely into these new (or renewed) priorities. Yoga doesn't (or shouldn't) concern itself with competition, politics, materialism, or popularity—in essence, illusion. It's an inner journey toward self-realization and an outer journey toward physical control, holistic health, and confidence that comes not from possessions but from self-possession.

The Least You Need to Know

- Yoga is really, really old but still really, really relevant.
- Different types of yoga—Hatha, Raja, Kriya, Karma, Bhakti, Jnana, Tantra, Mantra, and Kundalini—emphasize different practices but have the same goal: enlightenment.
- You don't have to be spiritual to practice yoga, but if you practice yoga, you'll probably end up being a little more spiritual.

In This Chapter

- ◆ Yoga don'ts
- ◆ Yoga do's
- ◆ Body and breath control
- ◆ Detachment and concentration
- ◆ Meditation and pure consciousness

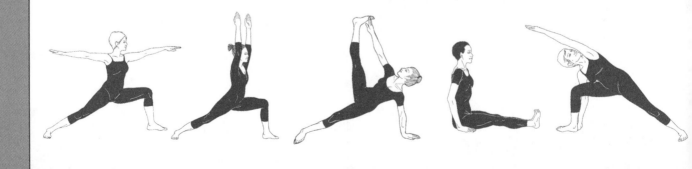

Chapter 6

Walking Yoga's Eightfold Path

If you're the kind of person who likes a nice, clean set of rules to live by, this is the chapter for you! In his *Yoga Sutras*, Patanjali, an Indian sage who was the first to record the previously oral tradition of yoga practice, explains the eight limbs, or paths, of yoga. These limbs provide a structure for your yoga practice and your daily life. They are designed to help you along the yoga path. One very important thing to remember about the eight limbs of yoga is that they are *not* commandments or laws! They are more like guidelines for living. But if you don't follow the guidelines, it doesn't constitute any sort of "sin." The Yoga Police won't come to your house and arrest you. Success with your yoga practice will simply be easier if you live your life according to Patanjali's suggestions.

However, if you don't want to meditate, give up meat, or relinquish your materialistic nature, don't pressure yourself. Remember that yoga is not only a practice, but something that happens to you. As you progress and grow, you might find that you're naturally less materialistic, you lose interest in eating meat, or you become drawn to meditation as the next logical step in your journey. These are some possible outcomes of studying yoga, but maybe those things won't happen for you. Maybe something deeper and even more profound is inside you that yoga has yet to help you discover.

Yet for those of you who want some commandments and want them *now*, it's also fine to view Patanjali's Eightfold Path more stringently. It all depends on who you are and what kind of thinking you're most likely to respond to. Here's a quick version of the Eightfold Path:

Eightfold Path at a Glance

1. Yoga don'ts (*yamas*)
   Nonviolence
   Nonlying
   Nonstealing
   Nonpursuit of lust/desire
   Nongreed
2. Yoga do's (*niyamas*)
   Purity
   Contentment
   Self-discipline
   Self-study
   Devotion
3. Yoga poses (*asanas*)
4. Breathing exercises (*pranayama*)
5. Detachment (*pratyahara*)
6. Concentration (*dharana*)
7. Meditation (*dhyana*)
8. Pure consciousness (*samadhi*)

Sound interesting? We thought so! We talk a lot about the later steps of the Eightfold Path throughout this book, but we'd like to spend a little more time explaining the first two steps because these set up a structure for thought, behavior, and action that can help you to stay on track and follow the yoga lifestyle.

Yoga Don'ts: Just Say No (Yamas)

First we'll talk about Patanjali's suggested abstinences. This is a difficult category for a lot of people who want to do yoga but don't want to be bound to any restrictions. Again, the abstinences, or *yamas*, aren't rules meant to limit you. They are suggestions meant to help you grow by purifying your body and your

mind. Practicing them can teach you self-discipline. You might also find that you already live by many of them.

Know Your Sanskrit

Yamas (pronounced *YAH-mahs*) are five abstinences or forms of discipline that purify the body and mind: *ahimsa* (*ah-HIM-sah*) means "nonviolence," *satya* (*SAHT-ya*) means "truthfulness," *asteya* (*ah-STAY-yah*) means "nonstealing," *brahmacharya* (*BRAH-mah-CHAR-yah*) means "chastity or nonlust," and *aparigraha* (*ah-PAH-ree-GRAH-hah*) means "nongreed."

Do No Harm (*Ahimsa*)

The first *yama* is about nonviolence. "That's an easy one," you say? Well, nonviolence means more than keeping yourself from beating up your obnoxious neighbor when he won't turn down his stereo. We can be violent in many ways, often without realizing it.

Ahimsa involves nonviolent actions, nonviolent words, and nonviolent thoughts. Nonviolent actions involve the obvious—don't physically hurt people. (Not even when they hurt you first.) Nonviolence isn't exactly about turning the other cheek. It's more like dodging the punch. For some, nonviolent action also means vegetarianism, because meat was once an animal, bird, or fish that was killed, and killing is violence. But if this step is too big for you, don't worry about it for now. Concentrate on eliminating violence in other ways. You'll come to understand the full range of opportunities for nonviolence at your own pace.

Nonviolent words are also important. Nonviolent speech means refraining from words that slander, degrade, or hurt another person. A good rule of thumb is to "honey-coat" your words, because you might have to eat them later! But that doesn't mean you should lie instead. You needn't tell your Aunt Maude that her polyester pantsuit is the loveliest outfit you've ever seen—she might give you one for your next birthday! And what if she asks you what you think about it? Simply say, "Aunt Maude, that outfit is definitely *you!*"

Nonviolent thoughts are equally important. Aunt Maude can't hear you thinking, "If I had taste like that, I would never leave my house!" The trouble with your thoughts, though, is that they pervade your entire being and are notoriously difficult to control. Having nonviolent thoughts means refusing to wish harm to anyone, even if you really think they deserve it. (Oops! That's bordering on a violent thought right there!) Let your negative thoughts go, wish your enemies well (if only in the privacy of your own brain), and your heart will lighten. According to yoga, we are energy and our thoughts can be sensed on an energetic level, so they are impossible to hide completely. People sense what you're thinking, so you're better off transforming your negative thoughts than trying to hide them. The beautiful thing about yoga is that your awareness heightens and you perceive the thoughts of others more clearly, too (of course, that could reveal some things you'd rather not know, but in the service of truth, we say it's worth it).

A Yoga Minute

According to the Institute of Science, Technology, and Public Policy, more than 40 studies have demonstrated that large groups practicing organized meditation (specifically, Transcendental Meditation in these studies) in one location reduce social stress and violence in urban, metropolitan, and even national areas. For more information on specific studies about meditation and reduced violence, see www.kosovopeace.org/research.html.

And one more thing about nonviolence: Engaging in negative talk and thoughts about yourself ("I am ugly," "I am lazy," "I can't do anything right") is doing violence to yourself. It counts—so don't do it!

Tell No Lies (Satya)

The second *yama* involves truthfulness. But what is the truth? You and I have different truths, so isn't truth changeable? According to yoga philosophy, truthfulness is the result of our mind, speech, and actions being unified and harmonious. Truth does no harm and results in personal integrity and strength of character.

Check out these scenarios and see if any of them are familiar:

◆ Someone confides in you and you promise you won't tell his or her secret, but then you don't "count" your spouse or your best friend. You've said the words, "I'm not supposed to tell you this, but …."

◆ You receive an extra $10 bill with your grocery change or at the bank and walk quickly away. After all, you need the $10 more than that big corporation!

◆ You occasionally bend or creatively interpret the rules on your income taxes just a little.

◆ You tell poor Aunt Maude you aren't feeling well and can't possibly visit her this week, even though you're actually feeling just fine.

Most of us have had at least occasional instances when it seemed more convenient, easier, or even kinder to bend the truth (or just snap it right in two!). It isn't easy to suddenly wake up one morning, vow to act completely truthfully, then stick to your vow. You can start by becoming more aware of what you're doing.

Ask yourself, "Is this harmonious with all parts of me? Does this do no harm?" If you aren't sure, maybe you should hold back. Dig deeper for the real truth in your daily life.

Just like everyone around you, you are so much more complex than your outward appearance, your job, the face you show the world, or the opinions others have of you. What seems to be the truth—what is obviously the truth, what you know is the truth—often is not the truth at all. Truth is tricky, but it's out there, buried under layers of misrepresentations, grudges, low self-esteem, unfortunate experiences, negative input, and discomforts. Striving for truth and bliss in your everyday life will help those layers fall away. Living truthfully takes some effort, but you can do it!

There are absolute truths that one perceives in the stillness of one's being. We're all searching for truth. The good news is that it's within everyone's grasp.

No More Stealing (*Asteya*)

So you think you don't steal? Just because you've never shoplifted a candy bar or a car radio doesn't mean you don't steal. The concept is simple, even if the implications aren't: If it's not yours, don't take it. (We assume we needn't mention that this *yama* includes no robbing banks or holding up armored cars!) That means no shoplifting and no taking credit for someone else's creations, ideas (plagiarizing), or for anything else anyone has done or said. Don't interrupt people and steal their center of attention. Don't steal your child's chance to do something on his own by doing it for him. Stealing can also be done indirectly. For example, buying an item from a street vendor who you believe is selling "hot" items. Although you might justify buying the item by

telling yourself how little you are paying for it or that you were not the one who stole the item, in essence, this is still stealing. You are feeding the system that allows stealing to continue.

Your actions—every action—has its resonating effect all over the world, and even into future generations, and we have more personal power than we think when it comes to correcting injustice, locally and globally. Yoga can help us become aware of this power at all levels in our lives and in the lives of others.

Cool It, Casanova (*Brahmacharya*)

Brahmacharya is about chastity. No, don't close the book and toss it aside! This *yama* doesn't mean telling your spouse the fun is over and you now need separate beds. *Brahmacharya* is about virtue—and not just when it comes to sex. Many great *yogis* are householders, which means they are married … with children.

Brahma means "truth," and *char* means "to move," so *brahmacharya* essentially means "to control the movement of truth." Lust and desire, in their many forms, obscure truth. Developing the inner strength to control our lusts and desires helps us see truth more clearly. In other words, *brahmacharya* is a movement toward responsible behavior and a higher truth beyond the physical, the force of "I want" in life. The *Bhagavad Gita* describes this *yama* in the following way:

> While contemplating the objects of the senses, a person develops attachment for them, and from such attachment, lust develops, and from lust, anger arises. From anger, delusion arises, and from delusion, bewilderment of memory. When memory is bewildered, intelligence is lost, and when intelligence is lost, one falls down again into the material pool.

Being virtuous means holding the opposite sex in high esteem and nurturing respect for someone you love. It also means holding *yourself* in high esteem and refusing to let your body be swayed by its every whim, desire, and want, whether that desire is for a person or for power or for a pound of Hershey's Kisses. Refusing to let your body be swayed by desire certainly doesn't preclude sex, a good promotion, or chocolate, for that matter. Instead, this *yama* encourages the kind of restraint and attitude toward those things we tend to desire that will help keep our minds clear and focused. Desire in itself is not negative. It is only when desire takes over as the driver of your life when you might run into trouble. Yoga helps to put you—the real you—back in the driver's seat.

The *brahmacharya yama* is often described as being about sex, and technically, it does preclude sexual lust—the one-night stand, using people (including yourself) sexually, and all the other things we typically associate with the word *lust*. Letting your desire for sex consume you is no way to become self-aware or calm and centered! But *brahmacharya* also encompasses lusts and desires of all kinds. At the very heart of this *yama*, desire itself, no matter its object, is what keeps us from seeing truth. To master our desires is to gain self-awareness.

> ## Ouch!
> Engaging in meaningless physical contact may only lead you away from the possibility of encountering someone who could become a life partner.

Don't Be Greedy (*Aparigraha*)

Go to your closet and count the pairs of shoes lined up in there—or the red sweaters or white shirts or ties. Or maybe you can't even open the closet because it's bursting with *stuff*. It isn't easy, in this materialistic world, to abstain from greed. With television, radio, and billboards continually telling us what we want and what we must have, it's hard not to believe some of it. But have you ever bought something you've always wanted, then felt strangely dissatisfied, as if the fun was in the wanting, not in the actual possessing? That is greed's payoff—emptiness.

Nongreed means living simply, possessing only what is necessary, and recognizing that possessions are merely tools to use in life. Accumulations, whether material things or unnecessary thoughts, tie you down to this world. Simplify your life as you simplify your thoughts.

Greed can also surface in less obvious ways. Talking too much, interrupting others, and dominating conversations while barely showing a flicker of interest in the participation of others are all ways greed creeps into our lives through language. Think before you speak, consider how your words will sound, and think about what effect they will have. Practice listening and being truly present in a conversation, absorbing everything other people are saying.

Thoughts can also be a source of greed. Why do the Smiths have a swimming pool and a fancy two-level deck while you have to sit on the back stoop under the sprinkler? Why did your best friend get diamonds for her birthday when you only got a toaster? Envy and jealousy clutter the mind and can become obsessions. How much better it is to turn those feelings around and feel truly happy for the person who has something you don't have! In fact, once you start to be happy for someone else simply because of their joy, you might become so fulfilled by your happiness that you lose your desire for whatever they have. How much simpler your life becomes when you can be happy due to something beyond your own needs!

Yoga Do's: Just Say Yes (Niyamas)

And now for the fun part! *Niyamas* are Patanjali's observances—what to do, as opposed to what *not* to do. The first *niyama* cleanses the way for all the others.

Know Your Sanskrit

Niyamas are observances or personal disciplines. There are five: *saucha* (pronounced *SAH-chah*) means "purity" or "inner and outer cleanliness," *santosha* (*san-TOH-shah*) means "contentment," *tapas* (*TAH-pahs*) means "self-discipline," *svadhyaya* (*svahd-YAH-yah*) means "self-study," and *ishvara-pranidhana* (*ISH-var-ah PRAH-nee-DAH-nah*) means "centering on the divine."

Be Pure (Saucha)

Purity is achieved through the practice of the five previous *yamas*, so the *yamas* and *niyamas* work hand in hand. The abstentions clear away negative physical and mental states of being, leading you straight to purity. Purity can apply to various aspects of your life. Cleanliness is very important to yoga. Keeping yourself clean by bathing; dressing in fresh, clean clothes; and keeping your surroundings clean are all part of pure actions.

What you eat is also important. Fresh, natural, and healthful foods are best. Foods obtained through nonviolent means are ideal because they can be eaten with full, unadulterated joy. That's why yogis traditionally eat only a vegetarian diet. Of course, if you want to get "yoga-technical," vegetables are alive, too (all life is to be respected, revered, and appreciated, and all life is interconnected), so respect each meal for the life given to sustain another.

Be Content (Santosha)

Just saying the word *santosha* (*san-TOH-shah*) invokes a feeling of calm. Practicing contentment means finding happiness with what you have and with who you are. Of course, you can always work toward improvement, but that doesn't mean you can't be content while you're improving yourself! Contentment helps you see that you're exactly where you're supposed to be right now. It doesn't mean you'll be happy when you can finally stand on your head, get that promotion, or find a soul mate. It means happiness in this moment, as you are.

Contentment means learning to reevaluate obstacles as opportunities. Limitations are just learning experiences. Easier said than done, we know! If you feel unhappy with your life, you might find it especially difficult to cultivate contented thoughts. Practicing contentment involves taking full responsibility for your life and the situations you're in. Find the positives in life's lessons and choose to grow from them. You're in charge of your own destiny, but that also means you can't beat yourself up for the "mess" you're in. Thank yourself for it. Laugh! Know that every situation or challenge presented is a doorway to greater growth.

Wise Yogi Tells Us

Feeling discontented? Try this exercise. Create a list of everything that makes you discontented. Then rewrite your list, finding a way to see each source of discontentment in some positive light. For example, rewrite "I hate my job" to "My job has taught me that I am more creative than I thought." When you're finished, throw away that first list—you don't need it!

Be Disciplined (*Tapas*)

For all the *yamas* and *niyamas* to be truly effective, you'll need a little self-discipline. That's not your strong point? If self-discipline were easy, what would be the point? It would hardly be discipline.

Anyone who exercises daily shows self-discipline. Dedicating a specific time each day to your yoga practice is self-discipline. But how many times have you started an exercise program, only to abandon it as soon as it got boring or tedious? Learning how to stick to something even when you don't feel like it will build your strength and wisdom. You probably manage the self-discipline to brush your teeth twice every day. Just extend that discipline, bit by bit, to other aspects of your life, one step at a time. Maybe tomorrow you'll brush your teeth and have a healthful salad for lunch. Maybe next week you'll be brushing your teeth, eating salads, and doing 10 minutes of yoga. By next year, there's no telling what you can accomplish.

Disciplined words mean speaking gently and sincerely, not angrily or hurtfully. *Act* rather than *react*, because you cannot control the actions of others. Self-disciplined thoughts replace the negative with the positive, resentment with forgiveness, violence with peace, and unhappiness with joy.

The *yamas* and *niyamas* themselves provide an excellent opportunity to practice self-discipline.

Wise Yogi Tells Us

Self-discipline is difficult for almost everyone, but changing your attitude might help keep you on track. The best way to do this is to focus on the positive: "I will spend 30 minutes practicing yoga today." "I will relax with deep-breathing exercises tonight before I go to bed." "I will have a soothing cup of herbal tea this morning." Focusing on the positive makes being disciplined more fun! Because really, discipline isn't deprivation, it's self-care.

Be Studious (*Svadhyaya*)

Svadhyaya doesn't just mean you should read a lot of books. It means studying yourself through introspection. Do you act according to your beliefs? Do you say what you mean? Are you walking your talk? Studious action means paying attention to your physical self. How are you sitting, standing, or walking? Do you feel graceful or stilted? Do you look the way you feel? If not, why not? Studious words and thoughts involve the study of various sacred texts—whichever are relevant to you—to inspire and teach you. Through self-study, you can see which thoughts, actions, words, and experiences actually make you happy and which block your happiness. Dedicated, nonviolent introspection will fill your life with clarity.

Be Devoted (*Ishvara-Pranidhana*)

The last *niyama* involves devotion. Focus on the divine, whatever that means to you—how it is in you and part of you and all around you. This yama often misleads people into thinking that yoga is a religion. Some people might perceive it that way, but this yama is simply a call to practice your own spirituality, whatever it is. Nurturing your spirituality is an important part of balancing your whole self, which is yoga's realm. If you are already religious, you can bring yoga into your practice, too. Some yoga teachers might even teach according to their individual religious beliefs, although yoga itself is not a religion. Yoga merely helps you open the door to your spiritual self and walk through. Get comfortable in there, and your life will open up in new ways.

Ishvara-pranidhana is an observance that works beautifully with any religion. Whether you're devoted to God, Goddess, Krishna, Buddha, or the Force, this *niyama* reminds you to relinquish ego and center on your highest ideal. Positive energy will flow from the divine into all areas of your life.

Are You Wearing Your Walking Shoes? More Yoga Pathways

But what about the rest of the Eightfold Path? Technically, so far we've covered only the first two limbs (the do's and don'ts). The remaining limbs of the Eightfold Path are also important and complete the framework for the modern practice of yoga.

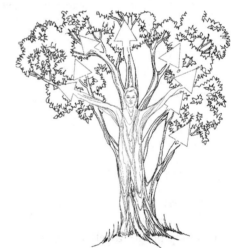

Growing with yoga's Eightfold Path.

Body Control (*Asanas*)

We've already talked about body control, or the *asanas*, as both an important part of yoga and its most well-known component. Remember that body control is not the only path, but merely one path yoga offers. Yet body control is very important and makes a great starting point for any aspiring *yogi*.

Asana literally translates as "posture" and is derived from the Sanskrit root *as*, which means "to stay." Patanjali describes an *asana* as having *sthira* and *sukha*, or steadiness and the ability to remain comfortable. Remember these two qualities when practicing your postures, keeping in mind the very important *yama* of *ahimsa*, or nonviolence: Never work to the point of pain, because that is doing violence to your body.

 Know Your Sanskrit

> **Sthira** (pronounced *STHIH-ra*) means "steadiness and alertness." **Sukha** (*SOO-kah*) means "lightness and comfort." Both are desirable qualities in yoga postures.

Breath Control (*Pranayama*)

Pranayama is another important path. *Prana* refers to the life force or energy that exists everywhere and is manifested in each of us through the breath. *Ayama* means "to stretch or extend." *Prana* flows out from the body, and *pranayama* teaches us to maneuver and direct *prana* for optimal physical and mental benefit.

After all, breathing is life. You can go for months without food, days without water, but only moments without breath. Breathing affects all our actions and our thoughts, too. Mastering your breath is an important step toward mastering the rest of yourself!

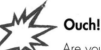 **Ouch!**

> Are you feeling listless, depressed, and under the weather? According to ancient yoga texts, you have too much *prana* outside your body. *Prana* is constantly moving and flowing into and out of us, and *pranayama* is a tool for maintaining your health and well-being. Keep yourself healthier and happier by using breath control to keep more *prana* inside (where it belongs)!

Detachment (*Pratyahara*)

The fifth limb of yoga is sense-related. *Pratyahara* is the practice of withdrawing the senses from everything that stimulates them. Normally, we live by our senses. We are drawn to look at beautiful or even ugly things. We listen, we taste, we touch, and we smell. This is the ordinary state of things, but it's also a state we can temporarily suspend in favor of a deeper awareness. *Pratyahara* cuts off the connection between the senses and the brain. This can happen during breathing exercises, meditation, the practice of yoga postures, or any activity requiring concentration.

 Know Your Sanskrit

> Pratyahara (*PRAH-tyah-HAH-rah*) means "withdrawal of the senses."

But what's the purpose of detaching ourselves from our senses? Aren't the senses good? They help us appreciate beauty, as when we watch a sunset, or warn us of danger, as when we smell smoke or spoiled food, and they permit us to communicate with each other. Unfortunately, our senses can also become so pleasurable that they control us instead of us controlling them. Maybe you enjoy your sensation of taste so much that you have become a little too obsessed with food. Maybe you love to talk but often talk so much that you forget to listen. Maybe you're addicted to television, caffeine, or sex. *Pratyahara* wipes the sensual slate clean.

Wise Yogi Tells Us

If the *yamas* and *niyamas* seem like a lot to remember, make yourself an abbreviated version of them—as plain (computer graphics?) or fancy (framed calligraphy?) as you like—and hang it up in your bedroom, bathroom, or wherever you'll see it each day. Or make a copy of the "Eightfold Path at a Glance" list earlier in this chapter. Soon you'll have them memorized, and they'll become a part of you.

Detachment is also a great technique for pain control and an excellent way to deal with uncomfortable symptoms or chronic conditions. Try this technique for attaining sense withdrawal:

1. Sit erect. Place your thumbs on your ears, closing them off. Your eyes should be closed. Place your index fingers near your eyelashes to hold them gently shut and prevent movement of your eyeballs. (This assists the eyes in staying focused on the sun *chakra*, or third eye. See Chapter 16 for more on the *chakras*.) Rest each middle finger on your nasal passages. Set your ring fingers on your upper lip and your little fingers on your lower lip.

2. Take a deep breath and gently press all fingers so your sense organs are suppressed. Turn inward, tuning out the external world. Focus your attention on your sun *chakra*.

3. When you can no longer comfortably hold your breath, release your fingers.

4. Exhale slowly. Inhale slowly. Repeat this gentle pressure for deeper reflections.

Concentration (*Dharana*)

Dhri means "to hold," and *dharana*, yoga's sixth limb, is all about learning to concentrate. Concentration involves teaching the mind to focus on one thing instead of many, as is our usual state of mind. *Dharana* is an exercise that can help with meditation. The goal is to become aware of nothing but the object on which you are concentrating, whether it's a candle flame, a flower, or a *mantra* you repeat to yourself. The purpose is to train the mind to ignore all the extra, unnecessary junk floating around, to learn to gently push away superfluous thought. *Pratyahara* (withdrawal of the senses) is often the result when *dharana* is achieved, and both assist with more productive meditation, or *dhyana*.

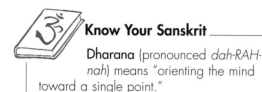

Know Your Sanskrit _____

Dharana (pronounced *dah-RAH-nah*) means "orienting the mind toward a single point."

Meditation (*Dhyana*)

Concentration is the exercise that leads to the state of meditation, and meditation techniques are, in essence, purity techniques. Meditation occurs when you've actually become linked to the object of your concentration so that nothing else exists. It's keen, heightened awareness, not nothingness. Your mind is completely focused and quiet but awake and aware of truth. Many methods exist to bring you to this state, but oneness with the object of your meditation and, subsequently, oneness with the entire universe, is the objective. And don't forget the wonderful fringe benefit of a calm and uncluttered mind that's able to think more quickly and see more clearly in all daily activities!

Know Your Sanskrit _____

Dhyana (*dee-YAH-nah*) means "meditation," and **samadhi** (*sah-MAH-dee*) means "becoming one with the object of your meditation."

Pure Consciousness (*Samadhi*)

All the limbs of yoga lead to *samadhi*, the final limb of the Eightfold Path. *Samadhi* means "to merge," and this state of pure consciousness means just that: a complete and total merging with the object of your meditation.

When in a state of *samadhi*, you understand not only that you and the object of your meditation are one, but that you and the universe are one. There's no difference between you and everything else. How does this feel? Like a loss of identity? Yes, identity is meaningless in *samadhi*, but you won't be sorry. Who needs an ego when you have *samadhi*? *Samadhi* is pure, total bliss.

The Least You Need to Know

- Yoga offers guidelines for living.
- The five abstentions are nonviolence, nonlying, nonstealing, nonlusting, and nongreed.
- The five observances are purity, contentment, self-discipline, self-study, and devotion.
- Yoga also involves body control, breath control, detachment, concentration, and meditation.
- Yoga is a journey into a deep, blissful oneness with the universe, leading to liberation and self-realization.

In This Chapter

- ◆ Hatha Yoga basics
- ◆ Opposites attract in Hatha Yoga
- ◆ Why yoga postures are so important
- ◆ Why the breath is so important
- ◆ How body obsession is a barrier

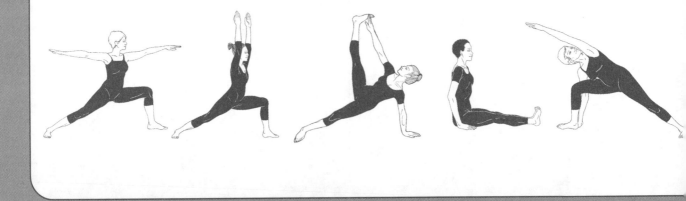

Chapter **7**

Hatha Yoga: Union with the Universe

We've explained how yoga has many paths and that Hatha Yoga's path is body mastery. Great! Now … what the heck does that mean?

Hatha Yoga's path to self-actualization is a method we Westerners can easily work with because we are so physically oriented.

Strike a Pose

The poses of Hatha Yoga are at the heart of its practice. Meditation and breathing are also key to a successful and well-rounded Hatha Yoga practice, but most people imagine yoga poses when they hear "Hatha Yoga," and rightly so. This discipline of teaching the body to move into specific positions and hold them while breathing is Hatha Yoga's power.

The poses of Hatha Yoga are by no means random. They are specifically designed to activate the internal, as well as the external aspects of the body. After your very first yoga class, you might feel like you've moved in ways you never even considered moving before. Joints we so often use in only limited ways get to experience their complete range of motion with yoga. Tiny muscles that usually lie unused get prodded into action. Organs stuck in a rut experience refreshment again. We stretch, we twist, we bend, we arch, we roll, we tuck, we reach, and we flex. And it feels great!

Our bodies are made for action. They aren't made for sitting at a computer all day, or even doing one single exercise or motion over and over and over again. They are complex and amazing organisms capable of the most incredibly minute actions as well as the most large and dramatic movements. The human body can manipulate cells on a slide plate under a microscope by hand, and it can also do a quadruple loop at the ice-skating rink or fly across a gymnasium doing handsprings and flips. But most of us don't use our bodies at these extremes. Hatha Yoga introduces us to the world of possibility within our physical selves.

Hatha Yoga is based around several types of poses. You might find that your yoga teacher or another book you read groups the poses together in different ways than we have chosen here, but essentially all yoga poses do certain things, such as bend forward or backward, twist one way and then the other, or invert the body. Some poses accomplish more than one of these things. Plow pose, for instance, is an inversion and a forward bend, while Wheel pose is both an inversion and a backbend.

To give you a roadmap for the pose chapters later in this book, here are some Hatha Yoga pose–type basics.

Standing Poses

Standing poses in general, and Mountain pose in particular, are at the core of many of yoga's most basic poses. Let's consider the importance of standing poses.

Standing poses develop and strengthen your legs, those all-important limbs and vehicles of motion. Standing poses also improve your balance, align your hips and spine, and maintain equilibrium throughout your body. Master the standing poses before you attempt to master the more complicated ones, such as balance poses and poses on the floor that require more advanced flexibility and/or strength. If you practice standing poses regularly, you'll notice an almost immediate improvement in your leg and hip flexibility, as well as increased strength and general stability throughout your entire body. Your balance and posture will improve, too.

Posture Perfect

Good posture is essential to proper form in the standing poses—and the seated ones, too. It also helps allow your body to achieve or maintain good health. Proper posture feels better, looks better, and *is* better for your body. Good posture also influences your feelings and thoughts. If you stand up straight and tall, you'll think more positive thoughts. It's true! Try it!

Good posture extends beyond the practice of your yoga postures. You spend a lot of your life standing, but do you stand in a way that is healthy for you? The next time the fact that you're standing comes to mind—whether you're in line at the grocery store, filling up at the gas station, or stir-frying vegetables at the stove—notice *how* you're standing.

Chances are, you'll notice that your posture is less than straight, tall, aligned, and balanced. Maybe you carry one shoulder higher or lower than the other. Maybe you shift your weight to one hip, or stoop forward, or lean your head to the left or right. Even if you're fairly balanced, you might not be standing as tall as you could be, and your muscles might be fighting gravity and bad habits rather than optimizing and balancing the body's strength and inherent balance with nature.

Posture is more important to your health than many people realize. Ask any chiropractor—if the body isn't aligned, the energy gets "clogged" in certain areas and doesn't flow freely. If part of you is energy-deprived, you're out of balance, and the more out of balance you become, the greater your chances of succumbing to stress, depression, and disease. Good posture helps a body heal itself, so help your body to be its best. In Chapter 11, poses like Mountain and Lightning Bolt can help you train your body to stand straight and tall.

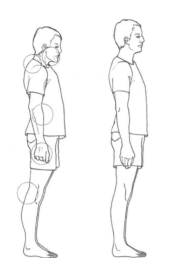

A misaligned body can impede the flow of energy. It doesn't look good and, more important, it can keep your body from achieving optimal physical and emotional health.

You might be tempted to flip to the back of the book to look for the poses you think look more difficult or impressive, but we urge you to stay right where you are! Standing poses, and Mountain pose in particular, provide an important training ground for all the yoga *asanas*. If you don't know how to stand like a mountain, all your other poses will be affected—and you might be surprised to learn that the more you practice Mountain pose, the more you understand that it is more difficult than it looks!

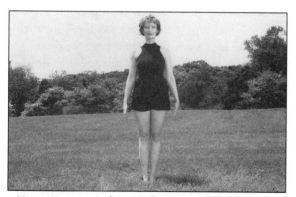

Mountain pose is the most basic standing pose and a core yoga pose that must be deeply studied before attempting more challenging poses.

Wise Yogi Tells Us

Here's an easy way to maintain good posture while standing: Pretend you have a loop attached to the crown of your head and a string tied to the loop. Imagine someone above you is pulling on the string. Feel how your entire spine and neck shift and stretch as the string pulls upward. That's what healthy posture feels like!

Warrior Spirit

One of our favorite groups of standing poses is the group of Warrior poses. These poses are popular because they are fun and empowering. But don't let the name mislead you!

We tend to think of warriors as wearing armor. In yoga, the warrior represents the strength of openness and the expansion of consciousness. It takes tremendous strength to live a life of nonviolence, which is the path of the yogi warrior.

When you practice the Warrior poses, visualize your entire center holding itself up. This internal lift strengthens and tones your muscles from the inside out. Also lift your abdomen while in the poses. You can still breathe fully and expand your abdomen while keeping it lifted; the lift supports, rather than impedes, the breath. Think strong foundation, fluid movement, and steady balance.

Ouch!

Don't get tense about the "warrior" idea. Some people hear the word *warrior* and their muscles immediately tense up as if they're preparing for battle. Yet the most effective warriors stay calm, clear-headed, and in a position to move in any direction as the situation requires. You can achieve this readiness without debilitating tension by concentrating on internally lifting the center of your body.

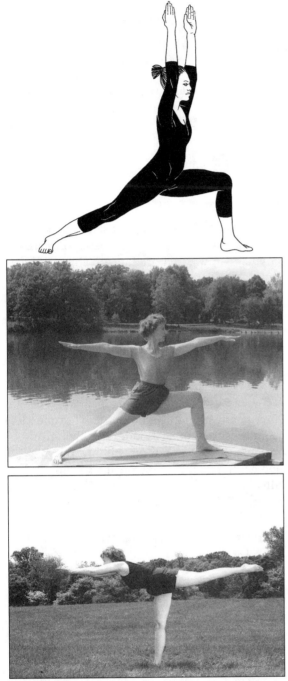

The Warrior poses help strengthen body, mind, and spirit as they energize your body, build confidence, improve balance, and provide strength.

Forward Bends

Standing poses easily morph into forward bends, although forward-bending poses apply to both standing and sitting poses. Forward bends stretch the back of the body. They are essential for lengthening the muscles of the back, legs, shoulders, neck, and spine. Forward bends also activate many of the internal organ systems by compressing the organs as the front of your body folds over itself. That same folding in can also help the mind focus inwardly for greater relaxation and a reflective, inner-gazing state.

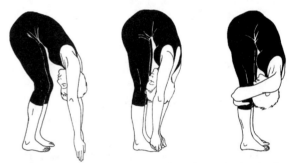

Standing Head to Knees pose lengthens the back of the body, helps stimulate internal organ function, and helps focus the mind on the inner self.

Backbends

Back-bending poses are the complements to forward-bending poses. Backward and forward bends balance each other in a yoga workout. Backbends stretch the front of the body, opening the chest, hips, and rib cage. They help in the release of emotions, the opening of the heart, and the stretching and strengthening of the muscles and opening of the torso, releasing tension in the body and the internal organs.

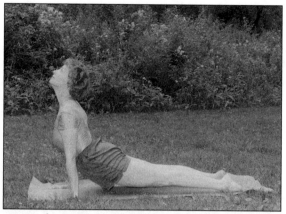

Upward Facing Dog is a basic back-bending pose that stretches the chest, strengthens the legs and arms, and helps open the heart for a freer flow of feeling.

Twists

We love twists, because twisting poses do amazing things for the spine. They open the joints of the hips and shoulders, add core flexibility, and can compress and stimulate internal organs in amazing ways. Just be sure you always counter a twisting pose that goes one way with one that goes the other way, to keep your bodymind balanced.

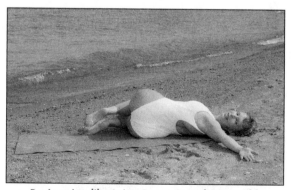

Basic twists like Lying Down Spinal Twist add flexibility to the spine and improve digestion and internal organ function.

Inversions

Inversions are lots of fun. Inversions give our body a break from its normal upright state and let you see the world upside down! Everything is turned topsy-turvy as your head goes down and your feet (depending on the pose) go up! Inversions help blood flow the opposite way in your body for a change, flooding your brain and upper body with nourishment and giving your poor legs and feet a break from all that downward flow. Some people believe that a few minutes in an inverted pose every day can actually lengthen your life. We don't know if that's true or not, but sometimes we take a break from writing long enough to do a nice shoulderstand or headstand, just because it feels so good and gets that brain working again.

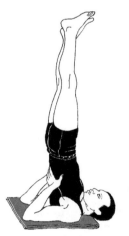

Shoulderstand pose inverts the body, promoting blood flow to the head, neck, and shoulders, and directs fluids out of the feet and legs. Try it as a great mental refresher, not to mention a break for aching feet.

On the Floor

While many yoga poses are based on standing poses, many have you down on the floor. Basic seated poses are important for yoga. They help you concentrate and isolate certain areas that need attention or need to be brought into balance with the rest of your bodymind. The primary poses are seated, meditative, and prone poses.

Seated Poses

Seated poses can involve many different kinds of poses, from easy to high challenging. Whether they involve a spinal twist, a hamstring stretch, or an abdominal strengthener, seated poses can benefit the body in a multitude of ways.

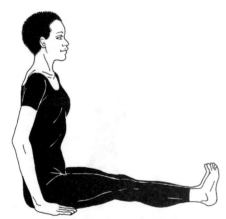

Staff pose is like Mountain pose for the floor. It encourages an inner strength and solidity, builds confidence, increases focus, and improves posture.

Meditative Poses

Meditative poses are just what they sound like: yoga poses suited for serious meditation. The most classic is the Lotus pose, but this challenging pose isn't for everybody, and beginners might want to wait and try it after they have more yoga

experience. Other seated meditative poses might be more comfortable and more conducive to quiet contemplation. Once you've mastered Lotus, however, it is an ideal meditative pose for stability.

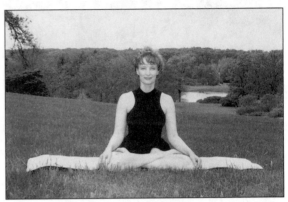

Lotus pose is the classic meditative yoga pose, designed to imitate the symmetry of the lotus flower and put the body in its most stable position for least distraction during meditation.

Prone Poses

Finally, prone poses are at the very heart of yoga, most particularly *shavasana*, or Corpse pose. This pose might look simple, but the deep meditative state it can help you achieve is what yoga is all about.

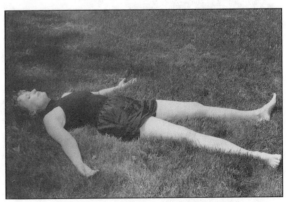

Corpse pose is a prone pose designed for deep and total bodymind relaxation.

Vinyasana, Ashtanga, and Power Yoga

A *vinyasana*, like Sun Salutation, is a series of poses linked together in a dynamic sequence. Practicing a *vinyasana* can be aerobically challenging and a lot of fun!

Ashtanga is a kind of yoga made popular by Sri K. Pattabhi Jois at the Ashtanga Yoga Research Institute in Mysore, India. This form of yoga links high-energy poses together in a sweat-inducing series of yoga challenges.

Particularly popular in the fitness-conscious West, power yoga (a version of *ashtanga*) has evolved into several different subforms that vary according to the teacher and the teacher's teacher. For one example, check out *The Complete Idiot's Guide to Power Yoga* (Alpha Books, 2000) by Geo Takoma and Eve Adamson. Power yoga is a great introduction to yoga for the highly athletic who might need to work more gradually into the slower and more contemplative forms of yoga.

To practice *vinyasana* and other yoga sessions, see Chapters 19, 20, and 21.

Know Your Sanskrit

Ashtanga Yoga is traditionally the yoga that specifically follows Patanjali's Eightfold Path as a way to enlightenment, but in the West we have come to associate the term with a highly athletic form of Hatha Yoga.

Know Thyself

What does self-awareness mean to you? Self-awareness means different things to different people, but here are some ways to look at self-awareness. Self-awareness is …

- Finding out that the alignment of your large toe is responsible for your headache. Discovering that your body is full of links, clues, and connections to your health and mental well-being.

- Pausing before your emotions take over your actions, and eventually finding out that your emotions can exist without taking over.

- Feeling truly connected to another living being—a parent, a child, a friend, a stranger in need, or that stray cat who keeps hanging around.

- Breathing deeply and slowly and noticing how different that feels.

- Looking in the mirror and seeing beyond your reflection; seeing the inner you written all over your face.

- Having vision and direction in your life and finding a deeper calling and heeding it.

- Recognizing that the Sun Salutation is reflective of the ebb and flow of life.

- Finding the clear steadiness of the eyes in an externally changing face; both inner and outer movement are ever possible.

- Experiencing pure joy simply by looking at something beautiful. You don't need to own it; you can be with it and then let it go.

- Finding inner peace. *Om.*

When the body is strong, controlled, and purified, *kundalini* energy can move freely up the spine and through the *chakras* without getting blocked anywhere along the way. If *kundalini* energy gets blocked, both physical and mental problems could result. The body that's physically prepared for the rise of *kundalini* energy will derive the ultimate benefit from its power. Hatha Yoga is that physical preparation.

Joining the Sun and the Moon

Hatha Yoga is about balancing the opposing forces of the body, just as opposing forces are balanced outside the body. Sun and moon, male and female, day and night, cold and hot—the universe is filled with opposites. Maybe you've heard of or seen the yin/yang symbol. This ancient Chinese symbol represents the universe of opposing forces. Notice how a white dot sits in the center of the black swirl, and a black dot sits in the center of the white swirl.

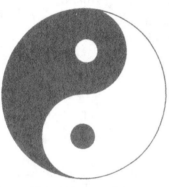

The yin/yang union.

Yin and yang are commonly associated with many different complementary qualities. Yin is primarily present in the moon, the night, cold, female energy, and heaviness. Yang is primarily present in the sun, the daytime, heat, male energy, and lightness. And because every force has an opposite and also contains a bit of its opposite within itself, male energy contains female energy, female energy contains male energy, night contains a bit of day, day contains a bit of night, and so on. So the universe goes—ultimately interconnected.

And so our bodies go, too. We are filled with opposites: a left and a right side, blood flowing to the heart and away from the heart, the delivery of nutrients and the removal of waste, inhalations and exhalations, hunger and satiety, sleeping and wakefulness, being with others and being alone, joy and sadness, birth and death, growth and decline. If any of the thousands of opposites and intricate balances within us become unbalanced, our bodies and minds won't work as efficiently.

Hatha Yoga balances us in many ways. Forward-bending poses are followed by back-bending poses, contractions are followed by extensions, upright positions are followed by inversions, and so on. The practice of Hatha Yoga also balances our mental and spiritual energies, for what we do with the body affects the mind and the spirit (that triangle again!)—ultimately interconnected.

Getting Subtle

On a subtler level, the movement of *prana* is balanced through muscular exercises called *bandhas*. As *prana* is drawn into the body through the inhalation of breath, *apana* is the energy generated in the body by exhalation that moves away from the brain and carries impurities out of the body. *Bandhas* are exercises, or muscular locks, designed to lock the flow of energy in the body.

The three primary *bandhas* are …

◆ At the chin (*jalandhara bandha*). This *bandha* strengthens and builds *prana*'s upward movement by bringing the chin to the chest.

◆ In the abdominal solar plexus area (*uddiyana bandha*). This *bandha* strengthens and builds *apana*'s downward movement by pulling your navel up and back toward your spine.

◆ In the area of the rectum (*mula bandha*). This *bandha* keeps *prana* from escaping from the lower body by contracting the perineal muscle (the muscle you sit on, in front of the rectum).

Know Your Sanskrit

Apana is the energy generated in the body by exhalation that moves away from the brain and carries impurities out of the body. *Bandha* means "to bind" or "to lock," and *bandhas* are muscular locks used during poses and breathing exercises to intensify the energy of *prana* and *apana* so it can eliminate impurities from the body. The three primary *bandhas* are chin or *jalandhara bandha* (*jah-lahn-DAH-rah BAHN-dah*), stomach or *uddiyani bandha* (*ooh-dee-YAH-nah BAHN-dah*), and anal or *mula bandha* (*MOO-lah BAHN-dah*).

Bandhas keep the system of balances in check by pulling everything toward a center point, intensifying the energy. Practicing these *bandhas* while sitting in meditation or holding a yoga pose can be a particularly powerful way of concentrating and intensifying *prana* in the body.

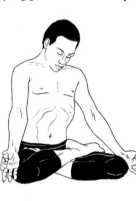
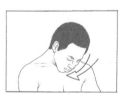

Practicing the *bandhas*.

The result is that *prana* and *apana* are retained within the body, joining together within *sushumna*—that hollow passageway through your spinal cord. Their mingling generates an intense energy that can help awaken the *kundalini* serpent power. This joining of opposites, of *prana* and *apana*, of sun and moon, of *ha* and *tha*, is at the heart of Hatha Yoga's

power. Maybe you aren't too concerned with awakening your serpent power, especially because you aren't sure exactly what it is—or even whether you want to know. Maybe you just want to feel more balanced, healthier, or more in shape. Most Westerners don't practice Hatha Yoga to the extent that they're even aware of the importance of *kundalini* energy, but traditionally, this awakening of the "serpent power" is one of the primary purposes of Hatha Yoga.

A Yoga Minute

In Hindu culture, cobras are considered reincarnations of important people. The Aztecs worshipped a snake god who symbolized light, luck, and wisdom. In Africa, some cultures worship pythons, and killing snakes is a crime. Egyptian kings wore snake representations on their crowns, and the crosier of *Asklepios* (the Greek god of medicine and healing) is still a symbol of the medical profession today.

Physical fitness—making the body feel good and look good—has traditionally been a peripheral benefit, but it has shifted to the primary focus for Westerners. If fitness is your motivation for beginning a Hatha Yoga practice, that's great. You'll benefit in many ways, no matter what reason brings you to the practice. But although fitness is important in Hatha Yoga, it means more than cut shoulders and washboard abs. Total fitness—of the mind, body, and spirit—is a far cry from body obsession. Body obsession is fitness gone awry.

If fitness is your goal, it doesn't hurt (and might even be ultimately helpful) to be aware of the power of balanced opposites inherent in your practice. This knowledge might steer you away from the path of body glorification—a possible side effect of heightened body awareness—and toward the more advanced paths of mental control (Raja Yoga) and spiritual awakening.

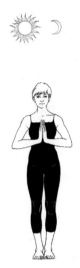

Hatha Yoga joins the opposites of sun and moon within the body. Here, the energies are drawn into the centered position of respect and thanks, namaste, or prayer pose.

Know Your Sanskrit

Namaste (pronounced *nah-MAHS-tay*) means "Obeisance to you" or "I salute the divine light within you" and is a *mudra* (hand position) in which the palms and fingers come together in the prayer position. Your hands are held with your thumbs against your chest in an attitude of focused devotion. *Namaste* can also be held loosely behind your back with your fingers pointed up.

Training the Body to Free the Mind

Think about how much time you spend worrying about your body! Check all the following statements that have ever crossed your mind:

- ❑ I'm too fat.
- ❑ I'm too thin.

- ❑ I'm having a bad hair day.
- ❑ My skin looks terrible.
- ❑ My body is unattractive.
- ❑ I have the best body in the room.

Our bodies are so much a part of us and so emphasized by our culture that it's extremely difficult not to put too much emphasis on physical appearance. Remember, though, that your body isn't all of you. In fact, your body is just one tiny part of you. You are the entire universe. You have the potential for perfection, contentment, and pure joy. Your body is just a convenient container for the luminous being that is you. In comparison to who you really are, even the most "perfect" body is a little, well … crude.

Wise Yogi Tells Us

Once you're comfortable in some of the yoga poses, try adding a new dimension to your workout: visualization. Visualization is the process of picturing something in your mind and letting it affect you. Visualizing something beautiful—an ocean, a sparkling lake, a magnificent canyon, a spectacular sunset—can make you feel peaceful and relaxed. Practice visualization while holding poses that are easy for you. Hold your image for as long as you can before other thoughts take over.

One Body ... or Three?

You have one body—or do you? Actually, according to yoga, you have three bodies: the physical body, the astral body, and the causal body. These three bodies can function separately, but they are intimately interrelated, too.

Maintaining an awareness of all three bodies will help you see more clearly who you really are. Self-actualization means knowing your *whole* self.

Here's a closer look at your three bodies:

◆ The *physical* body is the crudest of the bodies and the smallest. This is the you in the mirror. Yet even though it's crude, it's your best tool for growth. You can't deny you have a physical body, so yoga helps you make the most of it. The first three aspects of Patanjali's Eightfold Path strengthen and train the physical body: abstinences (*yamas*), observances (*niyamas*), and postures (*asanas*).

◆ The *astral* body is the vehicle of the spirit and corresponds with the mind. This layer exists within the causal body and encompasses the physical body. It is like the second layer, extending beyond the physical body but not to the limits of the causal body. The astral body is strengthened through the next three steps of the Eightfold Path: breathing exercises (*pranayama*), sense withdrawal (*pratyahara*), and concentration (*dharana*).

◆ The *causal* body is the largest, most widely reaching layer of you, starting with spirit. It's the subtlest body and holds the spirit as well as the other layers. This is where you started. Individuality (as we normally think of it) exists to a minimal degree in the causal body, which allows the spirit to shine and truth to be evident. The causal body is reached or experienced through the final two limbs of the Eightfold Path: meditation (*dhyana*) and superconsciousness or bliss (*samadhi*).

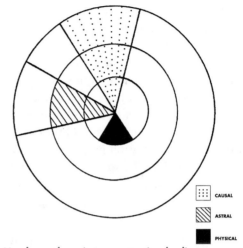

CAUSAL

ASTRAL

PHYSICAL

You have three interpenetrating bodies—yes, you (and you and you!)! These are the physical, causal, and astral bodies.

Hatha Yoga works under the assumption that the inner you is the you worth working on, but to get to the inner you, the outer you—in all its crudity—must first be controlled. Hatha Yoga works to get the physical body under control and in balance so it doesn't impede the other bodies—the astral and causal. Only then can the self-actualized, balanced you emerge in your full glory.

Hatha Yoga accomplishes this Herculean task of fine-tuning and delicate balancing by ...

◆ Building strength through exercises.
◆ Toning the organs and joints through exercises.
◆ Training the breath.
◆ Keeping the body infused with *prana*.
◆ Keeping the body clean.

Through these exercises, techniques, and rituals, the body is properly prepared for the rising of *kundalini* energy.

Hatha Yoga is about balance and emphasizes *pranayama* and *asanas*, or postures. Raja Yoga, or royal path, also incorporates Patanjali's

Eightfold Path, but with a greater emphasis on sense withdrawal, concentration, and meditation. Hatha and Raja Yoga exist in a symbiotic relationship. If you've mastered your body and your breath so *prana* is able to flow freely and unencumbered through your *chakras*, meditation is the natural next step in the progression. You have prepared your body to optimize meditation. In turn, meditation prepares your mind to stand back and let the spirit shine through.

As you look in the mirror, you might wonder about those different levels, those three bodies, and what they really are to the reflection you see. Actually, according to yoga, there are five sheaths of existence within the three bodies. What you see in the mirror is only one of those sheaths, or *koshas* (which can be translated as "envelopes") that make up the real you.

What's with all those layers? The concept isn't as complicated as it may seem. Just as a cell has a nucleus, just as atoms spin within molecules, just as our physical bodies have physical layers from multiple layers of skin to connective tissue to muscle, bone, and marrow, just as objects emanate haloed layers of electrical energy, our spiritual selves are layered, too. Each layer has a different quality, but the whole bundle equals *you*.

The Physical

- ◆ The physical body, *anna-maya-kosha* (pronounced *AH-nah-MAI-ah-KOH-shah*) or "food envelope," consists of your material body. This is what you see in the mirror.
- ◆ The vital body, *prana-maya-kosha* (*PRAH-nah-MAI-ah-KOH-shah*), is where *prana* lives and moves. It exists just beyond your physical body; it's your aura. Yes, prana also moves within your physical body, but it radiates around you, too, and this is what outlines your vital body.

Know Your Sanskrit _____

Koshas (pronounced *KOH-shahs*) are the five sheaths of existence that make up the body: the physical body, the vital body, the mind sheath, the intellect sheath, and the sheath of bliss.

The Emotional or Astral

- ◆ The mind sheath, *mano-maya-kosha* (*MAH-noh-MAI-ah-KOH-shah*), is the seat of the part of your mind that interprets all sensory input. This is where you become aware of emotions.
- ◆ The intellect sheath, *vijnana-maya-kosha* (*vizh-NAH-nah-MAI-ah-KOH-shah*), houses your intelligence and wisdom. This is where you become aware that you exist, at a deeper level, apart from your emotions.

The Causal (Where Everything Starts)

- ◆ The bliss sheath, *ananda-maya-kosha* (*ah-NAHN-dah-MAI-ah-KOH-shah*), contains the field of energy that links you with the universe and in which all is bliss. When we say "all is one, one is all" or make other references to how we are all one with the universe, we are talking about this final, outermost spiritual layer. Our physical bodies, our emotions, our thoughts are unique to us but the bliss sheath is the part of us that is the same as the universe, like the depth of the ocean beneath the individual waves. This was the source of the original you, the other sheaths are unfolding all the way down into an incarnation—again, that's you in the mirror.

Did you have any idea you were walking around with all those layers?

Achieving Vitality

Pranayama is the final, crucial aspect of Hatha Yoga all yogis will do well to practice. We talked about *pranayama* in detail in Chapter 6, so we'll just say a few more words here about *prana* and vitality.

Prana is vitality. Mastering *prana*, both physical and mental, is probably the single most important aspect of Hatha Yoga. *Prana* powers the universe with its energy, and it's the profound connection between you and everything else. Amazingly, something as simple as a breathing technique is the first step toward becoming aware of the movement of *prana* through your body and throughout the universe.

Even though *prana* can't be measured or observed, it can certainly be sensed by the yogi tuned in to its power. Wise yogis and others throughout history perceive *prana* on an intuitive level; those who use it will be astonished at its power. Try a little *pranayama* today, and you, too, will be on your way to greater awareness. *Prana* happens!

Stabilizing the Body's Energies

Finally—and this is really the point of bringing up all the body's layers and dimensions—what Hatha Yoga is all about is integration. In the state of *samadhi*, the self, including the body, blends into the universal energy we are all part of. All that bodywork is really just a way to learn how to transcend your body! Think of it this way: All your life, you've wanted to live in Florida, or Alaska, or California, or wherever. But you live on the opposite side of the country—say, in Providence, Rhode Island, or Amarillo, Texas. Finally, you're ready to start your big move, so you purchase a really nice car for your journey. As you drive across the country, you do everything you can to keep your car in top condition so you won't have any breakdowns or mechanical failures. You learn all about your car so you know what you're driving. And sure enough, you get there without a hitch, or if a tire does blow out or a belt does break, you know exactly what to do to fix it.

Hatha Yoga is the same way. The idea is not the car or the body, but the destination, and of course, finding joy along the way. You want to get to Florida, and you know the best way to get there is to have a vehicle in great condition. Keep your body in great condition. Know your body. Know your mind. Know yourself. You'll be less likely to wind up in the shop (the doctor's office) for repairs!

The Least You Need to Know

- Hatha Yoga is a balance of opposing forces.
- The primary Hatha Yoga poses consist of standing, forward-bending, back-bending, twisting, seated, meditative, and prone poses.
- A trained body won't get in the way of spiritual enlightenment and can even encourage it.
- *Prana* is in you, animates you, and flows through the universe.

In This Part

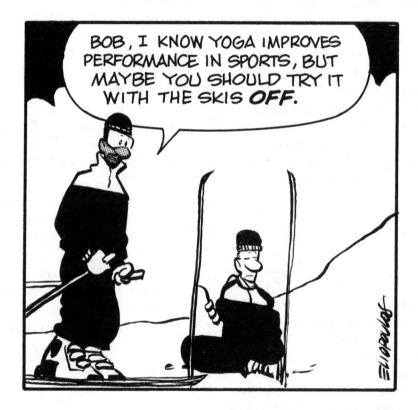

Part 3

Starting Your Yoga Practice

Here's your comprehensive guide to getting started. You'll learn how to approach a yoga practice with confidence and knowledge, how to find a yoga class and a good teacher, how to practice on your own at home, what to wear, when to practice, and how to fit yoga into your busy schedule. You'll also find tips for changing the way you think about exercise, from banishing the "no pain, no gain" adage from your mentality to learning how your breath can enhance your workout.

You'll have a chance to examine your motives and reasons for considering yoga by taking an essay test you can't fail. It will help to direct your thinking inward and allow you to better analyze your strengths and tendencies. Knowing your body and mind will help you craft a yoga routine that will work best for you.

In This Chapter

◆ Dressing for yoga

◆ Wearing the right attitude

◆ Being kind to your body

◆ Gently exploring your limits

◆ Using your breath to boost your workout

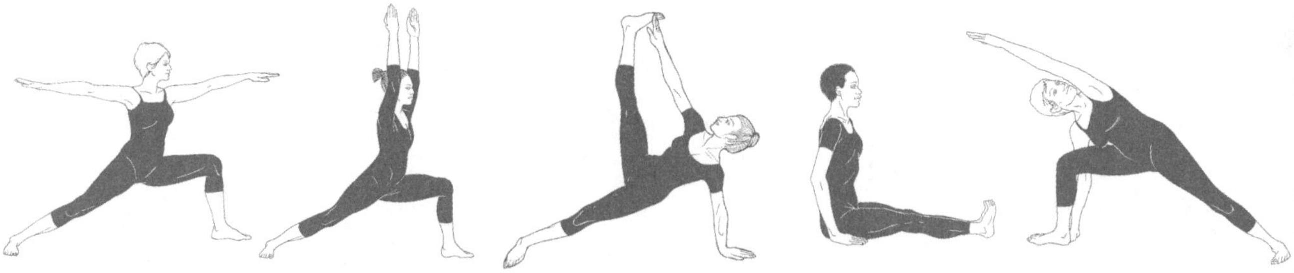

Are You Kidding? My Body Won't Do That!

Knowing how to practice yoga involves more than knowing how to do the poses. You won't be able to relax very easily in scratchy, stiff clothing that doesn't allow you to move freely. Likewise, the attitude you "wear" can hinder your practice. Learning to suspend your doubts, worries, and fears during your yoga practice is important for progress in your yoga journey. So is understanding when you are pushing yourself too hard, listening to your body to determine what it needs and what it doesn't need, and being prepared for deep breathing by knowing a few basic principles.

Loose Clothing and an Open Mind

You can't practice yoga well unless you're comfortable. The right clothing is important, because if you can't move easily, if your clothes are in the way, or if you are in any way unnecessarily distracted (say by a tight waist or stiff fabric), you won't be able to concentrate fully on your yoga poses.

There isn't any set yoga "uniform," but consider these points when deciding what to wear for your workout:

◆ Your clothes will be most comfortable if they are loose and flexible but not baggy. Tight clothes are restricting, and baggy clothes can get in the way of your movements. T-shirts and shorts or leggings, tank tops and biking shorts, or a not-too-baggy seatsuit are ideal.

◆ Dress for the temperature. If the weather is cold, choose long sleeves and comfortable pants that don't restrict your movement (sweatpants or leggings are both good choices). Remember to keep a blanket nearby in case you get chilly during meditative poses you hold in stillness for longer periods, such as *shavasana*.

◆ Clothes that bind are a distraction from your yoga practice. If the feel of your clothes is very noticeable around your waist or at your ankles or wrists, they are probably too tight. Also, binding clothes will restrict the flow of energy through your body.

◆ Take a look in the mirror while wearing your yoga clothes. Can you see the basic shape of your body, or are your clothes hanging and baggy? Your teacher will need to see how you are holding the postures to make sure you are doing them correctly. If you are doing yoga on your own, relatively form-fitting clothing will allow you to check your form and alignment in a mirror without trying to imagine your form in a pose under that oversize T-shirt and those baggy pants.

Wise Yogi Tells Us

If you have long hair, don't forget to tie it back before your yoga practice. There's nothing more frustrating than finally achieving a headstand after months of practice, only to get your hands tangled in your hair!

◆ Yoga is best performed in bare feet. The more you practice yoga, the more sensitive and in tune with your environment you'll become, and that includes your feet!

A Yoga Minute

Bare feet learn to hold the floor, balance the body, and participate fully in the alignment and movement of the postures.

◆ Don't forget to remove all metal jewelry before you practice, especially necklaces and bracelets. Yoga is about freeing the flow of energy in your body, and that energy could be disrupted by metal.

◆ Avoid wearing perfume, strongly scented deodorant, or cologne during your yoga practice. It can be unpleasant to others in your yoga class, especially during *pranayama* (breathwork), and some people are very sensitive to these smells.

◆ And what's the most important thing to wear? An open mind! The most perfect yoga outfit won't do you any good if you aren't mentally prepared. Before every yoga practice, take a few moments of quiet time to prepare for your workout.

Think about what you are about to do and what you want to accomplish. If you're just getting started, even if you aren't completely convinced yoga can do everything people say it can, willingly suspend your disbelief for just a little while. An open mind means a body open to new movements and achievements. You might surprise yourself by what you can accomplish when you aren't wasting your energy doubting yourself and your workout.

I Don't Think My Body Will Do That ...

Now that you're properly attired, you *look* like a yogi—but do you *feel* like one? Maybe you're reluctant to begin that very first practice because you know you aren't flexible or you're convinced you won't be able to achieve many of the postures you've heard about or seen.

The problem with an attitude of doubt is that it not only undermines your self-confidence, it also implies that you see yoga as a competition. We've said it before, but we can't emphasize enough how important this concept is, especially for competitive and goal-oriented people: Yoga is not a competitive sport! If you can't do the Lotus pose today, that doesn't matter one iota. Eventually, with regular practice, it will come. And even if it doesn't, it's still not a reflection on your ability as a yogi. You are much more than your body, and much more than the poses your body can achieve.

If you have a hard time relinquishing your competitive nature, try addressing your inner thoughts with these responses:

> **Your thought:** *I'm much more flexible than that poor guy next to me!*
>
> **Your response to yourself:** *My body is responding well today.*
>
> **Your thought:** *I'll never be able to do a headstand!*
>
> **Your response to yourself:** *I'll master this Shoulderstand any day now, as long as I keep practicing. Maybe then I'll think about trying to learn the Headstand.*
>
> **Your thought:** *I think the teacher likes me best.*
>
> **Your response to yourself:** *I've really found a teacher who understands me and my yoga needs.*
>
> **Your thought:** *At this rate, I'll never be as flexible as that girl in the front.*
>
> **Your response to yourself:** *That girl in front does that posture well. I'll try to visualize how it would feel to hold the posture that way, and maybe my body will understand the posture better.*
>
> **Your thought:** *I look really hot in this new workout gear* or *I look really good in this muscle shirt and bicycle shorts,* followed by *I wonder if there will be any cute guys/girls in the class.*
>
> **Your response to yourself:** *I feel really good in these clothes. I think they will be great for yoga.* (What do you think your yoga class is, anyway—a singles bar?)

Each posture you try should be a movement you're able to perform. Accept and respect your current level of fitness. Also accept how you feel from day to day. You might be able to do postures one week that you suddenly are unable to achieve the next week. So many factors besides how "in shape" you are determine your ability to achieve a pose. Your mood, your stress level, the time of day, how well you have warmed up, your current feelings about yourself, the natural ebb and flow of your energy level—all these conditions will affect your workout. Each day, find your own movement and level.

Then start at that level, progressing as your body allows. Some days you might move ahead noticeably in your flexibility or strength. On other days, you might feel as if you have regressed. That's natural, and the regression will soon correct itself, so don't let it worry you. A good teacher can help you determine how fast you can advance, but you can also listen to your body, because it will tell you, too—as long as it isn't being overruled by your ego.

Remember that yoga is about toning down the ego. Your ego is what tells you to try to outdo the girl next to you or to match the picture in the book precisely. Your ego encourages you to try postures that are beyond your current fitness level, to hold postures too long, or to try the most difficult version of a posture first.

When your ego acts up ("Why don't I look like that when I do the Shoulderstand?"), gently steer your mind in another direction. Remind yourself that this is your journey, and your progress is all that matters. The yoga road has no maximum or minimum speed limit!

Wise Yogi Tells Us

Your ego lets seemingly nonchalant comments slip out of your mouth, such as "I could do the Lotus pose the first time I tried," or "You found the Plow position difficult? That's strange …," or even, "I can't believe you could stand on one foot for so much longer than I could!" Let all that go. It doesn't help you. It only holds you back.

No Pain, Supreme Gain

If you've ever participated in any team athletics, whether elementary school dodge ball or professional basketball, you've probably been told by some coach or teacher somewhere along the line that if it doesn't hurt (or isn't, at the very least, mildly unpleasant), you just aren't working hard enough.

The interesting thing about yoga, and one of its distinctly non-Western qualities, is that it allows you to work incredibly hard without ever feeling pain, discomfort, or even displeasure of any kind. Sure, yoga can be challenging, and it can even make you sweat. But yoga should be innately enjoyable because of many reasons:

◆ It doesn't hurt. Causing yourself pain would be to ignore the observance of *ahimsa* (nonviolence).

◆ It boosts *all* of you. A successful yoga workout increases self-esteem along with fitness and awareness.

◆ It purifies your body, mind, and soul. Being clean feels good!

◆ Even at its most serious, yoga is just plain fun!

Yoga should never cause you pain. Pain means violence and possibly injury. Violence and injury mean a setback. Better to move slowly and steadily forward than to jump ahead in leaps and bounds, then fall back bedridden for a month. You'll gain so much more strength, flexibility, sensitivity, and awareness if you are so attuned to your body that you push it to its limit but never far enough to hurt anything. Respect your body, don't abuse it—it's an integral part of you, after all.

Of course, none of us is perfect, and in any physical activity, occasionally we all overdo it, especially when we're trying to outdo someone (even ourselves!). We know you're trying to listen to your body and not be competitive. But just in case, watch out for these signs that you might have injured yourself:

◆ Severe back pain and muscle spasms could be a sign of a back sprain, often caused by a sudden bending of the spine that tears ligaments.

A Yoga Minute

Surveys of industrialized nations show that more than 75 percent of the population over 45 years old suffers from lower back pain.

◆ Immediate, acute shoulder pain that gets worse over the course of a few hours might be caused by a tear in the tendons and/or muscles around the shoulder joint. A severe tear might inhibit movement and can be caused by a minor fall on an outstretched hand.

◆ Pain in the knee and an inability to straighten the knee, followed by swelling that lasts for two weeks or more, might be due to torn cartilage. This can happen when a bent knee is twisted.

◆ Foot pain from standing for excessive amounts of time or overusing the foot can result in a strain or sprain.

◆ Dizziness can be a sign of low or high blood pressure or blood sugar levels. If you become dizzy, sit down immediately. Check this condition with your doctor.

◆ Headaches can have numerous sources. One reason people get headaches is because of insufficient oxygen. *Pranayama* to the rescue! Breathing exercises might help your headaches, and the stress-reducing aspects of yoga can also be helpful for this common problem.

Of course, the best way to handle an injury is to prevent it. Stay alert to your body. Communicate with your muscles and joints. Be kind to them. Remember *ahimsa* (nonviolence)!

Finding the Edge vs. Feeling the Burn

"But if yoga is so easy on your body, how are you supposed to get anywhere?" you might wonder. Hey, we never said yoga was easy! Yoga isn't always easy, and sometimes it's downright difficult. Just because you aren't committing violence to your body doesn't mean a yoga workout is akin to a day of sunbathing at the beach. On the contrary: Yoga can be tough and intensely challenging.

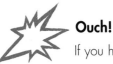

Ouch!

If you happen to overdo it during your yoga workout and find yourself in serious pain, do yourself a favor and *go to your health-care provider immediately!* Ignoring the pain won't make it go away and, in some cases, could result in a serious or chronic health problem. Just do it!

The difference between yoga and other types of exercise is that the challenge and the progression are deeply internal and subtle. Perhaps you've been trying to accomplish a pose in which you bend forward and touch your head to your knees. The first time you try it, you don't even come close. You can barely bend forward without your back causing you pain, so bend your knees and slowly work at bringing your head and upper body down. Slowly build so that your back strengthens and you can straighten your knees. Lean into your farthest point in the stretch and hold it. Remember to keep breathing, letting your breath travel through your body and into the pose. Holding the pose won't hurt, but you'll definitely feel something. Your muscles might shake a bit, and that's okay, as long as you aren't forcing the issue. You might even break a sweat. You're feeling the "edge" of your flexibility as well as an edge of your awareness. Your muscles are waking up and saying, "Hey! What is it you want us to do? This is weird, but okay, we'll give it a try." Your mind is waking up, too, and taking notice.

The next time you try this pose, you get a little closer—maybe three or four inches from your knees. The farthest point of the stretch is now a little farther than it was before. You stretch to this point and hold it. Now your muscles have become accustomed to a new "normal" level of flexibility. You find the new edge and test it—not to the point of pain, but just to see where it now lies. Your muscles feel it, and so does your mind.

A few weeks, or months, or maybe a lifetime later (how long it takes isn't important, because it's not a competition), you lean into the stretch and … wow! There it is! Suddenly your head is resting quite easily on your knees. You've stretched your boundaries and pushed your edge to a new level. At this point, you may simply feel triumphant, but you may also feel an awakening to a new level of yourself. No longer simply proud of your achievement, you're now aware of yourself in a new way.

Therein lies yoga's power—the physical process breaking into the mental process and lifting the whole of you to higher and higher states of awareness.

Keep in mind that every posture contains an "edge" or a point past which—for today, at least—you can't quite go. This is the point around which you want to linger, because it's the source of yoga's power. You'll soon see how productive it is to recognize an edge but not let it define you.

Don't Forget to Breathe

And once again, we remind you of your ever-present breath. Although breathing exercises are performed separately from the postures, breathing is also important during the postures. Of course, you have to breathe while exercising, but becoming aware of your breath, even breathing in a specific way according to the posture you are holding, will enhance your practice and help your body work better.

Here are a few breath-savvy concepts to keep in mind while practicing your *asanas:*

◆ Inhalation most often occurs when your chest opens, your limbs extend outward or upward, and your head is up.

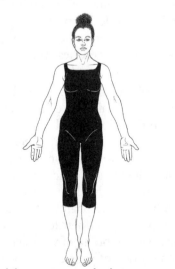

Inhale while opening your body into *prana* arch.

◆ Exhalation most often occurs when your chest contracts inward, your limbs move close to your body, your head is down, and your body curls into itself.

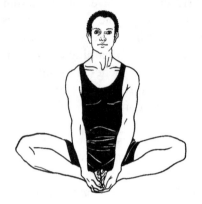

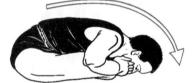

Exhale while folding the body into Butterfly pose.

◆ Retaining the breath after an inhalation helps stabilize and energize the chest area.

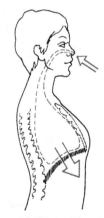

Inhale and hold the breath for a moment to energize the chest.

◆ Retaining the breath after an exhalation helps stabilize and energize the abdominal area and releases toxins from the body.

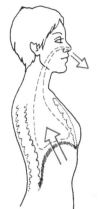

Exhale and hold before inhaling
again to energize the abdomen.

◆ Forward-bending poses are conducive to
exhalation, then retention.

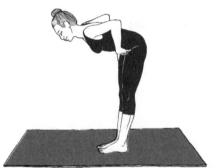

Bend forward from your hips as you exhale, then hold
for a moment to feel your body's stillness and strength.

◆ Back-bending poses are conducive to
inhalation, then retention.

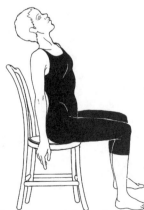

Bend back as you inhale, then retain the breath for a
moment to feel the power of *prana*.

Wise Yogi Tells Us _____

Your breath has four modes:

◆ Inhalation

◆ Exhalation

◆ Retained breath after inhalation

◆ Retained breath after exhalation

Learning how to use each mode when it is most
beneficial will greatly enhance your practice.

Breathing deeply and well during exercise
keeps a steady supply of oxygen in the blood so
muscles can work at their peak. Breathing keeps
the mind calm and focused, which will further
enhance your workout. And because the breath
is the vehicle by which *prana*, the universal life
force, enters the body, you'll certainly want to
breathe deeply during your workout. *Prana* is
the energy that keeps you vibrant and animated.
It's the key to a great workout, so get as much
into you as possible! Breathe! Breathe! Breathe!

Ouch! _____

If you become out of breath or
fatigued during your workout, stop!
Yoga isn't circuit-training, marathon-running, or
nonstop anything. Rest is encouraged within a
workout—as a transition from one type of posture to another, as a chance to feel the aftereffects of a posture, and to maintain awareness.
Bodies aren't meant to be exhausted but to be
gently and lovingly improved and maintained.

The Least You Need to Know

◆ Wear comfortable clothing during yoga.

◆ Don't be competitive—with others or with
yourself.

◆ Don't force any posture until it hurts, but
keep exploring your limits.

◆ If you have any lingering pain, consult a
doctor immediately; don't wait for it to
become chronic.

◆ Breathe deeply and often!

In This Chapter

◆ Choosing a yoga class and finding the right teacher

◆ Doing yoga on your own with books, videos, CDs/
audiotapes, and the Internet

◆ Making a schedule and sticking with it

◆ Squeezing yoga into your busy day

◆ Revitalizing with yoga throughout the day

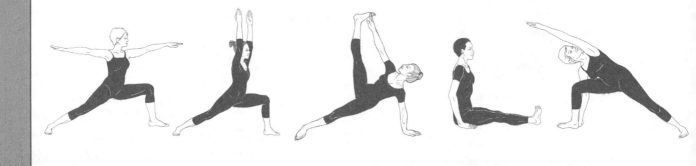

Chapter 9

Where and When Do You Practice Yoga?

So you've decided to give yoga a try. Great! Now what? Now is the time to make a game plan. Decide how you would like to proceed with your yoga. Do you want to take a class and reap the benefits of a qualified instructor? Do you want to try yoga on your own for a while, then consider a class later if you like what you experience? And how will you fit yoga into your hectic schedule? Do you have time for a class, for a morning or evening practice, or both? Can you make time?

Whatever course you choose to take, make sure you have the necessary preparation so you can get the most from your yoga experience. Your personality, your schedule, and your general inclinations will all have an effect on the type of yoga that will serve you most effectively.

Choosing a Yoga Class

Probably the best way to start out with yoga is to take a class. You can learn a lot from books and videos, but a real live teacher can address your personal challenges and direct you in ways a book can't. (But don't stop reading this book yet! We still have a lot left to tell you.) Consider the following reasons to take a yoga class:

◆ A teacher can see you from all angles, making minor adjustments in your posture to help you get the most from each position.

◆ A teacher can advise you on the best postures for your particular physical challenges, such as a stiff neck, lower back pain, or tennis elbow.

◆ If you have a class to attend at a prescheduled time, you might be less likely to put off or skip your practice. And regular exercise is the most beneficial for anyone.

◆ Other students learning yoga along with you can offer peer support and camaraderie, in addition to your teacher's encouragement.

◆ A class and a qualified teacher in conjunction with personal practice and lots of books on the subject will teach you more about yoga than any one of these methods alone.

Yoga classes vary greatly in their format and approach, so if you do decide to take a class, you'll first want to do a bit of shopping. The right yoga class is highly personal—what *you* love, your friends might not benefit from at all, and vice versa. If you are used to a high-energy, aerobic workout, you might initially be impatient with yoga's slower pace, although it will serve as an excellent balance for your life. If you're generally inactive, you might benefit more from a yoga class where steady, flowing yoga movements get the heart pumping.

A Yoga Minute

When you look for a yoga class, you have several factors to consider: the teacher's method and approach, the size of the class, class schedules, and location, to name a few. Plan on spending some time exploring the possibilities. It might take a while to find the right class and the right teacher for you, but many yogis believe that when the student is ready, the teacher will appear. Keep your mind and heart open.

You also might be confused about the wide array of yoga methods. The difference is largely due to who has most directly influenced the teacher or under which method the teacher was trained. Before signing up for a class, ask the teacher which school of yoga he or she practices, then ask him or her to explain the basic philosophy of that particular school or method.

Make sure any yoga class you consider meets the following criteria:

◆ The yoga teacher is a qualified instructor. Anyone can teach yoga, but not everyone can teach it well. Don't be fooled by health clubs touting "yoga" classes taught by club employees who might have read a book on yoga or who think all fitness is basically the same. Some health clubs offer excellent yoga classes, but you'll want to ask about the teacher's training.

◆ The class is small enough that the teacher can give you individual attention. You'll want help adjusting postures and creating a routine suited to your ability so you won't get injured, frustrated, or bored silly.

◆ The class is conveniently scheduled and easy to get to. Otherwise, you know what will happen. Eventually, going to class will be too much trouble and you won't go.

If you don't like your first class, your first teacher, or the way you felt after your first yoga workout, don't give up. Some people overdo it their first time out and vow never to practice yoga again. If you can't relate to your teacher; if you pull a muscle; or if the class environment is high-pressure, competitive, or unpleasant in any way, you just haven't found the right class or the right teacher for you.

Or maybe you weren't completely open to the experience—could your competitive nature have overshadowed the benefits you were receiving? Was the teacher encouraging a competitive attitude, or was the teacher inattentive to your needs? Maybe you couldn't understand what the teacher wanted you to do. (Teachers are human, too.) Many teachers are grounded in the noncompetitive philosophy, but some still see yoga simply as physical fitness, with all its competitive aspects. Many are excellent at doling out individual help and counsel, but others might have classes that are too large for a really personal approach.

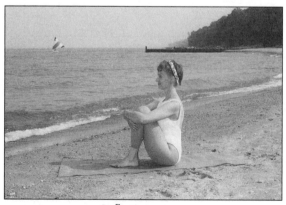

Reflective pose.

Finding Your Personal Guru

You've heard the word _guru_, we're sure, but you might be confused as to what a guru actually is. A guru is a spiritual teacher. You can have many spiritual teachers in your life, but traditionally, you have only one guru, and you attach, spiritually, not only to the guru but to the guru's lineage (in other words, the particular tradition out of which that guru comes, what he or she has studied, what "school" or "branch" of yoga he or she is associated with). Literally, the word _guru_ means "dispeller of darkness," and that is the guru's role: to help you dispel your own spiritual darkness.

Do you need a guru? Not necessarily, but perhaps. A guru/disciple relationship between mature individuals is really a journey of spiritual revelations and discoveries for both disciple and guru. The guru's "job" is to give you spiritual guidance and insight and to insist that you think for yourself. In fact, it is essential that a disciple have the freedom to follow or not follow that guidance. A good disciple will travel toward spiritual independence, but a guru makes a great traveling companion with an excellent road map to get you well on your way.

The concept of the guru is a little hard for us Westerners to swallow. After all, we like to be self-sufficient. We aren't a submissive, follow-the-leader type of culture, and the idea that we should surrender to some kind of a master—putting our physical, mental, and spiritual development in his or her hands—makes us uncomfortable. This isn't a difficult concept for many Easterners, whose culture has taught them, over the course of centuries, that the best way to truly learn anything—a craft, a posture, a philosophy, enlightenment—is by loyal devotion to a wise individual who has sage advice and knowledge to impart.

We Westerners like to question, and our doubting natures are only encouraged when we hear story after story about spiritual teachers and leaders who have gone astray. Our modern world is full of temptations, and sometimes gurus, priests, evangelists, healers, and others whose purpose is to lead others to a higher spiritual plane cave in to temptation. A true, enlightened guru will remain your spiritual guide for a lifetime, but these days, good gurus are hard to find! (And many a guru will counter that good students are equally hard to find!)

But you might not need a guru—at least not in the traditional sense. For some, a guru is a crucial part of the yoga journey, but for others, a teacher is the perfect guide. A qualified yoga teacher you truly connect with can be your most valuable resource. A great yoga teacher can change your life and improve your practice of yoga far beyond what you could figure out on your own.

A Yoga Minute

Spell the word *guru* out loud: G-U-R-U. That's right! Gee, you are you!

It is important to understand that we all have a guru within. Don't be discouraged if you haven't found the *acarya* or other guru who is right for you. Be patient, keep your eyes open, and keep practicing. Move away from mediocre instruction and toward a teacher who inspires you. Eventually, you might find your way to your guru. Ultimately, the guru is an internal one.

Know Your Sanskrit

Acarya (pronounced *ah-CAHR-yah*) means "teacher."

Going Solo at Home

If you aren't quite ready for the commitment of a class, or if for any other reason you don't want to or aren't able to take a class, do-it-yourself yoga can be very rewarding. Design your own workout from the poses in this book, find a comfortable practice area, dress in comfortable clothing, designate a regular practice time (whether once a week or twice a day—we suggest daily), and get ready for your very first *asana!*

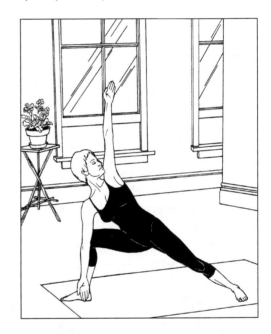

Setting Up Your Practice Area

One of the great things about yoga is that you can do it almost anywhere—in the bedroom, in the living room, even outside! Your environment should consistently include several things, however:

◆ **A soft surface.** Nonskid carpets are good surfaces for practicing yoga, but if your floor isn't carpeted or is slippery, use a small rug, a blanket, or a yoga mat (a thin rubber mat, sometimes called a "sticky mat," that can be placed on any surface for a comfortable, nonskid yoga practice area). You need the firmness of the ground, but the surface on which you work should be soft enough to be comfortable.

♦ **A source of warmth.** In the summer, you probably won't have to worry about keeping warm, but in the winter or in a drafty room, warmth can be an issue. Keep a blanket nearby to drape around yourself during still poses, breathing exercises, and meditation. Your muscles need to be warm to stay flexible, and you need to be comfortable to get the most from your practice. Practicing outside in the sun on a warm day is ideal. If you practice inside in the winter, consider a small electric heater for your practice area.

> **Ouch!**
>
> Keeping warm while practicing yoga is extremely important. If your muscles are cold, they can stiffen and lose flexibility, increasing your chance of injury. Warm muscles and joints are most conducive to a yoga workout. Also, in quieter poses and during meditation, you'll become colder more easily because you aren't encouraging active circulation.

♦ **Fresh air.** If you practice inside and weather permits, open a window and take a few deep breaths of fresh air before you start. Practicing outside will immerse you in fresh air. If the weather doesn't permit (if it's too cold or too hot outside), don't worry about the fresh air. You'll get some when the temperature is milder.

Practice in an area free of obstacles and distractions. Practicing yoga amid clutter and confusion is difficult and even counterproductive. As we've mentioned before, cleanliness is important to yoga, and that includes an uncluttered and clean environment. Although a seasoned yogi can find a sense of serenity in any setting (even your family room, where your teenager is playing video games and your twin toddlers are practicing for a career in large-building demolition), you might not be able to focus quite as well as you would in a quiet room all by yourself.

Even if the rest of your house is a perpetual disaster area, try to keep one special "yoga spot" clear, clean, pet-free, kid-free, and relatively quiet. Before you know it, the rest of your house will "magically" become less cluttered and more simply furnished. It's yet another positive influence yoga can have on your lifestyle.

Yoga from Tapes and Videos

Another great way to learn yoga is with a yoga video or CD/audiotape. With a video, you can see (or at least hear with a CD/audiotape) a teacher. You can watch the postures performed or hear them described, which can be easier to follow than a static picture in a book. The teacher on the video or CD/audiotape can offer advice and wisdom vocally. Some people comprehend information better if they see or hear it than if they read it, while others benefit much more from the written word.

If your teacher has made tapes or videos, you can use them to extend your in-person yoga practice by taking your teacher home with you via electronic media. Taking advantage of all possible levels of study will result in more learning opportunities.

One advantage of the audiotape/CD over the video is that your focus won't be glued on the television but can be directed inward instead. Only your hearing will guide you, so although figuring out how to do a posture might be more difficult, many simpler postures, and especially breathing and meditation work, are perfect for the audio medium.

Whichever method is most helpful to you is the one you should pursue. Don't worry about what anyone else does. This is *your* yoga. A visit to your local library, video store, bookstore, or even the back pages of this very book will reveal a wealth of available audio and video references you can borrow, rent, or buy. A library or video store will permit you to sample a variety of yoga teachers and programs without committing. Once you've found a few you like, consider buying the tapes/videos for your personal collection. Then, whenever the desire strikes (2 A.M. on a Tuesday or 11 P.M. on a Friday), you can do yoga!

Wise Yogi Tells Us

When practicing postures at home on your own, it might help to keep in mind these five steps to every pose:

◆ Visualize your body holding the pose.

◆ Gracefully flow into the pose.

◆ Become one with the pose—find the peace and balance.

◆ Gracefully flow out of the pose.

◆ Reflect and release. Let go. Feel the silence.

Wise Yogi Tells Us

No matter how different we are from each other, we all have one very important and illustrious quality in common: We're all human! Keep in mind these six universal laws for being human:

◆ You will be given a body.

◆ You will be taught lessons.

◆ There are no mistakes in life, only lessons.

◆ If a lesson is not learned, it gets repeated.

◆ The more often a lesson is repeated, the harder it gets.

◆ You know you've learned your lesson when your actions change.

Yoga from Books

We hope you don't have the impression that you *can't* learn yoga from a book. For some, it's the only way! Remember *svadhyaya*, the *niyama* that encourages self-inquiry? Reading books on yoga and practicing from a book are part of this observance, which helps you understand yourself. Many excellent books on yoga exist, illustrating thousands of poses, breathing techniques, and meditation techniques. Plus, you can go to the library and come home with 10 or 12 books on yoga—much easier (and perhaps cheaper) than sampling 10 or 12 teachers!

Books cover yoga in a variety of ways—from an array of suggested workouts to the history of yoga to essays on spirituality to suggestions for daily yoga-friendly living. It's important to spend time reading, studying, and filling your mind with the types of ideas and concepts that inspire you. If you study a posture on the written level, your mind will understand it in a different way and your body might even find it easier to follow.

If you thrive on reading, read to your heart's content—but don't *just* read. You also need to *act.* Get up and try what the book suggests. Following the postures from a picture and some text might be challenging at first, but once you find the posture, it will feel right, and pretty soon you'll have a sequence of poses memorized.

But don't stop there! The more you learn about yoga, the wiser you'll be. Find books with more *asanas* you haven't tried yet. Check out the *Bhagavad Gita* (that classic Indian epic about *Krishna*, Prince Arjuna, and the meaning of life). Find a teacher whose views make sense to you, and read everything you can by and about him or her. You might find that as your life changes, your yoga goals and interests change and grow. Just go back to the library or the bookstore and find another book more in keeping with your developing state of mind. And always maintain a balance between reading and doing, doing and reading. Mindbody. Bodymind.

What better first book than the one you have in your hands? We hope this book is piquing your interest as you begin your yoga journey with us. After you've mastered this book, you won't feel like a "complete idiot" about yoga (even though you never *were*). You'll be able to progress in your yoga practice with confidence and aplomb.

Yoga on the Net

For all you computer-heads and Internet lovers out there, despair not! The Internet is brimming with great yoga resources, from class information to "postures of the week" to peer support to spiritual guidance and inspiration. Of course, you always want to be careful when it comes to the people you talk to and where you send your money—use your common sense, then start surfing for yoga sites! Keep in mind that these websites do frequently change, as do their addresses. Here are a few to check out:

- ◆ **YOYOGA!** is Joan's (yes, the Joan co-authoring these very words!) marvelous yoga website with *asanas* of the week, yoga tips, massage tips, meditation tips, and other wonderful words of wonder, including the ever-popular "Yo Joan!" forum for all your yoga questions. Look up Joan at www.yoyoga.com.

- ◆ **Temple of Kriya Yoga Chicago,** where Joan studied, has a great website with plenty of resources and links. Check it out at www.yogakriya.org.

- ◆ **The Yoga Anand Ashram** site contains lots of great poses and meditation information with pictures and clear explanations. It covers many aspects of yoga, and the site is user-friendly: www.santosha.com.

- ◆ *Yoga Journal* is a popular yoga magazine and well worth the read. Browse through it at www.yogajournal.com.

- ◆ *Yoga International* is another excellent and popular yoga magazine. Check out highlights of current issues and back issues at www.yimag.org.

- ◆ **Yoga Site** is an "eclectic collection of yoga connections" and is full of yoga information, from philosophy to finding a teacher in your area. Great reading can be found at www.yogasite.com.

- ◆ **YogaChicago** is a bi-monthly resource guide to yoga activities in the Chicago area and elsewhere. If you live in the Chicago area (or not), check it out at www.yogachicago.com.

- ◆ **Next Generation Yoga** is a yoga studio in New York City devoted to yoga for kids, with age-specific classes for children from age two through age fourteen, as well as parent/child workshops, family activities, prenatal yoga, teacher training, and more. Check it out at www.nextgenerationyoga.com.

◆ **The Self-Realization Fellowship** is a worldwide religious organization dedicated to carrying on the spiritual and humanitarian work of Paramahansa Yogananda. Check it out at www.yoganandasrf.org/aboutsrf/index.html.

◆ **The Sivananda Yoga "OM"** page is the homepage of the International Sivananda Yoga Vedanta Center, a nonprofit organization founded by *Swami* Vishnu-devananda to spread the teachings of Yoga and Vedanta worldwide. Find them at www.sivananda.org.

◆ **Himalayan International Institute of Yoga and Philosophy** combines Eastern wisdom and Western knowledge. The institute offers a wide variety of seminars and programs. Visit the institute at www.himalayaninstitute.org.

◆ **Yoga Paths** is SpiritWeb's explication of the many forms of yoga. Find it at www.spiritweb.org/Spirit/yoga.html.

◆ **BKS Iyengar Yoga National Association of the United States'** website, where you can find yoga teachers who teach the Iyengar method of yoga, is www.iynaus.org.

A Yoga Minute

The world is full of wise yogis—even celebrities! These celebrities have all practiced yoga: Helen Hunt, Gwyneth Paltrow, Cameron Diaz, Jerry Seinfeld, Nicholas Cage, Woody Harrelson, Charlie Sheen, Emilio Estevez, Jamie Lee Curtis, Jeff Bridges, Jane Fonda, Drew Barrymore, Oprah Winfrey, Candice Bergen, Sting, Madonna, Karen Allen, and Quincy Jones.

When to Practice Yoga

Time, time, time … never enough of it, and it just keeps on passing us by. During the course of our busy lives, it's easy to become overwhelmed by the demands on our time. Family, friends, work, school, home … all require their share of our time. The furnace needs to be repaired, the dishes are dirty, the kids need to be picked up from soccer practice or ballet or the baby-sitters. You can't neglect time with your spouse, you have to finish the inventory at work, the baby needs some serious cuddling … and has anyone walked the dog lately?

Or maybe you're a student. You have five papers due in the next month. Calculus has completely eluded you. Seven chemistry problems are due tomorrow, and you're also supposed to have finished *War and Peace* by last week. Your roommate won't turn down the music, the library is closed because of a flood, and it's just starting to thunder, so studying outside isn't an option, and you hear a rumor that your history teacher is planning a pop quiz for tomorrow.

And we're suggesting you add some time for yoga?

Yep. And you'll be glad we suggested it, too. You do have time for yoga, even if it doesn't seem like you could possibly track down one spare second. All it takes is a little organization and some creative thinking.

Time to get organized! All great accomplishments start with some type of plan. An effective yoga practice has a plan involving two important aspects:

◆ How often will you practice each week?

◆ What will you do during the course of each practice?

The first question depends a lot on your schedule, your motivation, and your desire. If you take a class once a week, practice on your own during the week using the routine you and your teacher have crafted for you. Or if you do not have a teacher, set up a specific schedule of Hatha Yoga days. A regular schedule is the best way to reap yoga's benefits. Yes, even just once a week counts as a regular schedule (but you might soon find that once a week won't be enough, and you'll find more time, and more ...).

Ouch!

Always practice yoga postures on an empty stomach. Just before breakfast or dinner is ideal. Digestion will interfere with what yoga is trying to accomplish in your body, and a full stomach will make exercise uncomfortable. Your whole body, including your internal organs, should be focused on your practice, not on processing that spaghetti dinner!

When planning your weekly yoga schedule, remember that even though yoga isn't harsh on your body, you should still give yourself at least one day every week to rest. Rest is crucial for yoga. The time spent in *asanas* (postures) is balanced by the time spent resting, and it is this rest time when the body heals and replenishes its resources. Or rest every other day. Perhaps you'll do yoga for 20 minutes each morning before work on Monday, Wednesday, and Friday. Maybe you'll practice for 30 minutes after work and before dinner every Tuesday and Thursday and spend an hour at a yoga class on the weekend. Whether you do yoga first thing in the morning or right before bedtime, the key is to practice consistently.

Once you have a schedule, keep it in your head, write it down, post it on the refrigerator ... whatever it takes. Then follow your schedule! Remember *tapas*, the *niyama* about self-discipline? Here's a great chance to use it. You'll feel great about yourself if you faithfully stick to your yoga schedule.

Now what about the schedule for your routine itself? Your teacher can help you craft the perfect yoga practice for you, taking into consideration any special needs you have or problems you'd like yoga to address (bad knees, allergies, back pain, frazzled nerves). Or see Chapters 20 and 21 for ideas to comprise your yoga sessions.

Don't forget that every yoga practice should include the following:

- ◆ **A warm-up.** It's important to get your muscles warm and activated before you start stretching them. Warm-ups help prevent injury and make a wonderful transition from daily life to yoga mode. A short walk in the fresh air makes a great warm-up, because it sends blood to all your muscles and gets those joints moving. (The quality of your walk is more important than the length; use the time to prepare your body and mind.) You can get a similar effect simply by massaging your legs, feet, arms, and hands. Work those muscles and joints to get them ready for action. If you're lucky enough to know a massage therapist, a massage before (or after!) yoga practice can be therapeutic. You might also try a warm shower or bath, or a heating pad on stiff areas, to warm your muscles before your workout.

Wise Yogi Tells Us _____

The most spiritual time of day and the most ideal for practicing yoga is just before sunrise (about 5:30 A.M.). If you make it a habit to practice yoga before sunrise and then relax with a cup of herbal tea to watch the dawn, you'll find a new sense of peace pervading your days. And to think you've been sleeping through all that beauty!

- **A balanced set of poses.** Poses that bend or twist to one side should be balanced with poses that bend or twist to the other side. Forward bends balance backbends. Right-side-up poses balance inverted poses. Poses that stretch and expand are balanced by poses that curl and contract. Energizing poses balance relaxing poses. You get the idea.

- **Every yoga workout should conclude with the final relaxation, or Corpse pose.** In Corpse pose, mighty healing takes place … for your body and mind. Don't neglect this pose because you think you don't have time to just lie there. It's probably the most important of all the postures (see Chapter 18 for more on Corpse pose).

- *Pranayama,* **or breathing exercises.** After you practice your *asanas,* set aside a short time for the practice of a breathing technique or two. Replenish your body's *prana,* or life force!

- *Dhyana,* **or meditation.** You might not be ready to include meditation in your workout. If that's the case, that's fine. Diligently practice your *asanas* and *pranayama,* and you may find that meditation soon becomes a more compelling prospect. Or if you would like to try it but

are short on time, you might consider meditating at a different time of day. Whenever you meditate (after your *asanas* and *pranayama* or during separate sessions), remember that meditation is part of yoga, too, and will have a direct benefit on your workout. (Your workout will have a direct benefit on your meditation efforts, as well.)

Wise Yogi Tells Us _____

If you're feeling depressed or even just a little blue, which should you do—meditation or postures? If you guessed postures, you're right! The action of the postures is designed to move impurities and negativity out of the body. Meditation, on the other hand, involves stillness and concentration. If you are filled with negative feelings, meditation could actually concentrate them and make you feel worse. Meditation is best practiced in a positive frame of mind.

Here's a rhyme to help you remember:

> If you're down, move around.
> Feeling great? Meditate!

Sticking With It

To really get the most out of yoga, a commitment is in order. Although occasional yoga is better than no yoga, life changes and dramatic benefits will come more quickly and easily if you practice yoga regularly, whether that means a few times a week or a few times a day. Commitment-phobic, are you? Don't be! This is a relationship with yourself, so even though you might discover some surprises (what relationship doesn't have a few of those?), this commitment is well worth the effort you put into it.

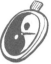 **A Yoga Minute**

Keep a yoga journal. Whatever questions or issues seem personally relevant or important to you should be the subject of your journal entries. Keeping written track of your practice in this way will not only encourage you to practice regularly, but will also serve as a valuable and interesting record for the more advanced yogi you will be in the future. Someday it might be fun and enlightening to see how far you've come and what path you took.

Still, even for the most well-intentioned person, cultivating a new habit can be difficult at first. If you're having trouble sticking to your yoga schedule, try the following strategies. One of them might be just the inspiration you need.

◆ **Let's make a deal.** First yoga, *then* breakfast. No yoga, no food. Or first yoga, then a long, hot bubble bath. No yoga, no bath. Whatever deal you make with yourself, be firm. Soon, you might find your deals have turned around: If I clean the whole kitchen, I get to practice yoga for 30 whole minutes!

◆ **It's a family affair.** Get your partner or kids involved! When you don't feel like practicing, someone else in the family probably will, and that can be enough of a motivation. (Who could deny a preschooler begging to "play" yoga?) Conversely, when your partner or kids are feeling less than motivated, you might be the one to encourage them (see Chapter 22 for more on partner yoga).

◆ **Associate yoga with another pleasurable activity, then always link them.** To use a previous example, every time you get up early to do yoga, you also get to relax with a cup of tea and watch the sunrise. Or whenever you do yoga, your family knows they can't bother you for an entire 30 minutes, or however long you can convince them to do without you. Maybe you can even work up to a whole glorious hour! Yoga will mean peace, relaxation—time for you, and you alone.

◆ **Keep a yoga journal.** For every day you practice yoga, take a few moments in the morning or evening (or whenever you have time) to write down how long you practiced, what time of day it was, exactly what you did, and, most important, how you feel about it. Did you make progress today? Did you feel like you experienced a setback? How do you feel now? Are you still carrying the feeling of your practice, or is it gone? How is your stress level? Don't feel you have to address all or even any of these questions—they are just suggestions.

◆ **Put yoga on your to-do list.** Put it right alongside all your other important daily duties, then check it off when you have finished. Subconsciously, you might not be giving yoga a high priority, and that's why it's so easy to forget it or put it off. Consciously placing yoga high on your list, equal to (if not higher than) such important tasks as getting the car fixed, turning in that report to your boss, or buying the groceries for your big dinner party, might be the motivation you need to accomplish your yoga practice every time it's scheduled.

Maybe another strategy will work better for you, and that's fine. Just have a strategy that will work for you. Commitments require a plan, but ideas without a plan rarely amount to anything. Take your yoga seriously, commit, exercise a little self-discipline, or simply allow yoga to be so fun and refreshing that you wouldn't possibly skip a workout! Soon you'll have no trouble making yoga a natural part of your life.

> **Ouch!**
>
> Your body reacts differently to stress than to relaxation. Compare these physiological responses:
>
> | Stress | Relaxation |
> | --- | --- |
> | Heart rate increases. | Heart rate decreases. |
> | Muscle tension increases. | Muscle tension decreases. |
> | Breathing rate increases. | Breathing rate decreases. |
> | Blood pressure increases. | Blood pressure decreases. |
> | Blood-clotting time decreases. | Blood-clotting time increases. |

Yoga Bytes at Home, School, and Work

If you're an extremely busy person, as most of us seem to be these days, you might find it difficult to find time for yoga. Perhaps you think your day is so densely packed with activity that yoga will never fit. Don't despair! The great thing about yoga is that you get big results even when you spend just a little time at it each day.

Three 10-minute (or even 5-minute or 3-minute) slots for postures, the first for warm-ups, the second for more strenuous postures, and the third for relaxation postures, are all you need to start practicing yoga, and you can spread them throughout the day if necessary. You might find that the increased energy you gain magically adds time to your day for even more practice!

You can even slip tiny little "yoga bytes" into your day to keep you focused and feeling great. Try squeezing in yoga during the following "free times" at home, school, and the office.

Yoga on the Home Front

Here are some yoga bytes to try at home:

◆ Get up 10 minutes before the rest of the family to practice. Morning is a great time to practice Cat pose. Get down on your hands and knees, then arch your back up as high as you can while lowering your head. Imagine you are a cat stretching after a long nap. Then relax your back and bring your head up. Do this a few times, breathing with the movements. This exercise keeps your spine limber and gets you ready to pounce on the new day!

◆ Practice right after your shower, before getting dressed. Try Lightning Bolt pose to get your energy soaring (see Chapter 11 for Lightning Bolt pose guidance).

◆ Practice Mountain pose while waiting for the pasta to boil (see Chapter 11 for Mountain pose instruction). Watch the bubbles slowly building and rising to the surface of the water. What powerful forces are heat and energy! Reflect on how to choose to use the "bubbles" that inevitably build up inside you.

◆ Practice while waiting for the laundry to dry. Stand behind a chair. Place your hands on the back of the chair. Take a large step back. While continuing to hold on to the chair, straighten your arms out and bend forward. Now lift one leg straight out behind you. Balance. Warrior pose! This pose strengthens the legs and stretches the spine.

◆ Practice deep breathing while running your bath water. (see Chapter 15 for more on how to breathe).

◆ Practice your regular yoga routine while the rest of the family is watching television. (Eventually, they might decide what you are doing is more interesting and join you!)

◆ Practice with the kids for a family-bonding yoga session. Kids usually love yoga, especially moving like different animals. Try Cat pose (described earlier in this list). Everyone purrrr like a cat! Then try Tree pose (see Chapter 11). Ask your kids what it's like to be a tree. Be a family of trees in different kinds of weather—a gentle breeze, a thrashing thunderstorm, a perfectly still day. Are your trees sturdy and strong, or young and flexible? Does the wind barely stir them, lash them all around, or knock them right down?

A Yoga Minute

Want to learn more about yoga with kids? Check out *The Complete Idiot's Guide to Yoga with Kids* by Jodi B. Komitor and Eve Adamson.

◆ Practice just before you go to sleep, but stick to relaxation postures such as Lotus pose (see Chapter 14), Child's pose (see Chapter 17), or *shavasana*, or Corpse pose (see Chapter 18). Otherwise, you might be too energized for slumber.

Know Your Sanskrit

Shavasana, also known as Corpse pose (*shava* means "corpse"), is perhaps the most important of all the yoga *asanas* and involves total relaxation while lying, "corpselike," on the ground. *Shavasana* is a surprisingly challenging pose. It isn't easy to lie still—and keep your body-mind still, too!

School Days

How about some yoga bytes for the stressed-out student:

◆ Are you nervous about a test you are taking? Breathe! Increase your exhalation so it's longer than your inhalation. Do this a few times. Come back to the test. This type of breathwork releases toxins from your body and centers your mind.

◆ Feeling a lot of tension in your back? Sit up straight. Keep both knees and feet together and facing forward. Twist your upper body. Bring one arm around the back of your chair. Do not overtwist your neck. Look behind you. This movement improves circulation to the spine and brain. It also improves flexibility and eyesight.

◆ As you walk across campus from class to class in the fresh air, take a moment to focus on your surroundings. Breathe in the fresh air. Feel the sun on your face and the wind in your hair. Instead of worrying about the test you just took, the quiz you are about to take, or the paper due tomorrow, let all your worries go—just for a minute!—and live wholly in the moment.

Yoga Makes Work Less Work!

Here are a few yoga bytes you might like to try at the office if your situation permits:

- **Practice on your coffee break instead of drinking coffee.** (Yoga is far more energizing, once you break that caffeine addiction!) Sit with your fingers wide apart on top of your knees. Inhale deeply. Open your mouth wide and stick out your tongue. Look up and exhale strongly. Repeat the process a few times—not in front of your boss, though! (unless you can get your boss to practice yoga with you!). This releases emotions, tensions in the face, and self-consciousness. It also helps to break a depression cycle.

- **Practice right before your lunch hour.** While sitting, as you take a long inhale, stretch one leg straight out in front of you and hold it up parallel to the floor. Pull your toes back toward your head. Hold for three counts. Lower your leg as you slowly exhale. Do each leg a few times. This improves your hip joints and strengthens your legs so your knees won't be as stiff when you stand.

- **At the end of a long workday, pause for a moment to get centered and refocus before you head home.** Stand up and stretch your arms up over your head. Look up. Bend forward and touch the ground. Bend your knees if you need to. You have just connected the sun to the earth. After an accomplishment like that, you're ready to head home.

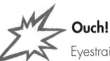

Ouch!

Eyestrain can result from staring at a computer all day. Try a yoga fix: Keeping your head still, look up as far as you can, focus on something, and count to three. Look down, focus, and count to three. Repeat six or seven times, focusing in different directions, then close your eyes and rest. When you open your eyes, they'll feel remarkably refreshed.

Yoga Renewal

Depending on what time of day you practice yoga, you can experience different kinds of renewal. We humans are deeply affected by the time of day. We all have a *circadian* (daily) *rhythm*, or physiological rhythms associated with the 24-hour clock. Have you noticed you have more energy in the morning, the late afternoon, or at night? Are you a "morning person" or a "night person"? Are you usually hungrier at a certain time of day, or sleepier, or happier, or more depressed? Probably, if you take the time to notice, you'll be able to determine how your feelings, emotions, and energies change throughout the day. So it only makes sense that morning yoga, afternoon yoga, and evening yoga will all be a little different. And remember, yoga is *about* rhythm and balance—of body, mind, and spirit. Our very lives move to the rhythm of our heartbeat and our breath.

Although each person's rhythms are different, people have a few similar tendencies. Keep these points in mind when deciding what time of day to practice yoga:

- ◆ Early morning yoga tends to be slower. Do not rush into postures. Gently and steadily move through your workout.

- ◆ Late-morning to midday yoga will probably be more intense. The body is awake now and ready to rock and roll (literally!). This is a perfect time for *vinyasana*, a way to practice yoga that involves a steady flow of yoga postures.

- ◆ Afternoon yoga is centering. The body naturally takes a siesta in the midafternoon, so a more intense workout might help you get through this time. If you end your workout with *shavasana* (Corpse pose), you'll be ready for the rest of your day.

- ◆ Evening or late-night yoga is unwinding. Let the strain of a busy day float away. If your day was unusually stressful, an intense Hatha Yoga workout will help release tensions before you go into a nice, long *shavasana*.

No matter when you practice, yoga will renew you.

Yoga has many purposes—among them, to energize, heal, relax, realign, and inspire you. But all of yoga's purposes lead to renewal, or a new you, free from stress and preoccupation with the self.

The Least You Need to Know

- ◆ Yoga is best learned from a good teacher. Finding a teacher who is right for your personality is important for a successful yoga practice.

- ◆ You can also learn yoga at home through books, videos, CDs or audiotapes, and the Internet.

- ◆ Establish a plan that works for you—how often you will practice yoga and what you will do in each practice. It doesn't take much time!

- ◆ When starting out, strategies such as getting the family involved or keeping a yoga journal can help you stick with your practice.

- ◆ You can easily fit in short yoga practices throughout your day.

- ◆ Your yoga workout will differ depending on when you practice.

In This Chapter

- Defining your yoga purpose
- Knowing your own style improves your yoga practice
- A yoga essay test
- Learning from your answers
- Ground rules for yoga practice

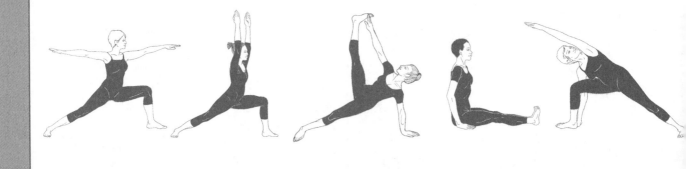

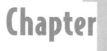

Crafting Your Personalized Yoga Practice

Just as it's important to have a plan for your yoga practice, it's also important to have a purpose. If you don't really know *why* you want to practice yoga, you won't really know *how* to practice yoga. You're an individual, and you bring a unique mix of motivations, emotions, tendencies, biases, needs, wants, and traits to your practice. Being familiar with all of these will not only help you determine which postures will be best for you, but will also be a great help to your yoga commitment.

Define Your Purpose

What are you looking to gain from your yoga practice?

- ☐ I'm primarily looking for a good fitness program.
- ☐ I'm in need of stress reduction.
- ☐ I suffer from a physical condition I believe yoga could alleviate.
- ☐ Eastern philosophy fascinates me.
- ☐ I want to increase my mind power.
- ☐ I like the idea of a holistic fitness program.
- ☐ I'm interested in yoga because I've seen how it has benefited others.
- ☐ All of the above!

If you really aren't sure, take some time to relax and dig deep into your mind. Think about why you want to be a yogi. You'll get some ideas if you just give yourself time to ponder the question.

Sense Your Style

Before you begin your yoga practice, you'll also want to get in touch with who you are. What is it about you, the individual, that will make your yoga experience unique?

- ☐ I am naturally energetic.
- ☐ I am resistant to exercise.
- ☐ I am an optimist.
- ☐ I am a pessimist.
- ☐ I am most concerned with:
  - ☐ The physical me.
  - ☐ The intellectual me.
  - ☐ The emotional me.
- ☐ I am easily excited.
- ☐ I am the calm, relaxed type.
- ☐ I consider myself self-confident.

Even if you aren't sure about the answers to these questions, give them some thought, too. Take the time to get to know yourself. The point of this entire chapter, and especially of the following "test," is to get you in touch with who you are so yoga can do its job.

Wise Yogi Tells Us _____

When you start to analyze yourself, your motives, your intentions, and your personality, try to be as objective as possible. Don't judge yourself. Just see yourself. Try to be like a mirror. A mirror doesn't say, "Hey, you look great today!" or "Whoa, you'd better not go out looking like that!" Your ego says those things. Be the mirror. Just reflect.

A Yoga Essay Test You Can't Fail

If you break out in a cold sweat at the thought of a test, think of this as a self-evaluation. No one else will read your answers (unless you show them to someone), so be as honest as you possibly can. Don't try to fool yourself. Your yoga journey will be better and more fulfilling if you really understand your goals, motivations, and desires.

Wise Yogi Tells Us _____

If you have a hard time analyzing your own personality, imagine you're someone else who's just met you. Try to look at yourself through the eyes of another person. What's your first impression of this new friend (you)?

For each question, write what first comes into your mind and—here's a new twist—keep on writing for a minute or two. Even if you feel you've answered the question in one sentence, continue and write anything that occurs to you, but try to keep closely focused on the question. This exercise is called "freewriting" or "stream-of-consciousness writing," and you might be surprised at what leaps out of your subconscious mind and onto the page! As for what's already in your conscious mind, you might not discern any leaping, but you might at least feel a bit of a foxtrot. We suggest that you use these self-evaluation exercises to begin your yoga journal. After you've been practicing yoga for a period of time, say six months, return to the self-evaluation and see if you'd still answer all the questions the same way.

Don't feel you have to hurry through this test. You don't even have to complete it in one session. But try to complete it before you dive into your yoga practice. Just as a doctor needs to understand all of a patient's symptoms before making a diagnosis, so you should fully understand your own physical, emotional, mental, and spiritual states before you start to improve them.

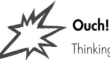

Ouch! _____

Thinking negatively about yourself—negative self-talk—can become a habit. Breaking this nasty habit can be difficult, but it's possible. First, make an effort to notice when you feel negative. Second, consciously try to rephrase your negative thoughts into positive ones. Eventually, you'll retrain your mind to accentuate the positive!

Remember the most important thing when completing this test: Don't censor yourself! Write what you really feel about each question. Seriously think about who you are and what you—not anyone else—thinks about the question. Don't even consider what you "should" think (whatever *that* means!). Just feel whatever it is you *do* think. Let it all hang out and then we'll take a look at who we're dealing with: you!

Because we don't provide you with lots of space here, feel free to record your answers on a separate sheet of paper or in a journal. We like to re-take this test every so often. If you keep your answers in a journal and take the test once or twice a year, you might find it enlightening to see how your answers change. Don't look at your old answers until you've re-taken the test each time.

1. If I had to describe myself to someone who doesn't know me, I would say:

   _____
   _____

2. I have an "outer me" I show to the world and an "inner me" that's more private. Here's how I'd describe the "inner me"—the qualities I have that people might not notice at first or that I consider mine alone and not necessarily for sharing:

   _____
   _____

3. (If you have anything even slightly negative in your answers to the first two questions, underline it.) Now: I could argue that the negative qualities I mentioned are also positive qualities when I look at them this way:

   _____
   _____

4. My best friends would describe me as:

   _____
   _____

5. When I'm confronted with someone who has different beliefs than mine, I feel:

   _____
   _____

6. If I could give one of my personal qualities to everyone in the entire world in order to make it a better place, I'd give everyone my:

   _____
   _____

7. The qualities in someone else that spark my admiration are:

   _____
   _____

8. This is the way I feel about my chosen profession, especially in terms of how it reflects my personality and satisfies my needs and ambitions:

   _____
   _____

9. If someone stole my parking space, would I be more likely to react physically (for example, jump out of the car and deck them), verbally (shout at them, swear profusely, or say something nasty about their appearance or intelligence), or emotionally (think to myself that the person is a jerk, imagine elaborate scenarios of revenge, or brood on the incident all day)? This is how I would be likely to act:

   _____
   _____

10. I think the greatest thing about the world today is:

    _____

    _____

11. I think some of the problems with the world today are:

    _____

    _____

12. I think the greatest thing about me is:

    _____

    _____

13. Here are my thoughts on the existence of a divine power:

    _____

    _____

14. If I could change one thing about the world, it would be:

    _____

    _____

15. If I could change one thing about myself, it would be:

    _____

    _____

16. I bought this book because:

    _____

    _____

17. I think it will be important for my yoga teacher to have certain qualities, such as:

    _____

    _____

18. I hope to accomplish the following from my yoga practice (ranked in order of importance):

    a. _____

    b. _____

    c. _____

    d. _____

    e. _____

19. I think yoga is different than other challenging physical activities like gymnastics or ballet or long-distance running in the following ways:

    _____

    _____

20. Considering all of these questions, I can think of five reasons why yoga might benefit me personally:

    a. _____

    b. _____

    c. _____

    d. _____

    e. _____

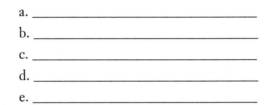

Wise Yogi Tells Us

If you find yourself reluctant to complete this test because you don't like to write, try speaking the answers into a tape recorder or even discussing the questions with a close friend. The point is to get yourself thinking about who you are, what you think, and what your personal journey is all about.

Let's Get Personal

See, that wasn't so bad! We hope you even thought it was kind of fun! And now that you're finished, it's time to score your test. Here goes: You get an A+. It's true! You answered every single question correctly.

If you find that, when evaluating yourself, most of your answers are negative ones ("I'm selfish," "I have low self-esteem," "I don't have very many friends," etc.), nip that negative self-talk in the bud! Whenever you catch yourself forming a negative thought, restate it in the positive ("I am aware of my needs," "I often put others first," "I have a few really good friends").

This test has no wrong answers, but that doesn't diminish your accomplishment. You have undertaken a fairly intense self-evaluation, and what you have learned will only make your yoga practice more fulfilling and effective. Continue to think about your answers to these test questions as you go through your day. Consider it the beginning of a beautiful friendship with your higher self.

The first step is getting to know all of you—even the parts of you you aren't so proud of. The next step is learning to be proud of the whole package. We hope you have a better idea of your own self-concept after taking this quiz, but even if you aren't completely pleased with what you discover, the most important thing you can do now is accept yourself. You are a unique individual, and you are human. You might think you're not perfect, and/or that nobody is perfect. We could argue that, deep down, everyone is perfect.

But we are all moving through life, exploring who we are, where we are, and why we are. We're all working toward self-discovery at our own pace.

Take it easy on yourself. You're working at your own speed and learning as you go, just like the rest of us. You are an amazing person, worthy of self-respect and self-love. In fact, you are miraculous. Feel good about who you are and where you are, and yoga will be a natural avenue of self-care.

Yoga Ground Rules

In the next chapter, we'll actually start learning and trying different yoga postures, or *asanas*. But before we do, let's examine a few ground rules that apply to every posture. Actually, these are not rules so much as sound advice and helpful hints to encourage you to optimize your yoga practice and make the most of each moment.

First, let's look at some general rules for poses. Before you start posturing, keep these important yoga tips in mind:

◆ Hold each pose for three breaths (both inhalation and exhalation) to start, and gradually increase the time you hold each pose, as you're able to do so.

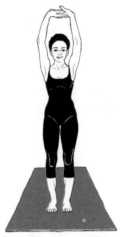

Don't rush through poses. Hold every pose for three or more slow, controlled breaths.

◆ Don't feel you have to look just like the picture! More important, find peace within each pose, and progress as your body allows you to.

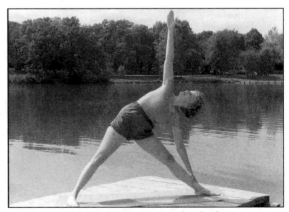

Can't manage a pose that looks quite like this? No problem!

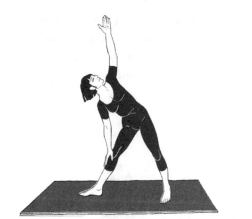

If your Triangle pose looks more like this, with your hand resting on your knee, you are still doing it correctly.

◆ For each pose, make sure you have a counterpose to keep your body balanced. For example, bends to the right should be balanced with bends to the left, forward bends with backbends, contractions with expansions, and so on.

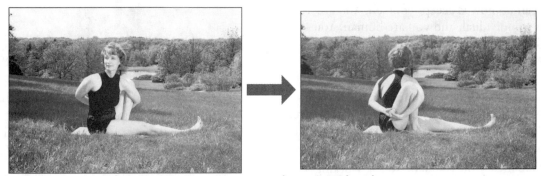

When you twist one way ... remember to twist the other way, too.

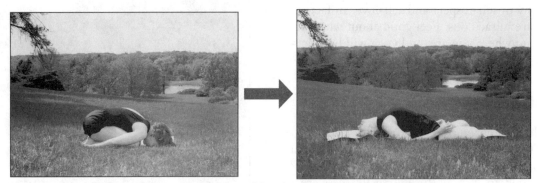

Child's pose is a relaxing forward bend to balance back-bending poses.
Fish pose is a relaxing backbend to balance forward-bending poses.

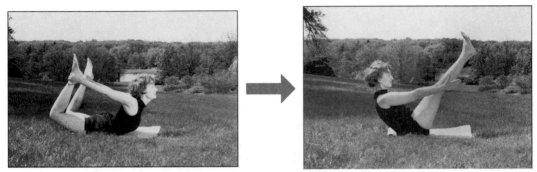

An expansion pose like Bow pose nicely balances a contraction pose.
A contraction pose like Boat pose nicely balances an expansion pose.

◆ Generally speaking, exhale as you go into forward bends and inhale as you go into backbends.

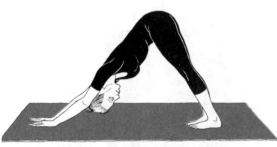

Exhale into Downward Facing Dog.

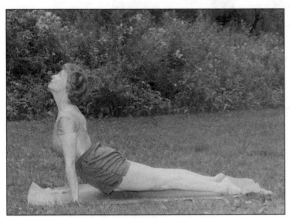

Inhale into Upward Facing Dog.

Listen to Your Body

We will remind you throughout this book to listen to your body. Pay attention to how your body is responding to each pose. Focus on how you feel, not on something else like the television or the radio. Listening to your body and responding to its needs is the best way to get the most out of each pose.

That's a short overview. Are you ready to begin? Let's stand up and get to it!

The Least You Need to Know

◆ Getting to know yourself better will make yoga better!

◆ Know thyself.

◆ Know thyself.

◆ Know thyself. (… And then it will truly be nice to know you, too!)

◆ Good posture, correct breathing, beginning at the beginning, and a concentrated focus will optimize your yoga workout—and your life!

In This Part

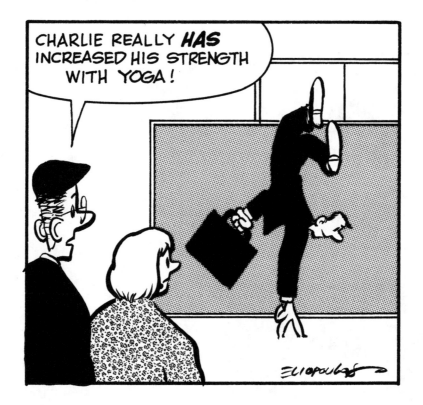

Part 4

Strength: Postures to Build Endurance

On to the workout! Part 4 consists of energizing poses you can try, master, and incorporate into your workout. Standing poses build strength, endurance, and steadiness. Balance poses improve poise and self-possession. Backbends release the flow of energy through your body. Twists and inversions rejuvenate and revitalize you. We'll give you lots of pictures and detailed descriptions so you know exactly how to do these strengthening and energizing yoga postures safely, accurately, and in the best design for bodymind balance. Let's go!

In This Chapter

- ◆ The importance of standing poses

- ◆ Lots of fun standing postures to try: Mountain, Triangle, Side Angle Stretch, Warrior, Lightning Bolt, and more!

- ◆ Balance poses, too: Tree, Eagle, Plank, Arm Balance, and more!

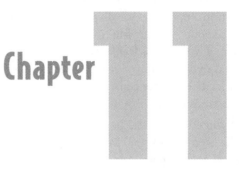

Chapter 11

What Do You Stand For?

Are you ready to start moving? Great! You might be eager to jump right in and try the Headstand or the Full Lotus pose, but learning the basics first is important. You wouldn't be able to play an advanced piano concerto competently without first mastering the scales. In yoga, those "scales" can be likened to the most basic of poses: Mountain pose, from which many standing poses begin.

Remember, standing poses are essential to yoga, and you might find you spend a good percentage of your practice in standing poses. Have fun standing, stretching, and strengthening with standing poses. Let's start by building a mountain.

Tadasana: Mountain Pose

Mountain pose is an important basic pose to learn well. It is deceptively simple in that it appears as easy as standing, but it actually requires great concentration because the entire body must be equally balanced. *Tada* means "mountain," and *sana* means "straight," so *tadasana* (pronounced *tah-DAH-sah-nah*) means standing straight like a mountain. As you stand in *tadasana*, try to feel the firmness and stability of a mountain.

Mountain pose benefits your body in many ways. It helps maintain balance and posture, which leads to internal balance, which leads to good health. You must have a clear understanding of this pose and be able to hold it well before you can hold any of the other standing poses well—including the Headstand, which is really just an upside-down version of *tadasana!*

When holding *tadasana*, it's important to breathe. Let your lower ribs expand on the inhalation. Imagine your diaphragm lowering to make room in your lower chest. You are a soldier of peace in *tadasana*, so there's no need to put up your armor or feel any tension. Try to notice the difference between tension and simple awareness.

As you complete the pose, distribute your weight evenly between your heels and toes, between each leg, and over each hip. Think *balance*. Let your belly expand and release its tension with each inhalation.

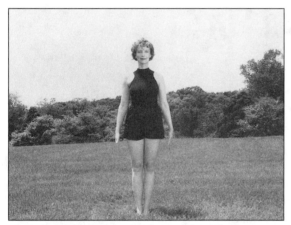

1. Put your feet together with your toes pointed forward. Your arms should hang by your sides with your palms facing toward your body.

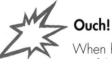

Ouch!

When holding Mountain pose, be careful to stay balanced. If you stand off-balance, your spine's elasticity and alignment will be compromised. Also, tilt your hips slightly in, which will naturally tilt your stomach back toward your spine. The heels on our shoes (even on our gym shoes!) constantly push our hips back and our stomachs out. Realign them with *tadasana*.

2. Lift your toes off the ground. Notice how the arches of your feet feel. Lift up slightly. Now, slowly place your toes back on the ground while you maintain the feeling of the lift in your arches. Feel the lift all the way up your entire body.

3. Feel your spine and the back of your neck lengthening. (Remember that string pulling up the crown of your head?) Pull up your thigh muscles and lift the front of your body. Relax your hands and face.

4. **Yoga Adventure:** Visualization is an effective tool for Mountain pose. As you hold this pose, imagine you are a mountain. Feel how steady, strong, solid, and balanced you are. Feel how you are both a unique, powerful manifestation and at the same time no different from the planet you rise out of.

5. **Yoga Adventure 2:** To give your shoulders, elbows, wrists, and upper arm muscles a nice stretch, try Mountain pose with your hands in prayer position, also called *namaste*, behind your back. Start by bringing your hands behind you at about hip level and touching your fingertips together. Gradually move your palms together so your fingers point up behind your back, and slide your hands up as far as is comfortable. Continue to hold Mountain and feel the sacred nature of this pose. The more you do this pose, the higher up you'll be able to bring your hands and the more flexibility you'll enjoy in your shoulder joints.

6. *Ta-da (sana)!*

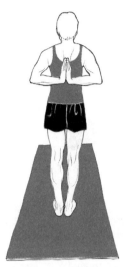

Holding your hands together in prayer pose, or *namaste*, behind your back while in Mountain pose adds balance, reverence, and a nice shoulder stretch to this basic pose.

Trikonasana: Triangle, the Happy Pose

Forming triangles with your body will teach it a sense of direction. The basic triangle, or *trikonasana* (pronounced *trih-koh-NAH-sah-nah*), is known as the happy pose because it opens your Venus *chakra* (the energy center located behind your heart) and allows joy to fill your body and radiate within you and from you. *Trikonasana* tones your spine and waist. It stimulates your bowels and intestines, strengthens your legs and ankles, improves your circulation, and develops your chest. It also strengthens your breath.

For those of you new to yoga, first try Standing Side Bend to prepare your body for Triangle. This pose has all the benefits of Triangle but is less intense.

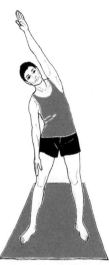

Standing Side Bend prepares your body for the more advanced Triangle pose by activating and energizing the muscles along the sides of your torso.

Once your torso feels more flexible and strong, move gradually into Triangle pose, moving down only as far as your body will comfortably allow. As you come back into *tadasana*, feel your chest opening. Breathe freely and deeply.

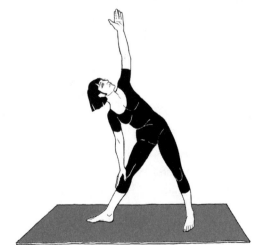

Modified Triangle is a perfectly correct form of Triangle for beginners. The more flexible your torso and shoulders become, the farther down toward the floor you can move.

1. Stand with your feet about three feet apart, your right foot pointed forward, your left foot turned out comfortably, about 90 degrees.

2. Bend to the left, reaching your left arm toward your left foot, and stretching your right arm straight up over your head. If you can, rest your left hand on your left ankle or calf.

3. Look straight ahead or toward the sky and stretch your neck. Feel the triangle formed by your legs and the ground, as well as the triangle shape formed by your entire body. Breathe deeply.

4. Slowly come back to a standing position, then repeat on the other side.

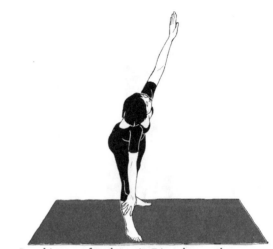

Reaching too far down in Triangle can throw your body out of alignment by pulling your hips back.

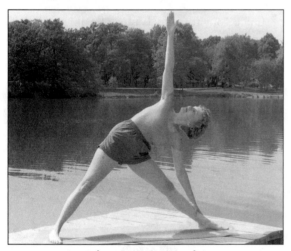

Joan demonstrates Triangle pose.

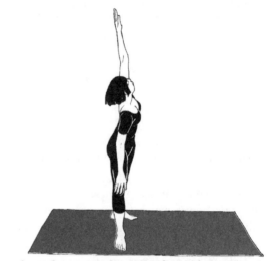

This is the proper alignment of Triangle pose. Notice how the hip and pelvis are pulled in and aligned with the rest of the body.

5. Don't worry if you can't reach your ankle at first. The length of your stretch doesn't equal the quality of your yoga, and in fact, extending beyond your body's capability can throw your hips out of alignment (see the following figures). Don't be so eager to touch your ankle that you tilt your body forward, cutting off your body's energy flow. Pretend your shoulders must stay pressed against an invisible wall behind you. You'll stay straight and your energy will soar!

6. **Yoga Adventure:** Take the Triangle pose a step further with the Revolved Triangle pose. After holding the pose for a few breaths, switch your arms. Bring the raised arm down, and hold the other side of your calf or ankle. Bring the arm that was holding your calf or ankle straight up above you. Breathe, then return to Mountain pose, and repeat on the other side.

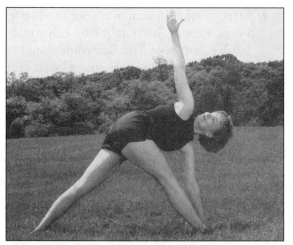

The Revolved Triangle pose might, at first glance, look like the regular Triangle pose, but look closer. The body is twisted around so the left hand is by the right foot. This is considered a more difficult pose because it incorporates a full spinal twist into the Triangle.

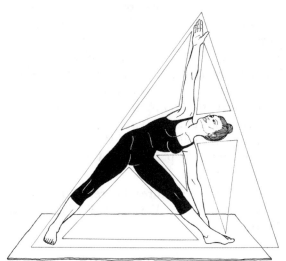

How many triangles can you find in this picture? Look at the lines made by the body and those suggested by the body. Perhaps you can find more than we did.

The next time you move into Triangle pose, consider how the triangle is used as a spiritual symbol in many different cultures: Pagan Goddess traditions used the triangle to symbolize the virgin, mother, and crone. In Egypt, the triangle represented the female principle, motherhood, and the moon. In Arabia, the triangle symbolized the three lunar Goddesses, and the Celtic shamrock was a three-way design originally representing the three mothers. The double triangle symbolizes creation in the Tantric tradition. The downward-pointing triangle is the yoni *yantra* or symbolic representation of feminine sexuality and the Mother Goddess, while the upward-pointing triangle symbolized the Mother Goddess's son and spouse to whom she gave birth repeatedly and who was her mirror image. And while Brahma, Vishnu, and Shiva later took the title of the Hindu trinity, it was originally a Goddess trinity.

We even use the concept of trinity today in everyday life, and we aren't just talking about the contemporary Western conception of the Christian trinity (Father, Son, and Holy Ghost). Consider also the notion of bodymind-spirit, a triangular relationship. Mother, father, and child are a trinity, and even the grammatical concept of "me, myself, and I" is a lovely and unified threesome. You can find triangles and three-way figures and concepts all over your life if you look. Think about that as you bend into a triangle.

Parshvakonasana: Side Angle Stretch

Parshva means "flank" or "side," and *kona* means "angle"—hence, *parshvakonasana* (pronounced *par-shvah-KOH-nah-sah-nah*) means Side Angle Stretch! This pose tones your legs, strengthens your knees, and lengthens your spine. It relieves back pain and sciatica problems, and stretches and strengthens the hips and stomach.

Exhale as you go into this pose, and inhale as you come out; breathe while you hold the pose.

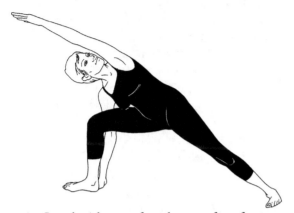

1. Stand with your feet three to four feet apart. Point your left foot forward and turn your right foot out so it is perpendicular to the left, the right heel lined up with the arch of the left foot.

2. Bend your right knee into a right angle with the floor and lean into the stretch so that the right side of your body moves toward the top of your right thigh and your right hand reaches toward the ground beside your right foot. Don't worry about touching the floor with your hand. Instead, concentrate on the side stretch of your body.

Ouch!

In Side Angle Stretch, be careful not to overextend your bent knee. It should be at or nearly at a right angle to the floor. Also, don't let your back leg flop. Keep it active by pushing down on your back heel. If you don't like the smell of your armpit as you look up against your arm, well … change deodorants! (Hey, at least you're working up a sweat!)

3. Stretch your left arm over your head so it forms a relatively straight line with your left leg and torso. Your left palm should face downward. Look up toward your arm and feel the stretch from your toes into your fingertips. Breathe deeply.

4. Return to Mountain pose, then repeat on the other side.

5. **Getting Started:** Side Angle Stretch feels amazing first thing in the morning when your muscles really need a good stretch to wake up fully. This pose is so energizing that it might eventually replace that morning cup of coffee!

Virabhadrasana: Warrior Pose

It takes the tremendous strength of a warrior to "conquer" inner peace. The Warrior pose, or *virabhadrasana* (pronounced *vee-rab-hah-DRAH-sah-nah*), fills the body with nobility and strength, calling upon the power and nourishment of the sun while firmly planting the feet upon the earth. *Vira* means "hero," and *bhadra* means "auspicious," so *virabhadrasana* means "heroic auspicious posture." Wow! Didn't you always want to be part yogi and part Conan or The Rock?

We demonstrate three different versions of *virabhadrasana* here: Warrior 1, Warrior 2, and Warrior 3.

Warrior 1

The first Warrior pose aids in deep breathing, relieves a stiff neck and shoulders, strengthens the legs, and trims the hips.

Be sure to exhale as you go into the Warrior pose, and inhale as you go out of the pose. Think "strength" instead of "tense." Be careful to relax your muscles while in Warrior. Keep your face and neck relaxed. Breathe normally.

Feel the warrior strength gathering inside you. Strength doesn't come from muscle contraction. Strength comes from within.

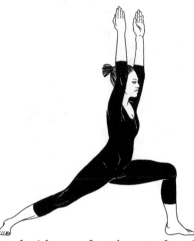

1. Stand with your feet three to four feet apart. Turn your right foot out so it is perpendicular to the left foot, left heel in line with the right arch.

2. Bend your left leg into or close to a right angle and rotate your body to the right, directly in line with your left leg.

3. Raise both arms over your head with your palms facing each other. Look straight ahead or upward at your hands. If your shoulders are relaxed, bring your palms together. For those with tight shoulders, it's best to keep your hands apart, which will help your shoulders stay down away from your ears.

4. Keep your back foot firmly planted and your back leg straight. Push down on your back heel. Take three rich, full breaths.

5. Remember that lift of your arches in Mountain pose? Notice what happens when you apply that technique here. Lift the toes of your back foot. Watch your arch slightly lift. Slowly place your toes back on the ground while maintaining the lift in the arch. As your toes touch the ground, let the lift of your arch ascend throughout the rest of your body. Breathe.

6. Return to the starting position and repeat on the other side.

7. **Yoga Adventure:** Bring your palms together and interlace your fingers over your head, while keeping your index fingers pointed straight up. Keep your shoulders down, away from your ears. Look up at your hands while keeping your neck strong. Imagine strength and energy shooting out of the tips of your index fingers. This variation intensifies the strength and energy of the Warrior 1 pose.

Warrior 2

The second Warrior pose has the same benefits as the first, but it also strengthens and shapes the legs, relieves leg cramps, brings flexibility to the legs and back, tones the abdomen, and strengthens the ankles and arms.

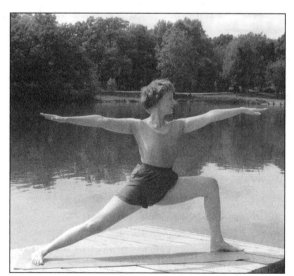

1. Begin as for Warrior 1, but keep your upper body facing forward as you bend your left leg into or close to a right angle with the floor.

2. Lift both arms straight out to form a "T" shape with your body. Look toward your left arm. Keep your shoulders down.

3. Hold the pose for at least a few breaths, return to the starting position, then repeat on the other side.

4. **Yoga Adventure:** Combining Mountain, Warrior 1, Warrior 2, and Triangle into a *vinyasana*, or a flowing sequence, is a great way to get your heart pumping and to energize your body and mind for a challenging day. Begin in Mountain, then flow into Warrior 1 according to the earlier instructions, then rotate your torso and bring your arms down into Warrior 2 position, then flow into Triangle pose, then back into Mountain. Repeat as many times as you like. Once you've combined these, add Warrior 3 to the sequence, flowing from Warrior 1 to Warrior 3, Warrior 2 to Triangle, back to *tadasana*, then turn the other direction, and start all over again on the other side. What a way to wake yourself up in the morning! Keep the movements flowing and full of energy. This Warrior *vinyasa* is a real confidence builder.

Warrior 3

Warrior 3 develops the strength and shape of your legs and abdomen; it also gives you agility, poise, better concentration, and improved balance. It is a more difficult pose than the first two Warrior poses. Be sure to exhale going into all the Warrior poses, and inhale coming out.

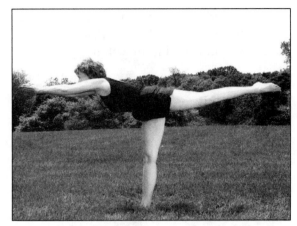

1. Assume Warrior 1 pose, then lean forward slightly, slowly straightening your front leg as you lift your back leg.

2. Extend your arms in front of you with your palms together, and look toward your hands. Work toward bringing your arms and lifted leg perpendicular to the floor. If you can't do that at first, no problem. This is something you will be able to do when you have gained sufficient strength and balance.

3. Return to a neutral position, then repeat on the opposite side.

4. **Yoga Adventure:** How long can you hold this pose? This balance pose is challenging both because you have to balance on one leg and because it takes strength to keep your arms and other leg lifted. Work on extending the amount of time you can hold this pose, for a superpowered, strength-building, balance-honing workout. Watch your breath! As the breath comes into balance, so do the balance poses. Don't hold your breath. Keep breathing, slowly and steadily.

Natarajasana: Shiva Pose

This challenging balance pose is named after Shiva, whose every step destroys and then subsequently recreates the universe. Shiva is sometimes called the cosmic dancer, and this pose is sometimes called Dancer pose. Visualize the ebb and flow, creation and destruction, and continual flux of the universe as you balance in this beautiful and difficult pose.

Begin in Mountain pose. Visualize a steady and firmly rooted center.

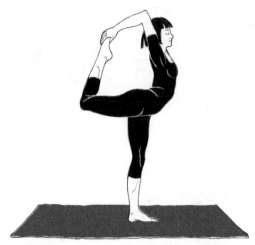

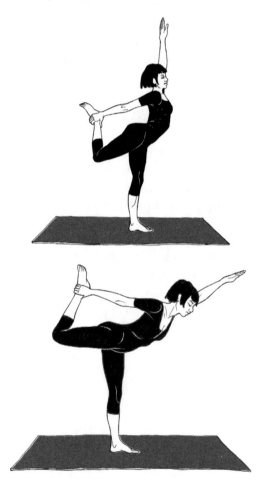

1. Bend one leg and grasp your ankle (as in Tree pose) and raise your opposite arm above you for balance.

2. Slowly bend forward and pull gently on your foot so your raised leg extends behind you, knee bent so your foot points upward.

3. Counter the balance by lowering your extended arm in front of you so that as your leg moves back, your arm moves in front.

4. Once you are very secure in this pose, you can reach both hands behind you to grasp your foot.

Utkatasana: Lightning Bolt Pose

Lightning Bolt pose, or *utkatasana* (pronounced *oot-kah-TAH-sah-nah*), is a powerful pose. *Utkatasana* means "raised posture." As you form the shape of a lightning bolt, you are filled with the dynamic energy of lightning. *Utkatasana* removes shoulder stiffness, strengthens your legs and ankles, lifts your diaphragm, massages your heart, tones your back and stomach, and develops your chest. It also warms up your body.

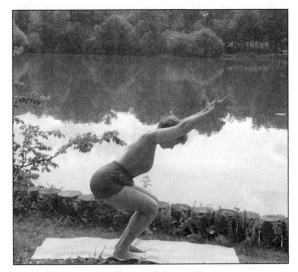

1. Begin in *tadasana*, Mountain pose.

2. Bend your knees and lift your arms over your head with your palms and arms shoulder width apart. Be careful to keep your knees from buckling inward; keep your feet together or slightly apart.

3. Extend your arms so they are straight and in line with your torso. Feel the shape of the lightning bolt and breathe deeply. *Zap!*

4. Return to *tadasana*.

5. **Getting Started:** For a less intense standing stretch that can help you get used to the from-the-hip bend of Lightning Bolt pose without the required leg strength, try Standing Forward Stretch. Stand straight and clasp your hands behind you at hip level. As well as you can while still remaining comfortable, bring your palms together and straighten your elbows so your arms point toward the floor. Pull your shoulders back to open your chest, squeezing your shoulder blades together. Lift your arms just slightly and, keeping your back straight, bend from the hips just until you feel a stretch in your hamstrings (the muscles along the backs of your thighs).

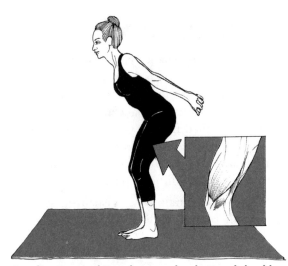

Standing Forward Stretch opens the chest and shoulders while stretching the hamstrings.

6. **Yoga Adventure:** Vary Lightning Bolt by turning it into a "Squat on Heels and Toes" pose. Stand with your feet hip distance apart. Squat, first standing on your toes, then squatting down. Come back up into Mountain pose. Next time, try squatting down while keeping your heels on the floor. This is more difficult, because it requires a fuller stretch of your quadriceps. These squatting variations develop the ankles, knees, and arches, while deeply stretching the quadriceps and knee joints. Be careful to keep your knees over your ankles. Don't let them droop in or out as you bend.

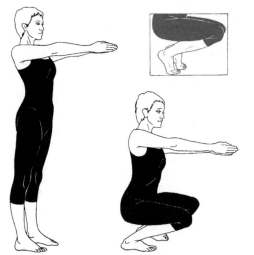

Moving into the "Squat on Heels and Toes" pose.

7. **Yoga Adventure 2:** Extended Lightning is a variation on "Squat on Heels and Toes" pose. Instead, from Lightning pose, slowly bend your knees and lower your hips toward the floor while keeping your spine straight. Keep your feet flat on the floor, eyes focused forward. Stay in this pose as long as you can keep your breath steady, then slowly rise back to standing, using your hands on the floor to help you if necessary.

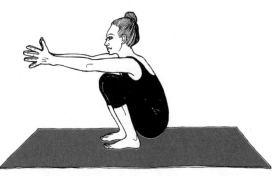

Extended Lightning strengthens the legs and feet and improves balance.

Balance Poses

We've emphasized before that balance is extremely important in the practice of yoga. When your body is balanced, a connection is formed between the two sides of your body (*ha* and *tha*, as in Hatha Yoga). But balance poses do more than coordinate your left and right sides. They help tie your entire body and mind together into a more integrated and fully functioning whole. Balance poses also increase self-confidence, because they teach you to stay centered, calm, and strong in precarious circumstances. If you accomplished Warrior 3 (in the earlier section), remember how great you felt? That's just a taste of the power of balance poses.

Vrikshasana: Tree Pose

Vrikshasana (pronounced *vrik-SHAH-sah-nah*) is one of the most basic balance poses. *Vriksha* means "tree," and a tree is soundly rooted in the earth but grows upward with branches reaching out to the sun. Wind might move the branches, but the tree stands firm. *Vrikshasana* tones the legs, opens the hips, and promotes physical balance. It also develops concentration and mindfulness.

Throughout *vrikshasana*, keep your breathing steady and regular so it doesn't interfere with your balance.

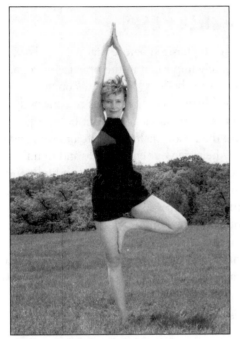

1. Begin in *tadasana*, Mountain pose.
2. Bring your hands together in front of your chest with your palms together in *namaste* (as if praying).
3. Bring your left leg up and balance the sole of your left foot on the inner thigh of your right leg, as high as you are able. If it's been a "vida loca" kind of day and you have a hard time balancing on one foot, keep your toes on the ground, turn your one knee out to open your hips, then simply balance the heel against your ankle. It's amazing how calming and balancing this pose can be!

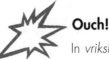

Ouch!

In *vrikshasana*, be careful not to raise one hip higher than the other. Keep your hips even by lowering the position of your foot on your inner thigh. Bend your straight knee slightly. If you become aware that you are hyperextending it, then, with awareness, stop hyperextending the knee: Straighten it with awareness. If your knees are sore after doing this pose, you probably are hyperextending.

4. Raise your arms over your head, keeping your palms together.
5. Return to *tadasana*, then repeat with the right leg.
6. **Getting Started:** If you find it too difficult to balance in *tadasana*, you can vary the pose slightly. Bring the sole of your foot to your opposite leg's inner calf instead of the thigh, or even rest it against your opposite ankle, to get a more secure feeling of the balance before hiking that foot all the way up to the opposite thigh. Also, you can leave your palms apart when you raise your arms. This great separation between your hands can help you balance more easily. When you feel more confident in the pose, you can bring that foot up and those palms together.

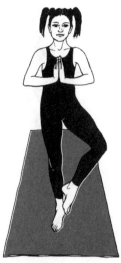

If you have trouble balancing, keep your raised foot just over the ankle of your standing foot.

Ardha Baddha Padmottanasana: Standing Half Bound Lotus Pose

The purpose of this more advanced variation of the Tree pose is to keep the trunk steady with the help of your arm. It has the same benefits as Tree pose but allows you to open your hips more fully, which in turn opens the Jupiter *chakra* (the energy center located on your spine behind your pelvis). It also allows a fuller chest expansion.

Don't be frustrated if you have trouble getting into Standing Half Bound Lotus pose. Standing Half Bound Lotus is similar to Tree pose, except your bent right ankle rests on the front of your straight left thigh. If your hips are not open enough yet and your knee isn't pointing toward the floor, it'll be difficult to connect your hand with your foot and could also overstrain your knee. Give yourself time and keep practicing the regular Tree pose. Eventually, your body will accommodate you.

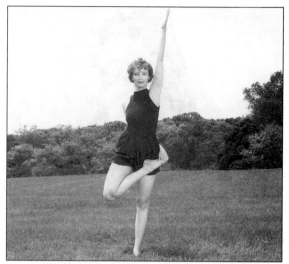

1. Bring your right arm behind your back and connect it to your right foot in front.

2. Lower your knee slightly toward the floor and raise your left arm over your head. Take three breaths.

3. Return to the starting position, then repeat on the other side.

4. **Getting Started:** This is a challenging pose. Poses that open the chest and increase shoulder and spinal flexibility will help get you to a point where you can reach your arm far enough behind you to grab your foot. Practice the Eagle pose (following), Side Angle Stretch (earlier in this chapter), Bow pose, Upward Facing Dog, and Butterfly pose to open the hips and both Standing and Lying Down Spinal Twists to help your body prepare for the Half Bound Lotus.

5. **Yoga Adventure:** For advanced students who have mastered Standing Half Bound Lotus, add an inversion to this already challenging pose. Once secure in Standing Half Bound Lotus, exhale and slowly bend forward to place your palm on the floor next to your foot. Hold for several breaths, then slowly return to standing upright.

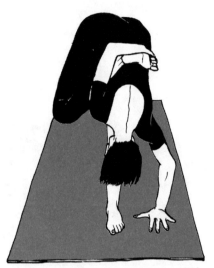

For advanced yogis, try this inverted version of standing Half Bound Lotus.

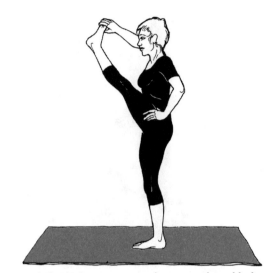

Extended Hand-to-Toe pose takes strength and balance.

6. **Yoga Adventure 2:** Standing Half Bound Lotus can morph into Extended Hand-to-Toe pose. This is another challenging balance pose. From Standing Half Bound Lotus, let go of your foot with your hand but keep your knee bent, your foot at your hip. Bring your hand around to the front and again grasp your toe. This time, slowly straighten your knee so your leg is outstretched in front of you. Lower your other hand to rest on your hip or stretch it out to the side for balance. Breathe and hold for a minute or so, then slowly release your foot and lower it back to the floor.

Once you become very secure in this pose, you can move your foot from the front to the side, but don't try this unless you are comfortable and stable with your leg in front and you're able to completely straighten your leg.

Garudasana: Eagle

The eagle is a sacred animal in many spiritual cultures, from Native America to ancient Hindu, and Garuda, a Hindu god, was thought to be half man and half eagle. Eagle pose is named after Garuda, who was said to be the carrier of the great Hindu god Vishnu and also the remover of obstacles. Try this pose when you are feeling mentally or physically blocked, and you just might find yourself soaring (metaphorically, of course) like an eagle. As with the Tree pose, *garudasana* (pronounced *gah-roo-DAH-sah-nah*) improves balance and concentration as well as develops the ankles and removes stiffness in the shoulders.

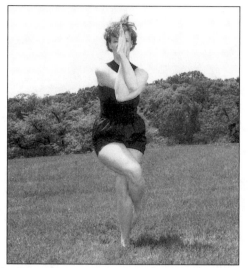

1. Begin in *tadasana*, but with your knees slightly bent.

2. Bend one leg over the other like you are crossing your thighs, then hook your ankle around the back of your other ankle. Try to stay balanced between your heel and toes.

3. Bend your elbows and bring one arm under the other arm, connecting your palms in front of your face. Even though your body is twisting, imagine your torso lifting and straightening. Breathe!

4. Return to *tadasana*, and repeat on the other side. This pose is usually easier going one way than it is going the other way. Reflect on which way is easier for you in regards to openness in your body. Continue trying it both ways, and eventually you'll balance.

5. **Getting Started:** The Eagle pose is a challenging pose. Don't force that ankle around your standing leg, or you could injure your knee! If your ankle doesn't hook around your standing leg easily, just place the top of your foot behind your ankle or your calf of your standing leg. Eventually, your flexibility will increase. Better to work within your own limits than to injure yourself!

Plank Pose

Now let's try getting down on the floor for a whole new angle on balance poses. The Plank pose develops strength in your arms and legs. It helps create a balanced and strong body. It is often used as a transition pose, leading or connecting one pose to another.

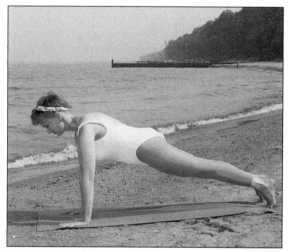

1. Begin in Downward Facing Dog pose.

2. Exhale as you lower your hips down so that your body is in a straight line from your head to your ankles.

3. Try to keep your body in a straight line from your ears to your ankles. You will discover where the weakest sections of your body are the longer you hold this position: They are the parts that start to sag toward the floor!

4. Breathe. Push your heels out to keep your lower back from caving in.

5. Come back down onto your stomach, or use this pose as a transition into the following Arm Balance pose.

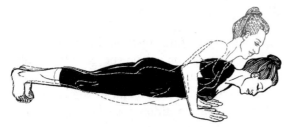

Don't let your torso collapse in Plank pose. Only hold the pose as long as you can hold it with correct form.

Ouch!

Keep breathing steadily throughout *vashishthasana*. Don't let your hips droop down, because this will cause strain to your back and put undue force on your arms. Keep your elbows straight, and keep your foot balanced on your leg. Don't let anything droop!

Vashishthasana: Arm Balance

Vashishthasana (pronounced *VAH-shish-THAH-sah-nah*) is a pose named after the Indian sage Vashishtha. *Vashishthasana* strengthens the wrists and arms and tones the lumbar and coccyx regions of the spine. It also develops concentration, nonattachment to either achievement or failure, and an undisturbed, steady mind.

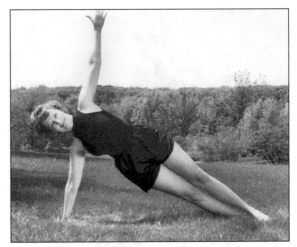

1. Begin in Plank pose.

2. Turn your entire body to the right, and balance on your right arm and foot on the side of your body. Your torso should be in a straight line, held in a diagonal to the floor by your right arm.

3. Lift your left arm up straight in the air with your palm facing forward.

4. **Getting Started:** Don't lock your elbow in this pose or you could injure it. Keep your arm straight, but keep strength and flexibility in your elbow so you could bend it easily at any time during the pose (just as you would keep your knees just slightly bent rather than locked when standing for a long time). Your muscles should be holding your weight, not your elbow joint. Depending on your fitness level and center of gravity, this pose can

require quite a lot of arm strength. If you find you are straining your wrist or elbow or if your arm starts to shake and you feel you can't hold the pose another second, for goodness' sake, stop! Or to vary the pose slightly while you work on building arm strength, bend your bottom leg and rest your lower knee on the floor while keeping your upper leg in line with your torso. To rest from this pose, turn your body into Downward Dog pose.

5. **Yoga Adventure:** For a fun variation of Arm Balance, try this challenging variation: From Arm Balance, slowly raise your straightened upper leg until it is parallel to the floor. Then, raise it higher and bring your raised arm down to meet your foot. Grab your toes and lift so your legs form a right angle to each other.

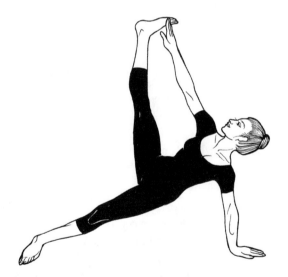

This variation of Arm Balance takes great strength and balance and fortifies the muscles in your arms, back, abdomen, and legs.

Ardha Chandrasana: Half Moon Pose

Half Moon is a beautiful pose in which your body imitates the shape of a half moon. This balance pose improves your coordination and your mental concentration, as well as helping to align your spine. You can do this pose with a yoga block or other support such as a book or small stool, or you can try it on the floor. The key is to keep your torso and limbs as straight as possible so your body and raised leg are parallel to the floor, while your arms and standing leg are perpendicular to the floor. This pose is easier to do in front of a mirror so you can check your alignment.

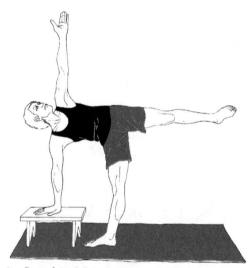

1. Stand in Mountain pose. Place a stool or other support (if using one) against the wall for support.

2. Inhale and open your feet so they are shoulder-width apart. Turn your left foot in and your right foot out into the foot position used for the first two Warrior poses.

3. Raise your arms straight out on either side so they are parallel to the floor.

4. Exhale and bend your right knee, placing your right palm on your thigh. Bring your left leg up as you begin to straighten your right knee. As your right knee straightens, your right hand comes down to the stool.

5. Align your arms so they are perpendicular to the floor and in line with each other, as well as parallel to your standing leg. Energize the fingers of your raised hand, pointing them up.

6. Continue looking forward for balance. Keep your gaze steady on a point of focus.

Birdland

Yoga poses often imitate the plants and animals in nature, so it's not surprising that many yoga poses imitate birds. The next three bird poses are all extremely challenging balance poses, but until you've become comfortable with balances, you might want to try them under the guidance of a qualified yoga teacher.

Bhujapidasana: Crow Pose

Crow pose looks difficult, but once you find your balance, it's really not as hard as you might think. It does take arm strength and good concentration, however. This pose nourishes and strengthens the hands, wrists, and arms in addition to cultivating great focus. Be careful not to drop your head too far forward or shift your weight one way or the other, or this crow will probably tip off the fence. Achieving this pose will make you want to crow!

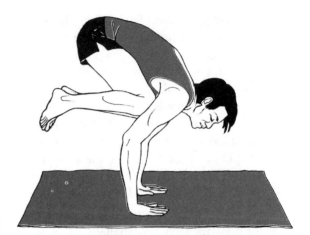

1. Exhale and squat down with your feet together and knees apart. Place your hands about one foot in front of your feet, fingers slightly spread, about six inches apart.

2. Gently rock back and forth on the balls of your feet to find your center of gravity.

3. Place your upper arms, right on the triceps (the muscles on the backs of your upper arms), firmly under your kneecaps. Continue to rock gently, keeping your feet on the floor, just to get a feel for where the point of your balance will be.

4. Focus on a spot on the floor just in front of your hands and gently ease your feet off the floor, resting your knees on your upper arms.

5. Don't be surprised if you can't do this pose right away, or can only balance for a few seconds. The more you practice the Crow, the more confident and balanced you will become. This pose is not a matter of strength; it's a matter of balance.

6. **Getting Started:** Crow pose is difficult, especially if you aren't used to putting your body into a squatting position. As a first step, get used to Crouching pose first. For this pose, squat as you would for Crow pose, with your feet together, knees apart, and hips dropped toward the floor. If possible, bring the soles of your feet all the way to the floor (this is difficult, and you might need to stay on the balls of your feet at first, which is also just fine). Reach your arms around and under your knees to grasp your ankles. Rest and breathe in this position to strengthen your legs and your ankle, knee, and hip joints.

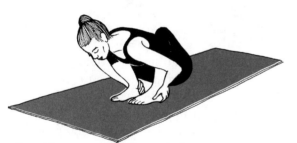

Crouching pose can help you feel more comfortable in an extreme squat before attempting a squat balancing pose like Crow pose.

Kukkutasana: Rooster Pose

Rooster pose is similar to Crow pose. However, in this highly advanced pose, your arms pierce the Lotus pose to stand on the ground like a rooster. This pose looks fancy and is lots of fun to do once you are able to master it comfortably. However, you must be able to sit comfortably in Lotus pose before attempting this pose (see Chapter 14). Rooster pose increases hip flexibility, shoulder strength, and concentration.

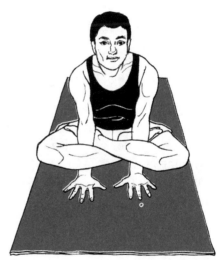

1. Sit in Lotus pose (see Chapter 14 for directions on getting into this challenging meditative posture), with each foot placed on top of the opposite thigh.

2. Slide each hand between the calf and thigh of each leg and place on the ground under your hips, rocking back to make a space. Inhale.

3. Exhale as you slowly straighten your elbows, pushing down on the floor to lift your body above the floor so your hands support your weight. You will have to adjust to find your center of balance.

4. Breathe and hold for a short time, then lower yourself back down.

Mayurasana: Peacock Pose

Peacock pose is another challenging pose that takes great abdominal and back strength. It is great for strengthening your body's core, honing balance and concentration, and improving arm and wrist strength, but it might take quite a while to master, so don't be frustrated if you can't do it right away ... or even a year from now! Again, we will remind you that yoga is a process.

This pose is particularly difficult for women. Because the balance in this pose is centered over the chest, where men tend to have their center of gravity, and because men tend to have more upper body musculature, experienced male yogis might find this easier to do than experienced female yogis, even those who are very strong. Women tend to have a lower center of gravity in the hip area, which can make this balance much more difficult to find. Women might have better luck doing the Lotus version of this pose because it brings the legs closer to the center of the body.

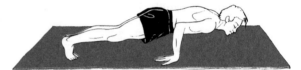

1. Begin by squatting down onto your knees. Place your palms on the floor together between your knees. At first, point your fingers to the side. Eventually, work toward being able to point your fingers back behind you.

2. Bend your elbows and slowly move your body forward until your elbows are over your abdomen and your upper arms hug the front of your chest. Slowly extend your legs out behind you, toes resting on the floor.

3. Easing forward, gradually and slowly move your head toward the ground until your feet lift off the ground. Keep your body, head to toe, in a straight line. Imagine you are a teeter-totter finding that center balance. Don't try to lift your legs off the ground, just let the balance of your upper body and gravity do the work.

Working toward stability and balance in your yoga practice can be a challenging and exciting journey that lasts a lifetime. Learning the basic standing postures is a great way to start, and balance poses will increase your stability. Practicing these basics will improve all aspects of your yoga practice and give you an inner peace and strength. Working toward more challenging poses keeps your yoga workout inspiring and stimulating.

The Least You Need to Know

◆ Standing poses like Mountain, Triangle, Side Angle Stretch, Warrior, and Lightning Bolt are important basics for strength and balance.

◆ Posture isn't just about looking good. It has a profound effect on your health and well-being.

◆ Practice the basic standing postures before you progress to more complicated poses.

◆ Balance poses like Tree, Eagle, Plank, and Arm Balance create stability and a centered sense of being.

◆ Balance poses can be quite challenging in our ever-changing world.

In This Chapter

◆ The health benefits of backbends

◆ Backbends help you laugh more

◆ Lots of great back-bending postures to try: Cobra, Bow, Upward Facing Dog, Fish, Camel, and Wheel

◆ Modifications, challenges, and other tips to improve your yoga practice

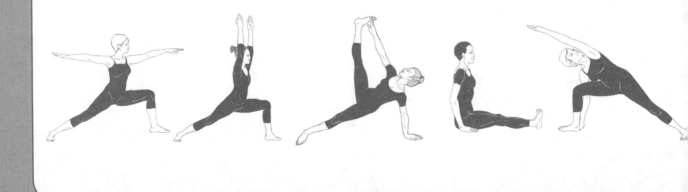

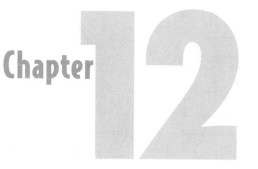

Chapter 12

Bending Over Backbends

A few people have naturally flexible spines and find backbends easy, but for most people, backbends are a challenge. We tend to spend more of our lives bent slightly forward, and our spines just aren't used to bending the other way. All the more reason to practice backbends—for the sake of balance.

Open Up and Laugh More

Whether or not you are naturally flexible, bending poses are extremely beneficial for improving your spine and toning your internal organs. The movement into and the holding of backbends releases your *chakras*, or the energy centers in your body, so energy and joy can flow through you unimpeded. After a few good backbends, you might just open up and laugh out loud.

Start by performing a simple stretch to open your neck, shoulders, and chest. Sit up straight in a chair and begin to arch your neck back (see the following figure). Inhale as you do this. Focus your gaze upward. Feel that openness in the center of your chest? It's as if you're lifting your heart—and your spirits as well! It's important to arch your neck only as far as you can support it, as in the first window in the drawing. Try forcing your lower lip over your upper lip, as you see in the second window. It's hard to frown in a back-bending posture!

Again, in backbends, you always want to be supported; avoid the impulse to crunch your neck back as the figure is doing in the third window of the drawing. A crunched neck (a crunched *anything*, for that matter) is very anti-yoga and can lead to discomfort and injury. Smiles come naturally in backbends. Doesn't it feel good?

Let's get bent!

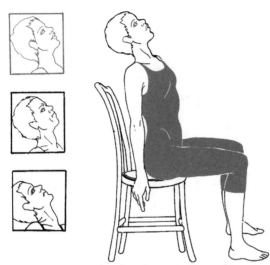

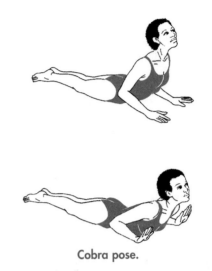

Cobra pose.

Opening stretch before bending. Avoid crunching your neck. The first box is correct, and the second two boxes show an increasingly crunched neck. Ouch!

Bhujangasana: Cobra Pose

Bhujanga means "serpent," and the cobra is a sacred and revered serpent in India. But what is a serpent? Basically, it's just one big spine! In Cobra pose, *bhujangasana* (pronounced *BOO-jhan-GAH-sah-nah*), concentrate on allowing the strength of your spine to move you. The Cobra pose helps align your spinal disks, open up your heart *chakra*, and strengthen your back. It also strengthens your nervous system and your eyes.

When practicing the Cobra pose, keep your elbows in toward the body. As your shoulders rise off the floor, don't scrunch them up around your neck. Keep your eyes open and peering upward to tone your peripheral vision (typically the first part of the eyesight to degenerate).

1. Lie on your stomach, flat on the floor, with your heels and toes together. Place your hands on the floor on both sides of your chest. Rest your forehead on the floor (you might want to use a mat for this one).

2. Inhale and lift your forehead, then your chin, then your shoulders, then your chest off the floor. Keep your hips pressed against the floor.

3. Look upward and breathe. Try sticking out your tongue and opening your mouth wide to help release your face. Then return to the starting position.

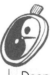 **A Yoga Minute**

Some doctors believe many cases of back pain are psychologically caused. Deep stress or emotional problems might manifest themselves as a backache.

4. **Yoga Adventure:** Does a snake have arms? Of course not! And you shouldn't rely on your arms for this pose. To see how much you are using your arms for support, lift your palms off the floor, as you see in the second figure in the drawing. How much of your body comes down? If it's a lot, your arms are doing a good portion of the work. Don't go up so high just yet. Let your spine strengthen and do the work.

5. **Yoga Adventure 2:** A variation of Cobra pose, this pose looks like a canoe. It's actually called *Poorva Nauasana* or the

Backward Boat pose. Straighten your elbows and rest your arms alongside your body. Then, inhale and lift your arms and legs off the floor. As you hold this pose, you can slowly move your arms out to the sides, as if you are flying, and around to the front (think Superman or Super-woman!), then slowly back around to the sides and alongside the body again. This variation on Cobra is a great torso strengthener and helps balance the muscles of the lower back.

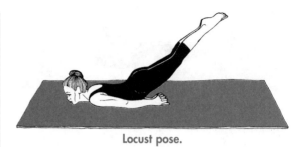

Locust pose.

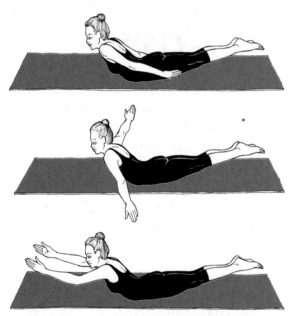

This Cobra variation strengthens the lower back and hones focus.

Shalabhasana: Locust Pose

When your back muscles have become strong from lots of back-bending yoga practice, try Locust pose, a challenging pose that uses the core strength of the torso, particularly the back muscles, to lift the lower half of the body off the ground. This pose is an incredible lower back, leg, and buttocks strengthener. It aligns the spine and helps balance the nervous system.

1. Lie on your stomach with your chin on the floor, legs together, arms alongside your torso, and palms on the floor.

2. Slide your hands under your torso and make fists under each upper thigh with your thumb pointing down, elbows as close together as possible.

3. Inhale and energize your legs and hips, straightening them so they rise off the ground and balance on your fists.

4. Continue to breathe and lift your legs and hips off your fists and upward. Keep your chin on the floor.

5. **Getting Started:** This pose is difficult, but the Single-Leg Locust pose is a great way to get the strengthening benefits of this pose before you are advanced enough to do the full Locust. For Single-Leg Locust pose, lie on your stomach as with Locust pose, but keep your arms alongside your torso, palms on the floor. Inhale, with your chin on the floor, and energize your legs and hips. Lift just one leg off the floor as high as you can without experiencing discomfort in your back. Breathe and hold for a few moments, then slowly lower leg to the floor. Repeat on the other side.

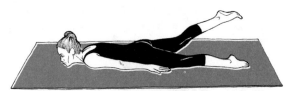

Single-Leg Locust pose is a great beginner's pose to build back strength.

Dhanurasana: Bow Pose

Dhanurasana (pronounced *DAH-noo-RAH-sah-nah*), a.k.a. Bow pose, is a high-energy pose. Imagine your body is like an archer's bow ready to launch an arrow. This pose keeps your spine supple, tones your abdomen, massages your back muscles, strengthens your concentration, and decreases laziness.

When in Bow pose, be sure to grab your ankles, not your toes or feet. If you can't grab your ankles, simply bring your hands back as far as you can alongside your body. Keep your elbows straight, not bent, and don't lift your shoulders up to your ears—keep them pressed down. Open your chest, lengthen your torso, and breathe!

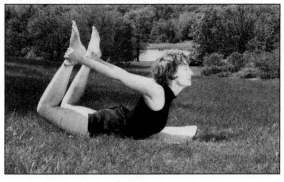

Bow pose.

1. Lie on your stomach. Bring both arms behind you and bend both knees.
2. Grasp your ankles with your hands.
3. Pull your body so it lengthens like a bow and look up. Continue extending for two or three breaths.

Half Bow

In Half Bow, the bow is strung one string at a time. When in Half Bow, be careful not to lean over to the side that is held straight. Balance both sides of your body, and be sure to breathe. You'll be able to tell how much caffeine you've had lately by how much your straight hand shakes!

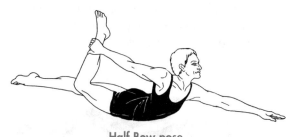

Half Bow pose.

1. Begin on your stomach as with Bow pose, but extend your left arm straight over your head, palm down.
2. Bend your right knee and bring your right arm back toward your right ankle.
3. Push your stomach into the floor with your tailbone tipped toward the floor. Lift your head and chest. Keep your focus on your outstretched arm.
4. **Getting Started:** This preparatory pose might look easier than the full Bow pose, but don't be fooled. You need the same concentration as with Bow pose. This pose is a preparation for Bow pose, so hold it for only a few breaths on each side. Then try going into full Bow pose for a longer sail!

Rocking Bow

Rocking Bow is the full Bow plus! It aids digestion, relieves constipation, and tones the intestines. The fuller the bow, the easier it is to rock and roll!

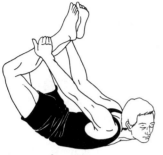

Rocking Bow pose.

1. Flow into Bow pose.
2. Using your breath, rock your body back and forth. Inhale as your body rocks back, exhale as you rock forward. Keep your arms straight.
3. **Yoga Adventure:** This high-energy, aerobic pose in motion is great for your whole body. Pick your favorite song with a medium to slow beat and see if you can rock and roll through the whole thing. If not, you can work up to it as you get fitter.

> **Wise Yogi Tells Us**
>
> Swami Vishnu Devananda says, "Om is a bow, the arrow is the Soul, Brahman [absolute bliss] is the arrow's goal."

Urdhvamukha Shvanasana: Upward Facing Dog

Urdhva means "upward," *mukha* means "mouth" or "face," and *shvan* means "dog." *Urdhvamukha Shvanasana* (pronounced *OORD-vah-MOOK-hah shvah-NAH-sahn-ah*) looks like a dog stretching upward. (Yoga shows great respect for dog poses—after all, what is "dog" spelled backward?) Upward Facing Dog is great for a stiff back. It strengthens the spine, alleviates backaches, increases respiration and circulation (especially to the pelvic area), and strengthens the eyes.

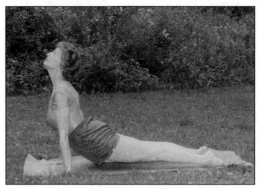

Upward Facing Dog pose.

1. Go into Cobra pose, then inhale deeper and straighten your arms, keeping your legs strong (this takes the pressure off your back).
2. Inhale and lift the front of your body off the floor as you look up. Continue to lift so your hips and legs are held just slightly off the floor, too. Your hands and the tops of your feet are the only parts of your body making contact with the floor in this advanced version. Let your arms do much of the work, not just your spine (as in Cobra pose).
3. Exhale as you come back down to the floor.

> **Ouch!**
>
> Be careful not to let your legs roll in while in Upward Facing Dog. Lift your inner legs. If you feel off-balance, concentrate on centering your balance on your feet. Weak legs will cause your back to curve in and hurt. Keep them strong!

Kapotasana: Pigeon Pose

Pigeons strut with their chests forward, meeting the world heart-first. This open feeling can be yours in Pigeon pose, a pose that flows naturally from Upward Facing Dog. Pigeon pose opens the chest, hips, and throat and increases flexibility in the spine.

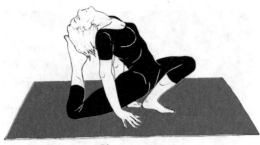

Pigeon pose.

1. Begin in Downward Facing Dog pose.

2. Exhale and draw one leg forward. Place your foot in front of your hips, knee bent and pointing forward. Support yourself by resting your fingers on the ground on both sides of your hips. This might be far enough for most of us and is an excellent version of Pigeon pose. If you would like to take this pose farther …

3. Inhale and bend the knee of the leg behind you as you reach back with your head toward your foot.

4. Eventually, work to the point where you can touch the crown of your head with the toes of the foot behind you. This is King Pigeon! *Coo!* (This means "Cool!" in Pigeon talk.)

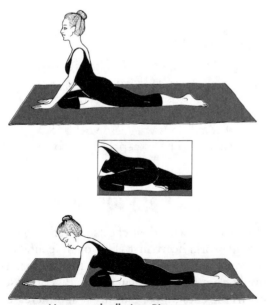

Move gradually into Pigeon pose.

Matsyasana: Go Fish

A fish must open its gills to breathe. *Matsyasana* (pronounced *mahtz-YAH-sah-nah*) fills the lungs with air, improving the yogi's ability to float in water. Fish pose energizes the calcium-regulating parathyroid gland (located in your neck), strengthens the abdomen, improves the voice by opening the Mercury *chakra* located in the throat, and relieves mental tension.

Half Fish Pose

Half Fish pose is a preparatory version of the full Fish pose that follows. Start with this pose and work your way up to the full Fish!

In the Half Fish pose, don't let your feet fall to the side. Keep your knees straight. Make sure the top of your head, not the back of your head, rests on the floor. Keep your elbows in, breathe regularly, and don't put your weight on your head. Let your elbows and arms support your weight.

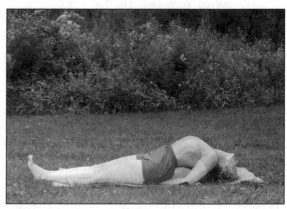

Half Fish pose.

1. Lie flat on your back with your feet together and your knees straight.

2. Place your palms facing down under your tailbone with your thumbs touching.

3. Inhale, then lift your upper chest and arch your back, supporting your weight with your arms and elbows. Allow your head to tilt back.

4. Rest the top of your head lightly on the floor. Feel the strength of the lift in your arms and chest. Hold for three breaths, then exhale as you come down.

5. **Getting Started:** If you have a stiff neck, jaw, or upper back, or if you feel uncomfortable resting your head in this position for any reason, place a folded towel, blanket, or bolster-type pillow under your neck and gently look up and back to accustom your neck and head to this position. No need to rush into the full tilt before you feel ready!

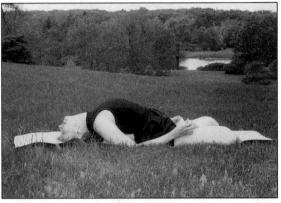

The full Fish pose.

1. Lie down on your back and bring your knees up, then cross your legs into the Lotus pose, with each foot lying sole-up on top of the opposite thigh. If you are not able to bring your legs into Lotus, simply cross your legs.

2. As you bring your crossed legs down to the ground, arch your back up. Let your head relax backward; the top of your head will just brush the ground or floor.

3. Reach your hands toward your feet, and if you can, hold your feet. If you can't reach your feet, place your palms on your thighs. The body is fully balanced in this position and does not need the additional arm strength as in Half Fish pose.

4. Breathe deeply in this position as your lungs are fully expanded.

5. Bring your knees and head up, uncross your legs, and lie back down with a flat back. Rest on your back for a few minutes.

Wise Yogi Tells Us _____

Backbends are so good at making it easier to breathe deeply—by opening up the chest and abdomen—that many people crave backbends! The deep breathing gets more oxygen to the brain. As a result, you feel stimulated, refreshed, and energized. Get a double benefit by completing your yoga backbends with a few balancing forward bends to relax the spine, along with a few moments of meditation on the swami's words.

Full Fish Pose

This pose is the same as the Half Fish pose, except your legs and feet are in the full Lotus position (see Chapter 14) and your hands hold your feet. If you cannot do the full Lotus, simply cross your legs. If you aren't in full Lotus position, you don't need to hold your feet. This variation further opens the pelvis and promotes energy flow through all your *chakras*.

Wise Yogi Tells Us _____

Whenever a particular pose opens a *chakra*, concentrate on that area while holding the pose. Feel the energy flowing through and from the target *chakra*. Your mind can help open your *chakras* even further.

Ustrasana: Camel

Ustra means "camel," and *ustrasana* (pronounced *oohs-TRAH-sah-nah*) imitates the body of a camel. Your shoulders and chest become more open and mobile through this pose. Your abdomen is stretched, digestion is improved, rib muscles are strengthened, and the pose can also help sciatica (a painful condition felt in the hip or thigh resulting from inflammation of the sciatic nerve—a long nerve that starts in the hip and runs down the back of the leg).

When practicing the Camel pose, pretend there is a wall in front of you and you are pressing your thighs toward it. Bend only as far backward as you can while keeping your neck properly supported by your neck muscles.

1. Begin on your knees with your feet behind you, legs and feet together or slightly apart.

2. Stretch your hips and thighs forward as you reach behind you with your arms. Imagine pressing your thighs against that imaginary wall in front of you. The spine extends and lifts upward as you lean back.

3. Let your body bend backward and your head tilt back. Look up. If you can't reach your heels, eventually you will. Take it gradually.

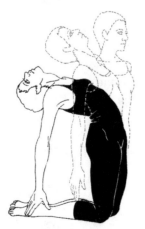

Camel pose.

4. Take several deep breaths in the pose, then exhale as you release and come forward to the beginning position.

5. **Getting Started:** If this pose is too difficult, you can place a chair or a footstool behind you and use it to support your elbows or hands (depending on the height of your support) behind you. Remember not to let your head hang loosely, but to support it with your neck muscles as you look up.

Cakrasana: Doin' Wheelies!

Cakrasana (pronounced *chah-KRAH-sah-nah*) or Wheel pose makes your body strong and mobile, like a wheel. It stretches and strengthens the stomach, improves the concentration by bringing blood to the head, and gives greater control over the body. It also prevents bad posture, tones the extremities, improves the memory, heightens energy and vitality, brings a feeling of lightness to the body, and improves circulation to the trachea and larynx. (The trachea, or windpipe, is the passageway between the larynx and the lungs, and the larynx is the area of the throat that contains the vocal cords.)

In Wheel pose, your hips might feel too tight to extend sufficiently. If your shoulders are tight or your arms are weak, you might be unable to push yourself up into position. Just keep working at it, and one day ... *POW!* There it is.

1. Lie flat on your back with your knees bent, feet flat on the floor.

2. Bend your elbows toward the sky and bring your palms to the floor next to your ears, fingers facing your feet.

3. Lift your navel (think of lifting your Mars *chakra*, located behind your navel), and push your torso up into an arch using your arms and legs. Your head should be off the floor, and your arms and legs will be almost straight.

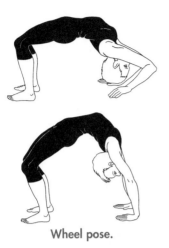

Wheel pose.

4. Hold for as long as is comfortable, then gently come back down.

Wise Yogi Tells Us

The Wheel pose is the most dynamic of backbends. It's the one that effectively stimulates all the *chakras* (also spelled cakras, which are often drawn as wheels), hence the name of the wheel pose: *cakrasana*.

5. **Getting Started:** If the full Wheel pose is too difficult, you can modify the position. In this variation, your stomach remains flat and your elbows and knees stay bent, so you aren't pushing yourself all the way up. You can leave your head resting on the floor between your hands.

6. **Yoga Adventure:** For an advanced version of Wheel pose, try Elbows-to-Ground pose. Slowly lower your body down onto your elbows, your hands pointing toward your feet. Then, slowly raise one leg up. Don't attempt this pose unless your balance in Wheel pose is very secure and you have good flexibility in your spine.

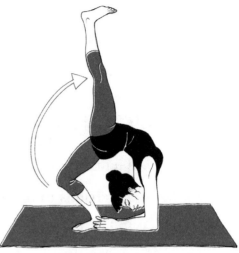

Elbows-to-Ground pose.

Backbends can open your torso and help you laugh more … and better! Don't we all need more and better laughs?

The Least You Need to Know

◆ Back-bending poses are important for increasing flexibility, as well as keeping various internal organs open and free.

◆ Open, toned organs result in open *chakras* and a free flow of energy throughout the body.

◆ Backbends are great for people who work at desks or computers all day; they correct that hunched-over posture.

◆ Backbends make it easier to breathe deeply and fully; they stimulate the body and get more oxygen to the brain.

◆ Backbends bring fuller laughs into our lives!

In This Chapter

- ◆ Gentle twists to realign your spine
- ◆ Inversions to invigorate
- ◆ Spinal twists to scintillate
- ◆ Modifications, challenges, and other tips to improve your yoga practice

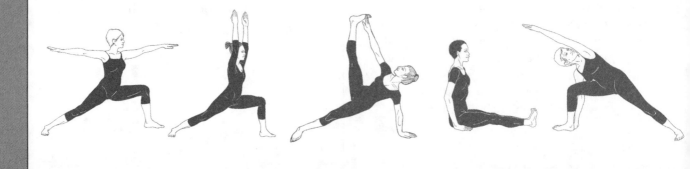

Upside Down and All Around!

Twists are wonderful ways to clear out your system. They free and realign your spine so that every part of your body works better. Twists massage the internal organs and help the body force toxins out. *Prana* is allowed to enter the spine and energize it. For balance, always remember to do *both* sides of a spinal twist.

And talk about a fountain of youth—inversions are amazing postures that balance all that standing and walking around right side up. Blood flows to the brain, gravity works the other way on every part of your body—in fact, after a good headstand, you'll feel almost like you've spent the day at a spa. So get ready to break out of the old habit of existing upright!

Maricyasana: Spinal Twist

Maricyasana (pronounced *MAH-rih-si-AH-sah-nah*) gives the spine a nice, lateral stretch, increasing spinal elasticity. The spinal twist also improves side-to-side mobility; decreases backaches and hip pain; contracts and tones the liver, spleen, and intestines; reduces abdominal size; improves the nervous system; prevents calcification at the base of the spine; frees the joints; and rouses your *kundalini* energy. Whew! It's energizing just saying all that!

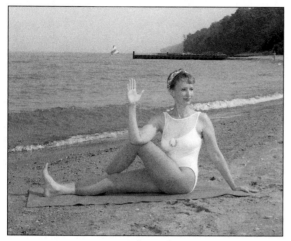

The Spinal Twist.

1. Sit on the floor with both legs out in front of you.
2. Bend your left leg over the outside of your right leg, then turn to the left.
3. Bend your right arm and place your right elbow on the outside of your left knee. Keep your shoulders down.

Ouch!

In Spinal Twist, don't overtwist your neck. Keep the twist the full length of your spine for full benefit. Some people overtwist their neck and neglect the full twist of their spine. Keep your bent knee facing upward to support a steady twist of your spine.

4. Lift your spine and twist, looking behind you as you push your chest forward (in the direction you are facing) to lengthen your spine.
5. Return to the starting position and repeat on the other side.

6. **Getting Started:** The movement of the Spinal Twist should be slow and deliberate, no matter how advanced you are. If you whip your spine around to the side, you could throw your vertebrae out of alignment. If you are having trouble getting the feel of it, count out five seconds as you twist around to look behind you, then take five seconds to twist back to center, five seconds to twist in the other direction, and so on.

Bound Knee Spinal Twist

This variation opens your hips as Spinal Twist does, but be sure to keep your back straight and shoulders down. And remember to enjoy this pose. This is a more advanced twist, and if you aren't enjoying it, skip it for now and try a different spinal twist instead.

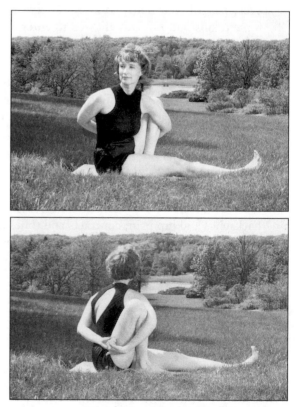

Bound Knee Spinal Twist.

1. From a sitting position with your legs straight out in front of you, bend your left knee and bring your heel in, right up against your body.

2. Turn to your right, bringing your left shoulder around your left knee.

3. Bring your right arm behind your back and connect your hands.

4. **Getting Started:** Can't quite connect your hands? Just reach them toward each other. You'll get there eventually. No hurry! As your shoulders open, your reach will expand, too.

Lying Down Spinal Twist

This variation tones the spine and strengthens the legs. It can also be quite relaxing as gravity helps you out.

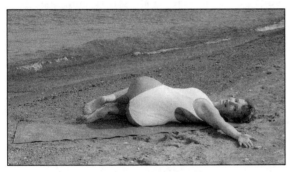

Lying Down Spinal Twist.

1. Begin by lying down with your knees bent and your palms together in front of your chest, as if in prayer (*namaste*).

2. Straighten your arms toward the sky, and let your knees and outstretched arms drop (control the movement) to the right.

3. Lift your left arm and bring it up and over so it rests on your left side. Your arms are extended so your body makes a T. Gently turn your head and look at your left hand.

4. Breathe. Enjoy. Relax.

5. Turn your head back to the right, bring your left hand back to your right hand, then gently bring your knees back to center.

6. Repeat on the other side.

7. **Yoga Adventure:** For an extra challenge, practice deep breathing while resting in Lying Down Spinal Twist. The twist adds resistance to the expansion of your lungs, strengthening all the muscles used for breathing.

Setu Bandha Sarvangasana: Bridge Pose

Now it's time to transition from twists into inversions, which we will do by skipping merrily over the yoga bridge. Yes, *setu bandha sarvangasana* (pronounced *SAY-too BAHN-dah SAHR-vahn-GAH-sah-nah*) means "Bridge Pose." *Setu* means "bridge," and *sarvangasana* is composed of *sarva* ("all"), *anga* ("limb"), and of course, *asana* ("posture"). *Setu bandha sarvangasana* does indeed look like a bridge, and it strengthens the neck and back; tones the entire spine; builds supple wrists; and bathes the pituitary, thyroid, and adrenal glands in blood and other nutrients. Bridge pose helps intestinal function as well. This pose is a good preliminary to Shoulderstand.

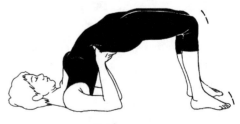

Bridge pose.

1. Lie flat on the floor, with your knees bent and your feet flat on the floor about hip distance apart. Keep your hands to your sides.

2. Grab your ankles and bring them directly under your bent knees. Lift your hips, creating a bridge shape. Place your hands under your lower back for support, pointing your fingers in toward your spine. Keep your elbows next to your body. Your head, neck, and shoulders should stay on the floor.

3. Tighten your buttocks muscles to support your lifted torso. Make sure your knees are aligned with your ankles, that they face forward, and that they don't fall in or out as you hold the pose.

4. **Getting Started:** If Bridge pose is too difficult, start with Half Bridge pose. Clasp your hands under your body, drawing your elbows in so your arms are straight and resting on the floor underneath you. Concentrate on lifting your body as high as you can. This pose builds strength and flexibility to prepare your body for the full Bridge pose.

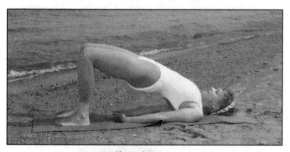

Half Bridge pose.

5. **Yoga Adventure:** For an even greater strength challenge, try Extended Bridge pose. Walk your feet out, away from your body, until your legs are straight. Keep those abdominals lifted and buttocks muscles working—you don't want your bridge to sag! Extended Bridge is a very difficult pose that takes a lot of torso strength. Be kind to your back. If it hurts,

bring your knees back to a bent position. Remember yoga's first principle? *Ahimsa*—nonviolence. We are shaping our bodies into postures nonviolently. Through this process, we build bridges of peace!

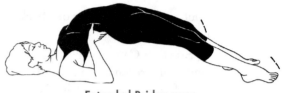

Extended Bridge pose.

Wallflower Stretch

Inversions can be a real challenge for some people who find it disconcerting to be upside down. To ease into inversions, or just to spend a really great 15 minutes after a hectic day, try Wallflower Stretch. Although not a classical yoga pose, this rejuvenating inversion takes very little effort but offers great benefits to your body, especially to tired legs and feet. Blood flows out of the lower extremities but the support of the wall makes this stretch so easy that anyone can do it, even those who have never tried a yoga pose before. All you need is a wall and possibly a folded blanket, towel, or small pillow. Wallflower Stretch also helps us see things in a whole new light. With our legs up the wall, our heads on the ground, and our arms and chests open to possibility, who knows what great inspiration could dawn!

1. Lie on the floor and scoot your hips up to a wall. Gently lift your legs and place them against the wall so your body forms a right angle with your legs up the wall and your torso on the floor. Keep your feet relaxed in a natural flexed position.

2. If it's more comfortable, place a folded blanket, towel, or small pillow under your head, neck, and/or hips.

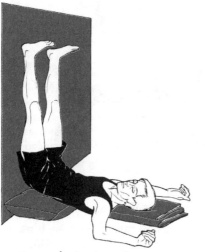

For a relaxing inversion, use a
wall to support your legs.

3. Inhale and open your arms, bringing them
   beside your head, palms open and relaxed.

4. Spend about 15 minutes here, breathing
   naturally and relaxing. Do a quick body scan
   to search out areas of tension and breathe
   into these areas to release the tension.

Wise Yogi Tells Us

Wallflower Stretch is a great stretch for
women who are suffering from PMS
and cramps. Although some yoga literature
advises against inversions for menstruating
women, this one is perfect because it is relaxing and rejuvenating but it doesn't invert the
abdominal area. Wallflower Stretch is conducive to inner reflection and a deep tranquility, in addition to a profound sense of
relaxation—all of which can help alleviate
some of the emotional upheaval and physical
discomfort that sometimes come with "that
time of the month."

Sarvangasana: Shoulderstand

Sarvangasana (pronounced *SAHR-vahn-GAH-
sah-nah*) is a great inversion that stimulates the
thyroid gland and the Mercury *chakra* (located
in the throat). It reverses the pull of gravity on
your internal organs and reduces the strain on
your heart, because your heart doesn't have to
work as hard to pump to the extremities when
inverted. The Shoulderstand helps with vari-
cose veins; purifies the blood; nourishes the
brain, lungs, and heart; strengthens the eyesight; and helps clear the mind.

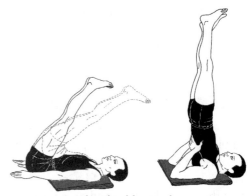

The Shoulderstand.

1. Lie flat on the floor, then bring both legs
   and hips up in the air. Lift up by contracting your abdominal and buttocks
   muscles. Although a little bit of a swing
   can help you get up there, let your muscles do most of the work.

2. Support your lower back with your hands
   so your upper arms are resting on the floor
   behind you, your elbows are bent, and
   your hands rest on your back with your
   fingers facing inward, toward your spine.

3. Bring your shoulders away from your ears
   and push your feet toward the ceiling,
   almost as if you were hanging by your
   feet. Breathe! (You'll probably notice that
   breathing feels different upside down.)

4. **Getting Started:** If you can't get up into a shoulderstand, don't force it. First practice Shoulderstand by bringing your legs back, as in the first drawing, then holding there for a while to accustom your body to the inversion. To protect your neck, it is best to go up into full Shoulderstand, especially the first time, under the guidance of an instructor. Typical problems during Shoulderstand are the tendency to crunch the neck, hold the breath, and twist the neck. Think of your neck lengthening as you hold the pose. Put a folded towel or blanket right at the tip of your shoulders to allow more room for your neck to stretch. Breathe! Don't allow your elbows to slide outward, and keep your neck lengthened and your feet together.

Halasana: Plough Pose

Halasana (pronounced *hah-LAH-sah-nah*) looks like a plough, and *hala* means "plough." Plough pose folds the torso, compressing the internal organs and digestive system. The effect is to suffuse the internal organs and organ systems of the torso with energy, stimulating the stomach and digestive tract, alleviating constipation, and energizing the spleen, liver, gall bladder, and kidneys. Plough also stimulates the spine, strengthens the nervous system, improves circulation, releases neck tension, decreases insomnia, promotes mental relaxation, activates the Mercury *chakra* (in the throat), improves communication, and stimulates the heart.

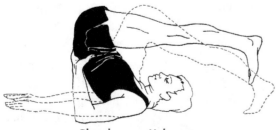

Plough pose, *Halasana.*

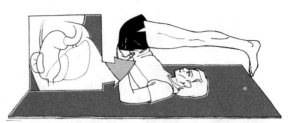

Plough pose compresses the torso, stimulating the stomach and helping activate the digestive system. Plough pose also energizes the gallbladder, kidneys, and spleen.

1. Lie on your back with your knees bent, feet flat on the floor, and hands at your waist.

2. Inhale and raise your legs, hips, and buttocks off the ground into Shoulderstand. Steady yourself in Shoulderstand. After several breaths there, begin to slowly bring your legs backward, keeping your legs together and straight.

3. Exhale as you lower your feet to the floor behind your head. As soon as you start to feel undue strain in your back, hold your feet and don't bring them down any farther. Touch your legs to the ground only when they are straight and you feel no painful strain in your neck or back.

4. Clasp your hands under your body, facing away from your feet.

5. **Getting Started:** In Plough pose, be sure to keep your knees straight. Don't twist your head or neck. It helps to learn from a teacher or experienced yogi before you try it. Don't force your toes to the ground; let gravity do this slowly. If your toes seem like they aren't even close, try Plough pose with a chair or large pillow behind you so your feet can rest on something a little higher.

6. **Yoga Adventure:** For an even greater challenge in Plough pose, try the Hands-to-Feet variation. This variation is identical to the first Plough, except that you stretch your arms along the ground until they touch your feet. This pose further opens and stretches the shoulders. Notice that this looks pose like an upside-down

forward bend. In fact, you might begin to notice that many "different" poses are really the same, just gravitationally different. (Meditate on that for a while!)

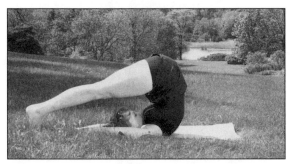

The Hands-to-Feet pose is a variation of Plough pose.

Dolphin Stretch

Dolphin Stretch is an energizing and arm-strengthening movement that helps prepare the body for Headstand. This movement builds shoulder strength, aligns the upper back and shoulders, and helps with mental clarity and focus. It is an excellent movement for building upper-body strength, and can make not only Headstand but also Handstand and Downward Dog feel more comfortable.

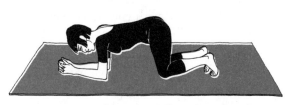

Begin the Dolphin Stretch from this position.

1. Begin on your hands and knees with your knees beneath your hips, your toes on the floor. Bring your elbows down to the floor, shoulder width apart. Clasp your hands together so your forearms form a V on the floor, keeping your elbows shoulder width apart.

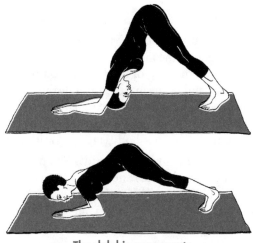

The dolphin movement.

2. Inhale and slowly straighten your legs, lifting your hips into the air. Drop your head down so the top of your forehead just lightly touches or hovers about an inch off the floor.

3. Slowly bring your heels down as far as possible. Don't worry if you can't put your foot flat on the floor; just feel a nice calf stretch.

4. Breathe steadily, then exhale as you lower your body and rock forward to bring your chin down to the floor to touch your hands.

5. Inhale as you come back up into Elbow Dog (Downward Facing Dog, but with your upper body resting on elbows and forearms instead of hands).

6. Exhale as you rock your body forward and touch your chin to your hands. Continue this movement back and forth, and imagine yourself a dolphin moving through the water. This is the way a dolphin swims through water. To understand the movements of the dolphin better is one more step in understanding nature better. This is the path of yoga. It is the path of self-realization. Aum.

Shirshasana: Headstand

Shirshasana (pronounced *sher-SHAH-sahn-ah*) is probably one of the most famous yoga poses and is considered the king of the Hatha Yoga poses (Shoulderstand is queen). Headstand stimulates the whole system, improving circulation and strengthening the nervous system, emotions, and brain. Plus, when your body is ready for it, it's fun!

But be sure your body is ready. You must have sufficient arm, shoulder, neck, and stomach strength, plus be well versed in *tadasana*, Mountain pose, so you can balance your weight evenly while upside down. Most of the weight is in your arms in this pose. Your arms, shoulders, and even the stabilizing strength of a strong abdomen support your bodyweight. Your head is a balance point in the pose.

The strength of these areas is developed in standing poses. Develop yourself on your feet before standing on your head.

Ouch! _____

Heads aren't meant to bear weight, and you could injure your neck if you put too much pressure on your head. Instead, your head is merely one of the minor supporting points in the supportive triangle you create with your arms.

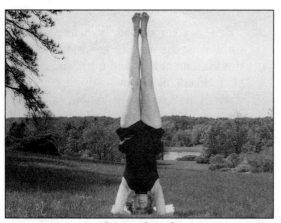

The Headstand.

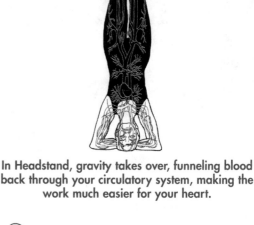

In Headstand, gravity takes over, funneling blood back through your circulatory system, making the work much easier for your heart.

Wise Yogi Tells Us _____

When first attempting Headstand, use a wall for support. The more comfortable and strong you become, the less you'll need the wall, until soon you'll be doing Headstands anytime, anywhere!

1. Get down on your hands and knees. Grab your left elbow with your right hand and your right elbow with your left hand.

2. Bring your elbows to the ground and release your hands. Keep your elbows this distance apart for best support.

3. Interlace your fingers so your arms form a point, then cup the top of your head in your palms at the top of the point, as if your head were inside the apex of a triangle.

Ouch!

As wonderful a pose as Headstand is, it shouldn't be practiced under certain circumstances. If you have high blood pressure, heart problems, or are pregnant, do not attempt Headstand or any of the inverted poses. You might still be able to do inversions with no problem, but talk to your yoga-friendly doctor first.

4. Slowly walk your feet in toward your body, straightening your back, then slowly raise your feet into the air.

5. Breathe! Try to stay balanced in Headstand for at least a few even breaths. Then come back down slowly. Remain with your head down for a few minutes before sitting up.

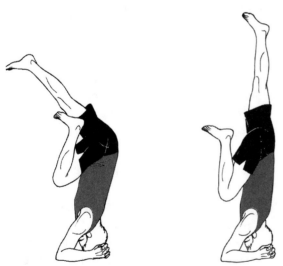

Maintain your balance when going into Headstand so that your hips and torso align with your head and shoulders.

6. **Getting Started:** Balancing in a headstand isn't just a matter of lifting your feet up and hanging out for a while—as your proficiency increases, so does your awareness. Your entire body will be making

minor adjustments, tiny movements, little shifts here and there—along your arms, shoulders, hands, neck, back, and legs—to keep you balanced. Notice how your body tries to compensate to keep you balanced. Your body knows. Learn from it!

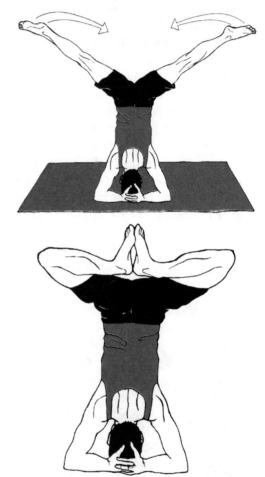

Once you become adept in Headstand, you may vary your pose by slowly moving your legs into different positions while maintaining centered stability.

7. **Yoga Adventure:** For very experienced Headstanders, try other changes in leg position, such as bending your knees, moving your legs apart, bringing the soles of your feet together, or the lovely and symmetrical Lotus headstand, *padma*

shirshasana (pronounced *PAHD-mah sher-SHAH-sah-nah*). While in Headstand, move your legs slowly and keep control over your balance. For Lotus Headstand, you must be able to bring your feet into the full Lotus position without the help of your hands. For any Headstand variation, be very careful when shifting your legs because any quick shifts in bodyweight, especially unevenly on one side, could cause muscle strain or vertebral damage to your neck, upper back, or lower back. Always move slowly to maintain your balance and keep your Headstand stabilized so your hips and torso remain in a straight line over your head. Headstand variations are definitely advanced postures, so please find a qualified teacher for personal guidance on these poses, okay?

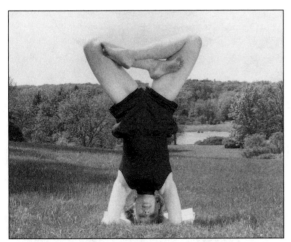

The Lotus Headstand—a
challenging Headstand variation.

Vrichikasana: Scorpion Pose

Scorpion pose mimics the unusual form and curve of the scorpion. This pose is extremely challenging and takes upper body strength, balance, concentration, and confidence. You should feel very comfortable with Headstand and be strong enough to hold it comfortably for about five minutes before attempting this pose.

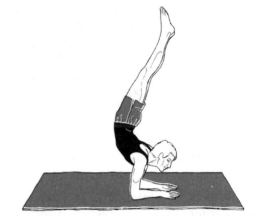

Scorpion pose takes great physical and mental
strength, but in turn, it imbues the bodymind with a
great sense of inner strength and balance.

1. Start in Headstand. Slowly release your hands and bring them apart, pressing your palms against the floor.

2. Slowly lift your head slightly off the ground and bend your knees, balancing so the curve of your torso offsets the weight of your lower legs.

3. If you feel very comfortable, try bending your knees so your toes touch your forehead, or straightening your legs all the way up.

4. **Getting Started:** Before attempting a pose like Scorpion, make sure you feel rock steady in Headstand. Be able to hold Headstand comfortably for at least three minutes. If you can hold Headstand for at least that long, then you are ready to attempt variations. Scorpion comes after mastery of Headstand.

Adho Mukha Vrksasana: Handstand

Adho mukha means "face down," and *vrksa* means "tree," so Handstand, *adho mukha vrksasana* (pronounced *AHD-hoh MOOK-hah vrik-SHAH-sah-nah*), is Tree pose turned upside down. To properly perform this face-down Tree pose or Handstand, your arms must be strong. Practice Downward Facing Dog (Chapter 17) to develop your arms and prepare your body for Handstand.

Handstand gives you tremendous energy. It strengthens your arms and shoulders, plus gives you all the blood-cleansing effects of inversions. If trying this pose scares you, work with a partner who can spot you. The Handstand, however, requires a lot of combined abdominal and upper-body strength. If you're not strong enough, concentrate on perfecting Headstand poses and Downward Facing Dog first.

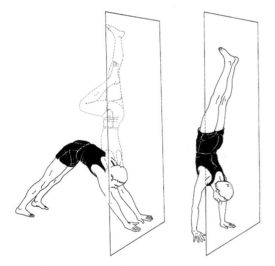

Moving from Downward Facing Dog into Handstand.

1. Perform Downward Facing Dog (see Chapter 17) in front of a wall, as the yogi is doing in the drawing. Place your hands on the floor, shoulder width apart, and about three to five inches from the wall. Slowly walk your legs in toward the wall.

2. Exhale and lift one leg straight up. Follow quickly with the other in a gentle kicking-up motion. Keep your arms and legs straight and firm. Push your shoulders away from the floor, and rest your outstretched legs lightly against the wall.

3. Hold the pose for as long as is comfortable. Breathe! Exhale as you come down.

4. **Yoga Adventure:** If you are a very experienced yogi who can balance easily in a Handstand, try this pose without a wall. But don't try this unsupported pose prematurely. Falling over the wrong way could cause you serious injury. If you do start to fall, bend your knees and roll out of the fall safely.

Now you have some basic (and some advanced) poses under your belt. Having fun? We are! Inversions can be incredibly refreshing and invigorating. Twists also keep the spine flexible and youthful, so dive into this yoga fountain of youth … head first!

The Least You Need to Know

◆ Spinal twists gently massage internal organs, strengthen the spine, and purify your system.

◆ Inversions—the Bridge, Shoulderstand, Plough, Headstand, and Handstand—are yoga's fountain of youth: They keep you young!

◆ Inversions send blood to the brain—that's brain power!

◆ Avoid inversions if you have high blood pressure, heart problems, or are pregnant.

In This Part

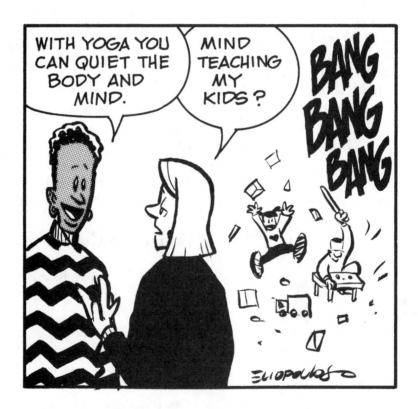

Part 5

Calm: Postures to Quiet the Body and Mind

The postures in Part 5 balance those in Part 4, calming and quieting the body and mind. First, we'll try some sitting poses including excellent poses for meditation, like Lotus pose. Sitting poses center the body and are conducive to a calm and tranquil mind. Next, we'll talk about breath and the yoga breathing exercises called *pranayama*. Learn how to infuse your body with life-force energy, *prana*, through these exercises. We'll tell you all about *chakras*, *mudras*, *mantras*, and *mandalas*, which can help you to refine, intensify, and optimize your yoga and meditation practice. Forward-bending poses are internalizing. As the body bends forward, folding in on itself, the mind can focus more easily inward. We'll show you some peaceful forward bends, both sitting and standing, for you to try. Finally, we'll devote a chapter to the most important of all the postures: *shavasana*. Also known as Corpse pose, *shavasana* is both the easiest and most difficult, because it involves simply lying on the floor in an attitude of complete and total relaxation. Just wait until you try to clear that active mind and keep that restless body still!

In This Chapter

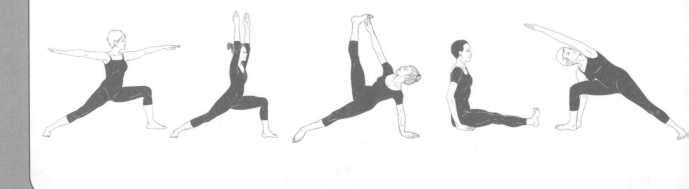

Chapter **14**

Are You Sitting Down?

It's time to take a load off! Lots of great and challenging yoga postures, as well as the meditative postures, are accomplished while sitting. Sitting poses are great because they keep your hips and legs flexible. You might even want to adapt some of the following poses for when you happen to be sitting on the floor outside of your regular yoga practice—just one more way to fit yoga into your day!

Flooring It

Everybody turf it! Yes, sit down on the floor. (Perhaps a welcome relief after a strenuous round of Sun Salutations.) You should feel comfortable in sitting poses, especially the meditative poses, because your body shouldn't distract you from your meditation. If you have a hard floor, a yoga mat or rug (one that won't slide around) will keep you comfortable. A carpeted floor is also fine. Don't use your bed—your practice surface should be comfortable but firm. You'll need the resistance of the floor for many of the postures, and a bed has too much "give." Ready? Set? Sit!

Dandasana: Staff Pose

A staff is a big stick used for support, like a walking stick. It is also a symbol of authority—he or she who holds the staff has the appearance of being large and in charge! Staff pose helps you internalize this feeling of confidence, increasing your concentration and clarity of focus. *Dandasana* (pronounced *dahn-DAH-sah-nah*) is also great for your alignment. Concentrate on your upper body becoming straight and powerful as a staff.

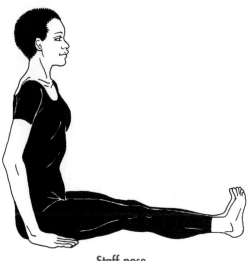

Staff pose.

1. Sit on the floor with your feet straight out in front of you. Keep your palms flat alongside your hips with your fingers pointing toward your feet. Keep your knees and toes together, your heels pushed out, and your toes relaxed. Keep your shoulders down and your chest open.

2. Push your palms lightly down against the ground to create space in your spine. Lengthen the top and bottom of your body. Center your weight over your hips. Breathe.

If Staff pose is uncomfortable, sit on a folded blanket until you become more flexible. Don't puff out your chest. Imagine, instead, that your head is being pulled upward, which will also keep your back from sinking down and your chin from coming up. Your chin needs to be in line with the floor.

Baddha Konasana: Butterfly Pose

Literally translated as "bound angle pose," this pose imitates a butterfly resting its wings on a lotus blossom. When holding *baddha konasana*

(pronounced *BAH-dah koh-NAH-sah-nah*), imagine the delicate beauty of this image of the butterfly. Butterfly pose opens your hips and Jupiter *chakra* (see Chapter 16) and loosens your knees and ankles.

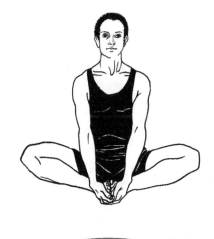

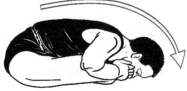

Butterfly pose.

1. Sit on the floor and bring the soles of your feet together, drawing them toward your body. Keep your back straight.

2. Open your chest and press your knees toward the ground as far as they will go. Don't bounce your legs up and down. Instead, allow gravity to gently release your hip joints.

3. Tilt your lower back inward to align the spine. Don't let your upper back hunch over. Keep your chin parallel to the floor.

4. As your hips loosen, you will eventually be able to bow forward with a flat back.

5. **Getting Started:** Some people find Butterfly pose easy because they have naturally loose hip joints. For others whose hips are less flexible, this pose can be

frustrating. If you fall into the less-flexible category, place a pillow under each knee. Press your knees into the pillows, rather than all the way down to the floor. The more you do this pose, the more hip flexibility you will gain.

Wise Yogi Tells Us

While practicing Butterfly pose, keep your entire back straight. If your upper back becomes rounded as you pull your feet in, leave your feet farther from your body; hold on to your shins or thighs if you can't reach your feet. Concentrate on the image of the butterfly. If you catch yourself frowning with unpleasant effort, loosen the pose a bit, think about beauty, and smile!

Virasana: Be a Hero!

A hero stands tall and proud, even when sitting on the floor! Hero pose refreshes your legs, stretches your knees, and balances your Saturn *chakra* (located at the base of your spine).

Virasana (pronounced *vir-AH-sah-nah*) also teaches you to expand your breathing space even while sitting. Imagine lifting from the top of your head and anchoring your hips to the floor. Let your breath expand everything in between.

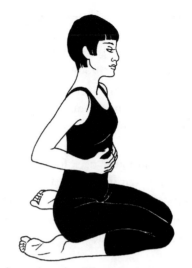

Feel your breath while sitting in Hero pose.

Hero pose can be hard on delicate knees if performed too quickly or attempted before your flexibility allows it. Go very gradually into this pose so you can feel at what point your knees are telling you to stop. If this is hard to do, sit on a telephone book. Every time you practice, tear out one page. In other words, go slowly. You'll get a little farther each time.

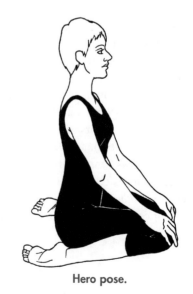

Hero pose.

1. Breathe deeply … heroes *always* breathe deeply. (That's how they stay calm in the face of adversity!) Feel your diaphragm lowering as your body fills with air.

2. Sit back on your heels, gradually separating your feet until you are sitting on the floor between your legs.

3. Keep your knees from buckling in, and move your lower back forward without inflating your upper chest.

4. Pull your calf muscles out and away from your sitting bones, still making sure your knees don't buckle in.

Gomukhasana: Holy Cow!

To us Westerners, the cow might seem less than glamorous. Sure, it may adorn the pot holders, aprons, and cookie jars in our country kitchens, and we might think cows are awfully cute, but we don't take them too seriously. In India, however, the cow is the most sacred of animals, worshipped for its giving nature—cream, butter, and dung, which is used as fuel for fire. Appropriately, Cow pose is meant to lead to a feeling of openness and giving. It also stimulates the nerves at the base of your spine, aids in longevity as it keeps your lower vertebrae from calcifying, opens your shoulders and chest, activates your Saturn and Jupiter *chakras* (located at the base of your spine and in your pelvic area, respectively), and helps raise *kundalini* energy. *Gomukhasana* (pronounced *goh-moo-KHA-sah-nah*) is composed of *go*, which means "cow"; *mukha*, which means "mouth" or "face"; and of course, *asana*, which means "posture."

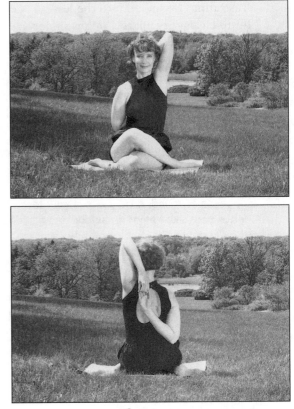

Cow pose.

1. Sit with your legs in front of you, then bring one knee on top of the other. Draw your heels toward your body in this cross-legged position.

2. Point one elbow toward the sky, with your palm facing back behind you. Point your other elbow toward the ground, with your palm facing out behind you. Bring your hands toward each other, clasping them if you can for an invigorating shoulder stretch.

3. **Getting Started:** Some people have less flexibility in their shoulders. If your hands don't touch in Cow pose, that's just fine. Use a strap or towel to get the same stretch and the same benefits.

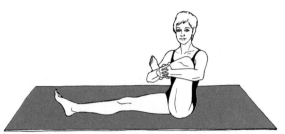

Cradle Rock opens the hips with a gentle, nurturing rock.

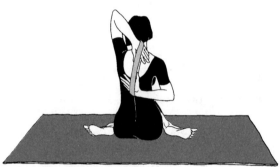

If your hands don't touch in Cow pose, use a strap or towel to feel the same stretch.

Cradle Rock

Cradle Rock is a gentle and relaxing movement that opens the hips in preparation for seated poses. It also encourages a self-nurturing and peaceful state of mind.

1. After completing Cow pose, inhale and stretch your legs in front of you.

2. Exhale as you bend one knee and grasp your ankle and calf with your hands. Gently rock your leg and calf in your arms, letting your hip joint release and relax.

3. Repeat with the other leg.

Meditative Poses

Technically, you can meditate just about anywhere and in any position, but ideally, try to meditate in one of several meditative poses. Why? There's nothing magical about the meditative poses, except that they arrange your body in a way ideal for meditation. Your spine is aligned so energy can flow freely, and your body is relaxed and comfortable. Meditative poses feel so wonderful that you barely notice your body. If a meditative pose is uncomfortable or painful, you aren't quite ready for it yet. Try a different one.

Mudras are special hand positions you can use while meditating to channel energy back through the fingers into the spinal column's *chakras*, directing and rebalancing *prana* in the body. Choose from the *mudras* in the following illustration; mix and match to enhance your yoga practice of meditation.

 Wise Yogi Tells Us

Placing your hands on your knees with your palms down gives you a sense of grounding and centering energy. Placing your hands on your knees with your palms up gives you a sense of releasing energy, opening, and liberation.

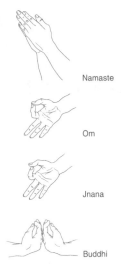

Namaste

Om

Jnana

Buddhi

Mudras for meditation.

Sukhasana: Easy Pose

Sukhasana (pronounced *soo-KAH-sah-nah*) is a great meditation pose for beginners. *Sukha* means "joy," and this pose feels so good that it fills you with joy! *Sukhasana* facilitates *prana-yama*, quiets the mind, and stills the body.

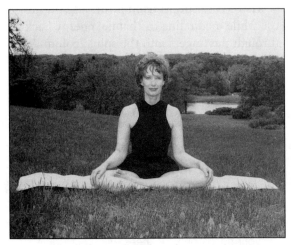

Easy pose.

1. Sit in a simple crossed-leg position, with either leg on top. Try to sit more often with the leg that is least comfortable on top, to balance your body. Rest your hands on your knees and breathe. Don't be concerned if your knees do not yet rest on the ground. This will come in time as your hips open.

2. If your back starts to arch, put a pillow under your tailbone to align your spine. What joy!

Vajrasana: Kneeling Pose

Vajrasana (pronounced *vahj-RAH-sah-nah*) is also called the Zen pose, because this is the meditation pose used by *Zen Buddhist* monks. *Vajra* means "thunderbolt" or "diamond." *Vajrasana* aids circulation to the feet, lifts the spinal column, and relieves pressure on the diaphragm.

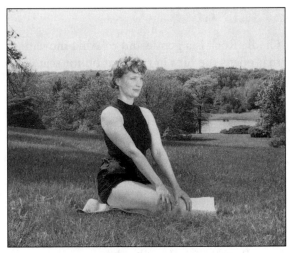

Kneeling pose.

1. Again, breathe! Sit back on your heels, keeping your heels and knees together.

2. Keeping your spine straight, place your hands on your knees. If your knees hurt, go back to Easy pose. If they don't hurt, enjoy *this* pose.

A Yoga Minute

Buddhism is a religion with many sects that teaches right living, right thinking, and meditation as a means to enlightenment. **Zen** is a sect of Buddhism in which enlightenment is sought through sitting meditation or contemplating enigmatic riddles called *koans*, rather than through the formal study of religious texts. For more on Zen, look for *The Complete Idiot's Guide to Zen Living* by Gary McClain, Ph.D., and Eve Adamson.

Padmasana: Lotus Pose

At last, the venerable Lotus pose! You've heard about it, maybe you've seen it, and perhaps you've even tried it. *Padmasana* (pronounced *pahd-MAH-sah-nah*) represents a lotus flower open to the light (*padma* means "lotus"). It keeps the spine from sagging and keeps you comfortable in meditation for longer periods of time than other positions. It also keeps your body from toppling over if you fall asleep during meditation (many wise souls have!). The Lotus position keeps your chest open, gives your diaphragm lots of room, and opens your Venus *chakra* (located behind your heart).

Wise Yogi Tells Us

The lotus flower is considered sacred because it is beautiful, symmetrical, and has a long root that reaches down into the depths of a pond. The lotus flower has its roots in the muddy earth, but it works its way through the mud and eventually blooms into a perfect white flower facing the heavens!

It's easy to be so concerned with trying to achieve Lotus pose that you forget the point of being in the pose: to be comfortable in your body. Because yoga is such an internal process, even if you're sitting in a perfect Lotus pose in what appears to be quiet meditation, inside you might not be practicing yoga at all. You might be distracted, worried, or suffering. You might be stuck in the mud! True meditation is joyful.

If your ankles or any other part of you (including your feelings) is in agony or pain, meditation will be much more difficult to achieve. Find an easier pose or postpone meditation in favor of more active postures. (Exercise is great when you're feeling low.) Come back to meditation when your mind is ready—and only then—in a position your body loves.

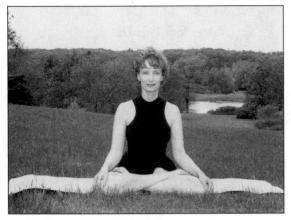

Lotus pose.

Ouch!

If your ankles, hips, or knees begin to hurt, practice nonviolence by returning to Easy pose. Lotus pose requires strong ankles and open hips. Practice yoga's standing postures to build ankle and hip strength, then come back to Lotus pose when you're stronger.

1. Sit on the floor and begin to breathe deeply.

2. Place your left ankle on top of your right thigh so the sole of your foot faces upward. Then move your right ankle to the top of your left thigh so the sole of your other foot faces upward (or the other way around—and next time, try to switch which foot is on top).

3. Shift a little to center your weight on your hip bones, then place your hands, palms up or down, on your knees. This pose should feel very stable.

4. Ideally, your body will form a tripod, with both knees and your body touching the ground. If you can't get your knees down toward the ground, you can sit on a cushion or pillow. This can also make the pose easier for people with less-flexible hips.

Baddha Padmasana: Bound Lotus Pose

Bound Lotus is the same as the Lotus, except that your right arm goes behind your back and holds your right foot, while your left arm goes behind your back and holds your left foot. This pose is even more stable and symmetrical than Lotus pose. Whichever arm crosses on top, go the opposite way next time. *Baddha padmasana* (pronounced *BAH-dah pahd-MAH-sah-nah*) deepens all the benefits of Lotus pose, and you'll be able to breathe more deeply. This is considered a more advanced pose than the advanced Lotus pose. Butterfly pose (described earlier in this chapter) is an excellent hip warmup for the flexibility needed for stability in Lotus and Bound Lotus poses.

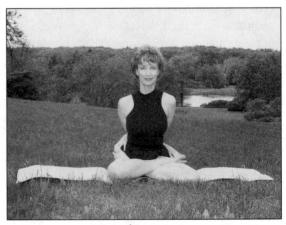

Bound Lotus pose.

Lotus and Beyond

Lotus pose creates such a stable, secure, and balanced base that it is used as part of many other poses. As your yoga practice progresses, you will find you can combine other poses with Lotus pose.

Neck Stretch

This stretch helps tone the muscles in the neck that connect to the collarbone, balancing our neck muscles. Remember, Hatha Yoga is about balance!

1. Sit in Lotus pose or any relaxed seated pose.
2. Inhale and gently tip your head back slightly, pulling gently on the muscles above your collarbone with your fingertips.
3. Breathe and relax in this position for several moments.

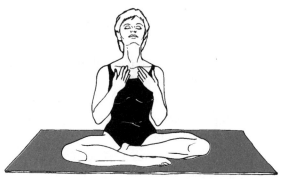

Seated Neck Stretch.

Tolasana: Scales Pose

Scales pose builds strength in the arms, shoulders, wrists, and hands. It also strengthens the abdominal muscles.

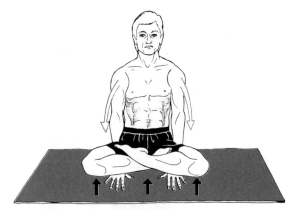

Scales pose.

1. Sit in Lotus pose with your palms pressed firmly on the ground on both sides of your hips.
2. Exhale as you energize your arms and contract your abdominal muscles. Push down on the floor, lifting your feet and hips slightly off the ground. Hold as long as you can.
3. Repeat with your legs crossed the opposite way.
4. **Getting Started:** You can do this pose while sitting in Easy pose if Lotus pose isn't comfortable for you yet. Make sure to contract your abdominal muscles contract as you lift, to help bring your legs and hips off the ground.

Lion in Lotus Pose

The Lion pose is a fun pose for kids as well as adults, but Lion pose is more than just fun. It gives all the facial muscles—from the tip of your tongue to the top of your forehead—a fantastic stretch. Although you can do Lion pose while sitting in Easy pose or other sitting poses, including sitting in a chair, we like Lion in Lotus pose because the body position looks and feels so much like a lion.

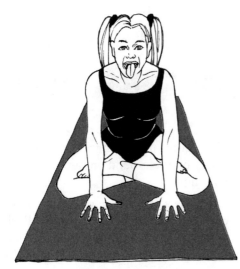

Lion in Lotus pose.

1. Relax into Lotus pose. Inhale.

2. Exhale as you tip forward on your knees, placing your hands on the floor, fingers spread out, about two feet in front of your knees, shoulder width apart. Keep your legs in Lotus pose.

3. Inhale deeply, then as you exhale, open your mouth and eyes as wide as you can. Stick out your tongue as far as you can. Raise your eyebrows. Open your face as completely as you can.

4. Relax your face as you inhale. Repeat again on the exhale.

5. Rock back into Lotus pose and breathe normally for a few moments, relaxing the muscles of your face.

Trataka: Seeing the Light

Trataka (pronounced *trah-TAH-kah*) cleanses the eyes by focusing them on a candle flame until they start to water. Although you can do this eye exercise in any sitting position, Lotus pose makes for a strong and stable sitting position. *Trataka* is said to strengthen the eyes and, in some cases, induce *clairvoyance*. *Trataka* is a meditation technique with the candle flame as the point of focus.

1. Sit in Lotus pose and place a lighted candle several feet in front of you at eye level.

2. Gaze at the candle flame, but don't bring your eyes too close to the candle.

3. The candle flame should be steady, so it is important not to have a drafty room when practicing *trataka*.

4. After a few minutes, rinse your eyes in cold water.

Spend some time in seated yoga postures every day, stretching, strengthening, and meditating, and you'll see real changes in your physical and mental well-being. Who thought you could gain so much from just sitting around?!

Padandgushtasana: Tiptoe Pose

Tiptoe Pose is a challenging balance pose that develops and strengthens your knees and ankles. It also promotes overall balance, stability, and confidence.

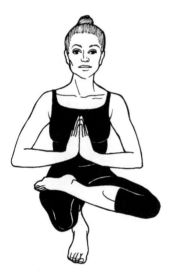

Tiptoe pose is challenging but helps develop strength, balance, and confidence.

1. Squat down with the weight balanced on the balls of your feet and your toes.
2. Pick a point of focus in front of you, and keep your eyes centered there for balance.
3. Once you have mastered this, try squatting down and then bring one leg up onto your thigh. Balance in this position for several steady breaths.
4. To come out of the pose, simply uncross your legs, sit down, and stretch your legs out.

The Least You Need to Know

◆ Sitting postures strengthen and increase flexibility in your hips and legs.

◆ *Mudras* are hand positions that enhance meditation by rechanneling energy that emanates from the fingers back into the body where it can stimulate the *chakras.*

◆ Meditate only in a posture that is perfectly comfortable. Some suggestions: Easy, Kneeling, and Lotus.

◆ Lotus pose can be a stabilizing base for many other yoga poses.

◆ If you're down, move around. Feeling great? Meditate!

In This Chapter

Chapter 15

Controlling the Power of Breath

Of course you can breathe … or can you? Maybe you can breathe well enough to get by without collapsing, but are you using your breath optimally? Probably not. Most people don't breathe as fully or deeply as they could, because it takes practice and concentration. Once you've learned the fine art of breath control, however, you'll certainly feel the difference.

An integral part of Hatha and other forms of yoga is *pranayama*, or breath control. In fact, the manipulation of breath to control the physical manifestation of *prana* in the body is Hatha Yoga's realm. People in all cultures have learned to manipulate *prana*, either consciously or unconsciously. Faith healers, hypnotists, prophets, shamans, and spiritualists use *prana*, although they might call it by another name. Yogis learn to use *prana* purposefully to push the mind to a higher state of consciousness. Speech can be charged with *prana*, which is why some people captivate us when they talk.

Prana, the Universal Life Force

The deeper the breath, the deeper the life force. In Chapter 6, we described *prana* as the life force or energy that exists everywhere and is manifested in each of us through the breath, but *prana* isn't exactly the same thing as breath or oxygen. *Prana* exists in all living things. It doesn't have consciousness—it's pure energy. Every cell in your body is controlled by *prana*. *Prana* animates all matter. *Prana* can be a difficult concept to comprehend; it might help to understand what it is if you understand what it *isn't*.

Once a body completely dies, administering oxygen won't bring it back to life, so obviously, oxygen doesn't equal life. Life is animated by more than oxygen—it's animated by *prana. Prana* is also not the matter it animates, nor the spirit it propels. *Prana* is universal energy that's in the air, in all matter, and is used by the spirit. You breathe in *prana* along with air, and *prana* regulates your body, from your nervous foot tapping the floor to your thoughts about your weekend plans.

Let's try getting in closer touch with the breath and the way prana infuses your individual body. Lie down on the ground on your back. Bend your knees to make your back more comfortable, and place your hands gently over your lowest ribs. This is the area of your body that houses the diaphragm, that powerful, plate-shape muscle that contracts and expands as you breathe. Inhale and imagine your diaphragm pulling down to expand the space for air in your lungs and expanding your rib cage in all directions. Exhale and imagine your diaphragm pushing up to guide the air out of your lungs.

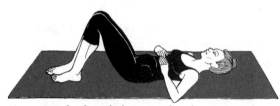

Lie on your back and place your hands over your lower ribs to feel the breath flowing in and out of your body.

The Anatomy of a Breath

We're now going to turn a little bit of attention to anatomy—anatomy according to yoga, that is. But don't get scared off; the concepts are easy to follow. Trust us.

Basic anatomy classes will tell you how breath flows in through the mouth and nose on the inhalation, expands the lungs, suffuses the blood with oxygen, how oxygen is pumped into the bloodstream and through the body, how the arteries channel carbon dioxide back into the lungs, and how that carbon dioxide leaves the body through the exhalation.

But ancient yoga anatomy theorizes that during this process, *prana*, or life-force energy, also moves in and out of the body with each inhalation and exhalation. According to yoga, *prana* moves through the body along two energy pathways on both sides of the spine. *Pingala* is on the right side and represents the sun. *Ida* is on the left side and represents the moon. In the middle is a passageway called *sushumna*, which runs through the spinal cord. Just picture a subway: The energy that keeps it running smoothly is *ida* and *pingala*. The *kundalini* is the train sitting at the bottom of this subway waiting to be energized.

The yoga interpretation of the body has a basis in Western anatomy, too. According to physiology, both afferent and sensory nerves exist in the body:

- **Afferent nerves** carry messages to the brain and correspond to *pingala*.
- **Sensory nerves** carry messages from the brain to the rest of the body and correspond to *ida*.

The spinal cord or center of these two currents (afferent/*pingala* and sensory/*ida*), *sushumna*, also controls the currents that move through the body's nervous system. In yoga, there are 10 currents, called *nadis*. *Pingala*, *ida*, and *sushumna* are the major three.

Picturing the physiology (Western-style!) of your thoracic cavity (the cavity containing your lungs and heart) might help you visualize what's happening as you breathe during *pranayama*. When you inhale, your 24 ribs and 2 lungs expand. Your diaphragm, the large, flat muscle at the base of your thoracic cavity, moves down to make room for air rushing in. Imagine that it looks a little like an upside-down plunger, helping to pull air in. Deep breathing means filling your lungs from the bottom up. You have a lot of room in there for air!

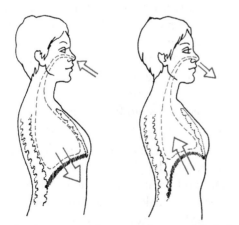

The diaphragm muscle moves down on inhalation and up on exhalation. Take a deep breath and feel the muscle in motion!

When you exhale, your ribs and lungs contract. Your diaphragm rises, pushing the air back out, again like a plunger. When you breathe, imagine the breath is flowing deep into your abdomen, then slowly filling up the abdominal cavity, lower thoracic cavity, and last of all, the chest. On the exhalation, imagine the air flowing out from the chest, the lungs, past the diaphragm, and out of the deepest regions of the abdomen. This is deep breathing!

Try not to move your chest or shoulders when you breathe. All movement should be in your abdomen or lower rib area. Put your hand on your abdomen and try to expand and contract from there. And keep those shoulders still! Rising and falling shoulders are usually an indication of shallow breathing.

Clearing the Way

For those prone to congestion and allergies, breathing exercises can be difficult. How can you breathe through your nose if you are all stuffed up?

Try blowing your nose before breathing exercises, or performing the traditional yoga cleansing practice called *neti* (pronounced *NEH-tee*). *Neti* involves various methods for cleansing the nasal passages. Clear nasal passages mean freer breathing!

One method is to sniff water into the nostrils and spit it out of the mouth, called *vuytkrama* (*VOOT KRAY-mah*)—but please don't drown yourself! Use room-temperature water. You can also buy *neti* bottles or *neti* pots; use these to pour water into one nostril, which will then come out the other nostril. The tilt of the head forward will help flush the nostrils. It might take some moving around to get that tilt right, but be patient and soon your nose will be flowing nicely. *Neti* is good for relieving nasal congestion or even putting the brakes on an allergy attack.

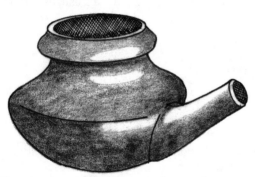

Use a *neti* pot to help clear out the nasal passages in preparation for *pranayama* breathing exercises.

Breath Control = Mental Control

Your breath and your mind have an intimate relationship. Just think about all the ways your breath is affected because your mind is experiencing something completely unrelated to breathing. Spend an entire day tuning in to your breath. Notice how it quickens or slows according to what you're doing, saying, or thinking. Your breath can even be affected merely by who you're near.

Just imagine watching an exciting movie. You're sitting still in your seat eating your popcorn. You aren't doing anything at all to get out of breath. As the opening credits roll, you see the name of your favorite actor or actress and your breath quickens in anticipation. When the movie gets suspenseful, you hold your breath. When the action speeds up, so does your breathing. Your breath responds to the movie's happy ending by becoming steady, smooth, and regular. As the credits roll, if the movie was a satisfying experience, you might even feel winded, as if you had been through a workout.

What your brain perceives, your breath mirrors and your body experiences. Imagine harnessing this power! Just as the mind influences the breath and body, so can the breath influence the mind and body. Controlling the power of breath is the technique of *pranayama*.

There are actually five manifestations of *prana* that act as vital energy in the body, depending on where they are. Each type complements one of the five nerve centers and is associated with one of the body's primary energy centers or *chakras*:

- ◆ **Prana** (*PRAH-nah*), not the *prana* that is the universal life force, but a sort of "sub-*prana*," rules the respiration process. It manifests in the heart *chakra* in the chest, flows into the body through inhalation, and moves up toward the brain. We know this is confusing. Just see it as one more layer of esoteric yoga anatomy!

- ◆ **Apana** (*ah-PAH-nah*) controls excretion, including the kidney, bladder, colon, genitals, and rectum. It's generated in the body by exhalation and flows down toward the rectum and out of the body, ridding the body of impurities. It manifests through the Saturn *chakra* in the lower abdomen.

◆ *Samana* (*sah-MAH-nah*) governs the digestive system, including the stomach, intestine, liver, and pancreas. It manifests through the Mars *chakra* behind the stomach.

◆ *Udana* (*uh-DAH-nah*) lives in the throat and controls swallowing. It also serves as the force dividing the astral body (the vehicle of the spirit) from the physical body at the time of death. It's the vital energy of speech and manifests through the Mercury *chakra* in the throat.

◆ *Vyana* (*vee-AH-nah*) flows throughout the entire body, regulating blood flow as well as muscle and joint movements. It's the vital energy of circulation and manifests through the Jupiter *chakra* located on the spine near the genitals.

What does all this mean for you? In short, the more *prana* you bring into your body, the better your body and your mind will work, and the better you'll feel. *Prana* gives you instant energy and supports long-term good health. It is the ultimate feel-good medicine and a powerful preventive health-care tool.

Blow Your Mind

So how do you get that *prana* inside you where it belongs? By learning *pranayama*, or yoga breathing techniques. *Pranayama* isn't difficult, but it takes concentration. There are many exercises to try, and following are a few. Experiment with each and consider incorporating a few of them into your yoga workout, between poses, before or after your workout, or whenever you need instant energy or calming.

You can practice breathing exercises just about anywhere, but they'll be more productive if you practice them in certain positions. All the following exercises will work better when your

spine is aligned and your lungs are able to expand to their maximum, not when you're slumped over in a chair watching television. Let your body position make things simpler. For each exercise, sit with your spine straight, on the floor or in a chair. Or choose one of the meditative postures from Chapter 14.

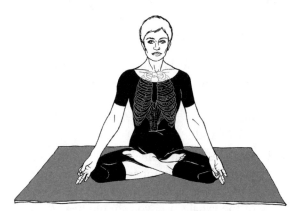

Lotus pose is a good pose for *pranayama* practice.

Om Exhalation

This technique extends the breath, softens it, and makes quieting the mind easier. Soon you'll feel a oneness drawing you closer to *samadhi*.

1. Inhale deeply, imagining your breath is moving all the way to the root of your spine.

2. Open your lips and begin to make the Om sound while exhaling slowly: *Ooooooooooooooommmmmmmmm*, spending approximately 20 seconds on the oh sound and about 10 seconds on the mmm sound.

3. Feel as if your entire being is enveloped in the sound. Let it surround and fill you.

4. Repeat several times.

Ujjayi: **Drawing Breath**

Jaya means "success on the spiritual path," and *ujjayi* (pronounced *oo-JAH-yee*) means "she who is victorious." The *ujjayi* technique aids in recalling and working with your dreams. It is also cooling to the head, aids digestion, soothes nerves, and tones the body. This breathing exercise produces sound in the throat with the inhalation.

1. Inhale slowly, keeping your lips closed and closing off the glottis, the opening between the vocal chords. Make a soft, humming sound: *hahhhhhhh*. Think Darth Vader breathing.

2. Imagine you are inhaling all the way to your heart. The upper portions of your lungs are full. You should feel the passage of the exhale, and you should hear it from the roof of your mouth.

3. Repeat several times.

Bhastrika: **Bellows Breath**

Bhastrika (pronounced *bah-STREE-kah*) is a powerful technique. Progress with it slowly to make the foundation strong. Bellows Breath brings heat to the body and is excellent for weight reduction, because it exercises the stomach and organs of the abdominal cavity. It clears energy, purifies the physical body, and opens up restrictions in the spine, permitting a freer energy flow. Put more emphasis on the exhale than on the inhale in this breath, just as a bellows "exhales" more forcefully than it "inhales."

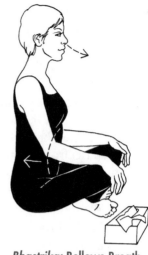

Bhastrika: Bellows Breath.

1. Exhale deeply and sharply, feeling your diaphragm muscle (refer to our definition earlier in this chapter) pull in your navel.

2. Inhale smoothly and exhale rapidly through your nose by continuing to force air out with sharp movements of your diaphragm. Don't worry about the inhale, which will take care of itself. Concentrate slightly more on the force of the exhalations.

3. Don't hold your breath between breaths. Aim for deep, quick movements of the diaphragm muscle. Remember, the inhalation will take little effort, especially as you practice this exercise and feel how the inhalation is a natural reflex following the exhalation.

4. Do 10 cycles, then hold your breath for a few seconds.

5. Repeat as many times as possible. If the strength of your exhalation begins to weaken, reduce the number of breaths in a cycle.

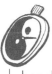

A Yoga Minute

We inhale oxygen and exhale carbon dioxide. Trees and plants inhale carbon dioxide and exhale oxygen. Perfect harmony!

Kapalabhati: Skull Shining

Kapalabhati (pronounced *KAH-pah-lah-BAH-tee*), or Skull Shining, is similar to Bellows Breath, except the inhale and exhale are evenly balanced with equal emphasis. This exercise has similar benefits but is like a calmer, easier, slower version. It is, therefore, more calming than bellows breath, which is more energizing. Because the skull consists of sinus passages, the technique is called Skull Shining, as it shines or clears the sinuses. It is also said to make your nose prettier!

1. Feel your diaphragm muscle pull in your navel as you exhale deeply and sharply. Then pause, holding your breath, after the exhalation for just a second or two.

2. Inhale deeply, then exhale again with equal force, pushing the air out as you did before. Again, pause after the exhalation for a few seconds.

3. Pause between cycles. Do as many cycles as you can, spending one minute on each. Gradually increase the time of your meditation after the cycle.

Shitali: Cooling Breath

Shitali (pronounced *shee-TAH-lee*) is great for summer! This technique is healing to the body and cools it from excessive heat. It clears the eyes and ears, satisfies hunger and thirst, activates the liver, and improves digestion. *Shitali* involves rolling the tongue, then inhaling through it like a straw.

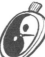

A Yoga Minute

Although tongue rolling has always been considered a simple, inherited genetic trait, recent evidence suggests otherwise. Many studies of identical twins have found that only one of the twins was able to roll his or her tongue. Some who couldn't roll their tongues have been able to learn how. In general, however, tongue rolling appears easy for some and virtually impossible for others.

1. Roll your tongue into a tube and keep the tip of it slightly outside your mouth. (If you can't roll your tongue, just try to raise the sides as well as you can, or just stick it out!)

2. Draw in breath through your curled tongue as if you're sipping through a straw. Fill your lungs.

3. When your lungs are full, bring your tongue into your mouth and close your mouth. Hold your breath for a comfortable amount of time. As you do so, relax your tongue, mouth, and face.

4. Lower your chin slightly and retain the breath for a few seconds.

5. Exhale slowly through your nose.

6. Repeat several times.

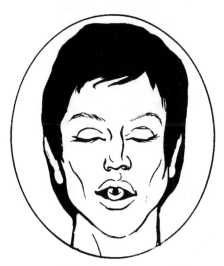

Breathing through your rolled tongue cools your body.

Nadi Shodhana: Alternate Nostril Breathing

Nadi shodhana (pronounced *NAH-dee shoh-DAH-nah*) balances the male/female or *ha/tha* within. This means it balances the emotional and physical natures. For example, when your emotions become overwhelming, this technique brings you back to a balanced state. Gradually, the amount of time when both nostrils are closed should increase comfortably. Keep your finger movement to a minimum.

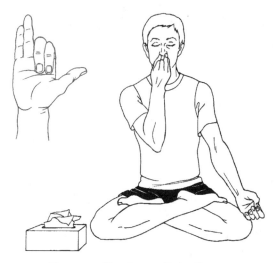

Finger position for *nadi shodhana.*

1. Sit in a meditative posture or comfortably in a chair or cross-legged on the floor. Close your eyes.

2. Cover your right nostril with your right thumb. Inhale through your left nostril.

3. Close your left nostril with the ring finger of your right hand. Your two middle fingers should be turned in toward your palm.

4. Hold both nostrils closed for as long as you can comfortably. Then release the right nostril and exhale through it.

5. Inhale through your right nostril, then close it again.

6. Hold both nostrils closed for as long as you can comfortably. Then exhale through your left nostril.

7. Inhale through your left nostril, close, exhale through your right nostril, and so on.

8. Repeat several times.

Bhramari: Bee Breath

Bhramari (pronounced *brah-MAH-ree*) is good for insomnia and is often used in conjunction with Alternate Nostril Breathing. It literally means "she who roams" (as a bee roams), and you'll make the soft, humming sound of a bee with this technique. Bee Breath helps awaken *kundalini* energy.

1. Sit in a meditative posture or comfortably in a chair or cross-legged on the floor. Close your eyes.
2. Close off your right nostril with your right thumb. Inhale through your left nostril.
3. Fill your lungs, close both nostrils, and retain your breath for a few seconds.
4. Open your left nostril and slowly exhale through the left nostril using your throat to make a soft *eeee* sound through your exhalation. The sound is produced within the head, resonating on or behind the soft palate.
5. Keep the exhalation going as long as possible.
6. Repeat with other nostril, starting with the left nostril for the inhalation.
7. Gradually intensify the breath and increase the sound of the *eeee*. (The bee is getting closer!)
8. Repeat several times, alternating nostrils.

Murccha Kumbhaka: Third-Eye Breathing

Murccha kumbhaka (pronounced *MER-chah koom-BHAH-kah*) focuses all your attention and energy on your third eye, the *chakra*, or energy center, located between and just above your eyebrows on your forehead. (For more on this and other *chakras*, see Chapter 16.) This exercise produces a focused, blissful feeling.

1. Gently and slowly inhale, then hold your breath.
2. As you hold your breath, concentrate on your third eye, the spot on your forehead about an inch above the place exactly between your eyebrows.
3. Hold your breath for as long as is comfortable, while staying focused on the third eye.
4. Exhale very slowly through your mouth, staying focused on your third eye.
5. Repeat several times.

Kevali Kumbhaka: Hold Your Breath (but Not Until You Turn Blue!)

Just like anything else, breath control and capacity increase with practice. In *kevali kumbhaka* (pronounced *kay-VAH-lee koom-BAH-kah*), you practice holding your breath. Don't make yourself dizzy, though, and don't hold your breath until you faint. Just hold your breath until you feel like you need to let it go again. The more you practice this technique, the longer you'll be able to hold your breath, which increases your lung capacity and makes your breathing more efficient.

1. Inhale deeply through your nose, then hold your breath.
2. Hold for as long as is comfortable.
3. Exhale gently, slowly, and fully.
4. Repeat several times.

> **Ouch!**
>
> Just as you will benefit more from yoga if you don't push your body to achieve a difficult posture before it's ready, also try to be aware of your breath capacity. Don't practice one-minute inhalations and two-minute exhalations your first time out! You might faint or hyperventilate. As always, go slowly and listen to your body. It will tell you when you're going too far.

Pranayama Plus

Many *pranayama* breathing exercises are performed while in a meditative seated pose, but others combine with yoga movements, are performed lying down, or otherwise enhance the *prana* flow by combining the movement of breath with the different movements and body positions.

In fact, every movement and change of position you make affects the way *prana* moves through you. We think you'll enjoy these alternative *pranayama* exercises as much as we do!

Modified Mountain Breath

This pose is simple, but it helps you become more keenly aware of the way your breath feels in your body and how that feeling changes with simple changes in movement.

1. Stand in Mountain pose, feet together, arms hanging at your sides, legs energized, feet planted firmly.

2. Breathe normally, but focus your awareness on the way your breath feels as it expands your rib cage from all sides and the way it feels as it flows out of your body and your diaphragm collapses.

3. After a few minutes in Mountain, inhale and raise your arms above your head into a simple arms-raised version of Mountain pose.

4. Continue to breathe, but focus again on your rib cage and diaphragm, noticing how the breath feels different than it did before. How does the space in your chest change? How does the energy change? How does the flow of air change with each inhalation and exhalation? Notice how simply raising your arms can change so much about your breath.

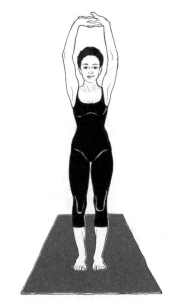

Feel how breathing changes simply by raising your arms.

Namaste Breath

This exercise is a great way to energize in the morning and center yourself to prepare for the day ahead.

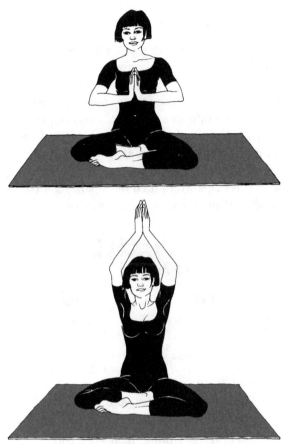

Namaste **Breath.**

1. Sit in Lotus or Easy pose and relax for a moment.
2. Bring your hands together in front of your chest in prayer position (*namaste*).
3. Inhale strongly and lift your arms straight up over your head.
4. Exhale forcefully and bring your arms back down in front of your chest.
5. Continue to inhale while lifting your arms and exhale while lowering your arms, keeping your palms pressed together.
6. Repeat 12 times, pause, and sit for a moment, noticing how you feel.
7. Repeat 12 more times, pause, notice how you feel, then repeat for a third set of 12.
8. Have a great day!

Sun Breath

This exercise emphasizes the breath in an expanded or rising position and then in a contracted or seated position. As your body rises and sets like the sun, your breath expands and then contracts, letting *prana* move in and out of your body. Think day and night, light and dark, warm and cool, yang and yin. It's no coincidence that this exercise borrows the first two positions from yoga's popular Sun Salutation. When you practice Sun Salutation, remember to use the breath the way you use it in this exercise.

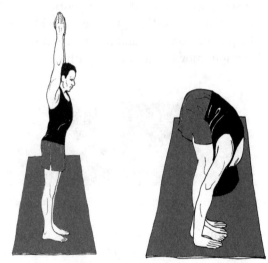

Sun Breath helps you feel the way your breath moves with a pose that expands on the inhale (left), then contracts on the exhale (right).

1. Stand with your feet together in Mountain pose.
2. Inhale and raise your arms above your head, expanding your rib cage in all directions and reaching as high as you can for a full, opening stretch.

3. Exhale as you bend over and reach toward the floor, collapsing your rib cage and pushing the air from your body with your diaphragm. Feel your torso contracting and bend forward as far as you can.

4. Repeat several times slowly, then return to Mountain pose and notice how you feel.

Weighted Breath

This exercise is like weightlifting for your diaphragm! You'll lie in Corpse pose but use a soft weight that will be comfortable on your stomach, such as a sandbag or a plastic-covered disc weight wrapped in a pillowcase or blanket, to help emphasize and add resistance to the diaphragm movement of the breath.

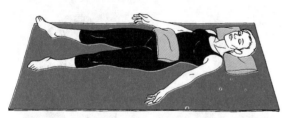

Weighted Breath strengthens your diaphragm muscle.

1. Lie in Corpse pose on your back on the floor, feet apart, and palms facing upward.

2. Place a weight on your stomach just under your ribs. Begin with a light weight of two to five pounds and work up to a ten-pound weight.

3. Concentrate on relaxing your entire body, but as you inhale, focus on lifting the weight with your diaphragm. As you exhale, feel how the presence of the weight helps press the breath out of your lungs.

4. Continue for several moments, then remove the weight and breath normally in this relaxation pose. Feel how different the breath moves without the presence of the weight.

Yoga Ball Breath

Many yoga classes now employ props to assist in holding a correctly aligned position. One of our favorite props is the yoga ball. Lying on a yoga ball instead of the floor opens the chest and the emotional center. Conscious breathing in this position helps suffuse the heart and the emotional center with *prana*, energizing and freeing your compassion and empathy. This pose also helps strengthen the small, stabilizing muscles of the torso as you balance on the ball.

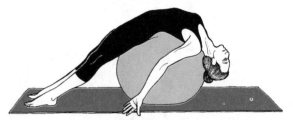

Breathing over a yoga ball opens the emotional center, suffusing it with energy and releasing compassion.

1. Squat down and lean your back onto a yoga ball.

2. Feet on the ground, relax your legs, rolling the ball back until it sits in the middle of your back and you find a comfortable, stable balance for your body.

3. Adjust yourself so your spine is centered on the ball. Separate your feet and plant them firmly on the floor for stability and balance.

4. Bring your attention to your breath. Feel how your diaphragm moves and how your rib cage expands and contracts while you rest on the yoga ball.

5. As you breathe steadily, focus on the opening of your chest and imagine love and compassion flowing freely from your heart.

6. Stay here for several minutes, enjoying the feeling, then slowly roll to seated on the floor and lie back on the floor in Corpse pose. Feel how your body adjusts to accommodate the shape of the floor after lying on the yoga ball.

Crocodile Breath

This pose helps you breathe through your back. It's easy to feel like your breath is solely a matter of expanding your rib cage forward and your diaphragm up and down, but noticing the way your lungs expand in all directions can free your breathing in amazing ways. As you lie on the floor in Crocodile pose, focus on how your torso expands outward from your back and let your whole body breathe! This exercise also uses the resistance of the floor to strengthen your diaphragm, as the front of your body moves outward with the inhalation against the floor.

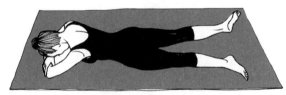

Crocodile Breath encourages "back breathing," because it uses the resistance of the floor to strengthen the diaphragm.

1. Lie face down on the floor with your forearms folded in front of you, forehead resting on your forearms. Your chest should be just slightly off the floor, but you shouldn't have to hold it up. Relax. Your legs should be straight and slightly apart. Heels relaxed inward brings more focused attention to the lower abdomen.

2. Inhale slowly and deeply. Feel your rib cage expanding out of your back as you inhale. Exhale completely and feel your back sink back down.

3. Inhale again, but this time, focus on the front of your body and feel the resistance of the floor as your body expands with the inhalation. Let the resistance of the floor help press the breath out of your body with the exhalation.

4. Repeat, focusing alternately on the back and the front, for about 20 breaths.

5. Roll over onto your back into Corpse pose and breathe normally, feeling the difference in your breath.

We're confident you're feeling more energized by now. What a great way to prime your body for yoga postures—and life!

The Least You Need to Know

◆ *Prana* is the universal life force that permeates and animates everything, including you.

◆ *Prana* flows into the body via the breath, so controlling the breath controls the flow of *prana*.

◆ *Pranayama* are breathing techniques that, when practiced, result in better control of the mind and body. Practice *pranayama* with good posture for optimal results.

◆ Pranayama can also work in different positions and in conjunction with different movements. Let *pranayama* inspire you as it energizes your life.

In This Chapter

◆ All about *chakras:* wheels of life-force energy

◆ Meditations on *mudras*

◆ Chanting with *mantras*

◆ *Mandala* circle power

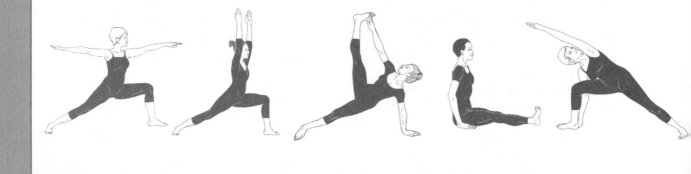

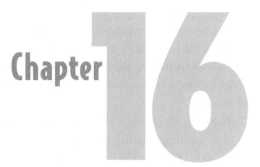

Chapter **16**

Chakras, Mudras, Mantras, and Mandalas

We mention *chakras* many times throughout this book, but in this chapter, we go into more detail about what they are, what they do, and how you can use them to optimize your physical, mental, and spiritual health. We'll also talk about several other tools and techniques you can use as part of your yoga practice to help center your mind, encourage focus, and improve energy flow through your body.

First, let's meet your *chakras*.

Meet Your *Chakras*

In yogic thought, the body contains energy centers, called *chakras* (literally "wheels"), that store energy, or the life force, *prana*. As energy moves through the body via meridians or energy channels, it collects and pools in the *chakras*, sort of like lakes along a network of rivers and underground streams. Westerners would interpret the *chakras* as nerve centers, but they are much more than this. They are centers of psychospiritual energy that don't precisely correspond to any tangible physical structure.

Although the body contains many energy centers and sub-energy centers, there are seven primary *chakras* along the midline of the body. Different people have different names for these *chakras* and place them in slightly different locations, but in essence, most agree that these seven *chakras* begin at the base of the spine (where the *kundalini* energy we talked about in Chapter 15 lies coiled and waiting to be activated) and continue along the spinal cord, ending in the seventh *chakra* at the crown of the head.

Different traditions associate different things with each *chakra:* which body parts, emotions, and thoughts each *chakra* governs; which colors each *chakra* radiates; which areas of our personality each *chakra* represents. We like to refer to the *chakras* according to their associated planets, excepting the top two *chakras*, whose names are descriptive.

There are no pervasive Western names for the *chakras;* people name them after colors, *mantra* syllables, the elements, and so on. Yoga scholar Georg Feuerstein names *chakras* things like "root prop wheel," "jewel city wheel," and "wheel of the unstruck sound"—names we certainly enjoy. None of these naming systems are arbitrary; the *chakras* do indeed correspond to many different energies. We find the planet-name system to be evocative but nonesoteric—and fun, too!

Here are the seven *chakras* as we experience them. Remember that although we feel the *chakras* centered in certain anatomical areas, the *chakras* exist in us and beyond our physical bodies as wheels of energy, so the descriptions of where the *chakras* are centered are approximations:

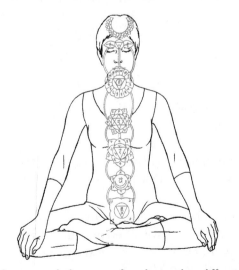

The seven *chakras* are often depicted as different *mandala*-like shapes drawn along the human spine. (More on *mandalas* later in this chapter.)

- **Saturn** *chakra.* Located just above the anus at the base of the spine, this *chakra* involves elimination and the sense of smell. This is where the *kundalini* lies. When awakened through yoga, this energy travels up the spine through all the *chakras.*

- **Jupiter** *chakra.* Located around the lower regions of the body near the base of the spine, this *chakra* involves water, sexuality, passion, the creation of life, and taste.

- **Mars** *chakra.* Located behind the navel, this *chakra* is associated with digestion or "gastric fire," your sense of self, and your actions.

- **Venus** *chakra.* Located behind the heart, this *chakra* is the center of your compassion and emotions.

- **Mercury** *chakra.* Located in the throat, this *chakra* is the center of communication.

- **Sun** *chakra.* Located in the middle of the brow, this *chakra* is also known as the third eye, or center of unclouded perception.

- **Thousand Petalled Lotus** *chakra.* Located at the crown of the skull, this *chakra* is the center of self-realization, perspective, unity, and enlightenment.

 A Yoga Minute

Every *chakra* has a corresponding color:

Thousand Petalled Lotus	Violet
Sun	Indigo
Mercury	Blue
Venus	Green
Mars	Yellow
Jupiter	Orange
Saturn	Red

All *chakras* must be activated or awakened for true enlightenment, which is not an easy process. Awakening your *chakras*—releasing the energy that flows through your spine—can take years, perhaps lifetimes! It's hard work to *en*-lighten up!

Ouch!

Feeling frazzled and unfocused? Try a pose that awakens your Saturn *chakra*, located at the base of your spine. Overemotional or unforgiving? Try a pose that stimulates your Venus *chakra*, located behind your heart. Angry or hostile? Try a pose to stimulate the Mars *chakra*, located behind your navel. Having a problem communicating? Work with your Mercury *chakra*, located in the throat. Each Hatha Yoga posture is designed to awaken different *chakras*, so practicing the right poses can be the best prescription for what ails you.

Poses to Power Your Chakras

Certain yoga poses can make releasing and opening the *chakras* easier. In this section, we'll show you a few poses for opening your *chakras*, which floods them with *prana*, energizes them, and helps balance your entire bodymind. Add a few *chakra*-releasing poses to your yoga routine and feel the power of *prana!*

Prana Arch

In this pose, the front of your body opens, releasing tension in your chest, neck, and abdomen. This pose is particularly effective for releasing the *chakras* in the chest and throat. Breathing deeply through this pose encourages

the flow of *prana* through the *chakras*. *Prana* Arch helps your body balance any slumping you might normally do, correcting your posture in a way that opens your chest and throat and frees energy. Good posture gives all your internal organs more room to work and makes you feel more confident, too.

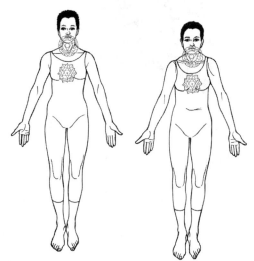

Slumped posture crowds your internal organs and impedes the flow of *prana* through the heart and throat *chakras*. Correct posture in *Prana* Arch pose opens the heart and throat *chakras*.

1. Stand in Mountain pose with your arms hanging loosely at your sides.

2. Inhale as you look up and just slightly behind you. At the same time, lift your hands, palms facing forward, away from your body and out to the sides, as if preparing to give someone a big hug.

3. Contract your buttocks muscles to support your lower back. Don't lean back farther than is comfortable. Breathe deeply several times. On the exhale, lower your arms and head, coming back into Mountain pose.

Open Pose

This pose is great for opening the *chakras* in the lower half of the torso. It is also excellent for relaxation and meditation.

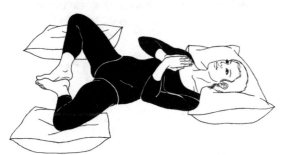

Open pose releases the lower *chakras*.

1. Lie down on the floor on your back with a pillow under your head.
2. Bend your knees and bring the soles of your feet together, letting your knees drop to the floor. If this is uncomfortable, or if your back overarches, place a pillow under each knee.
3. Bring your palms together in front of your heart in *namaste*. Breathe deeply several times, focusing on releasing your lower *chakras*. Feel the *prana* flowing through them.

4. If this pose brings strong feelings or emotions to the surface, let them come and feel them. Then, when you're ready, let them go. Keep breathing and relaxing until you feel calm, energized, and ready to move on.

The Healing Power of Chakras

Chakras do more than store energy. Each *chakra* controls a different system of your body as well as a different realm of your emotions. When a *chakra* becomes blocked, you could suffer from health problems—physical or emotional—in that area. For example, a sore throat or an inability to adequately communicate your feelings could signal a blocked Mercury *chakra*. Indigestion or an inability to act on your feelings could mean a blocked Mars *chakra*.

Chakras at a Glance

The following table shows you exactly what each *chakra* governs. Knowing what is linked to what can help you pinpoint a problem—a blockage or an overflow of energy somewhere—but how do you fix it? Try the earlier *chakra*-opening poses, or simply focus on a *chakra* and its associated color during *shavasana* or sitting meditation, to help release, activate, and empower that *chakra*.

Chakra	Color	Location	Physical	Emotional
Saturn	Red	Base of spine	Elimination or releasing, sense of smell	Instinctual responses and drives
Jupiter	Orange	On spine behind the genitals	Reproductive organs, taste, body's water content	Sexuality, passions, creativity
Mars	Yellow	Abdominal region behind the navel	Digestion, taking in or consuming	Actions, sense of self
Venus	Green	On spine region behind the heart	Cardiovascular system	Compassion, emotions associated with others
Mercury	Blue	Region of throat	Throat, tonsils, voice	Ability to communicate
Sun/third eye truth,	Indigo (deep blue)	Forehead, middle of the brow	Mental processes, thought, brain	Ability to perceive recognize delusion
Thousand Petalled Lotus	Violet	Crown of your head	Integration of the whole self: bodymindspirit	Enlightenment

Target Your *Chakras* with Yoga Poses

Depending on which *chakras* are blocked, certain yoga poses can help release and balance those *chakras*. For example, Triangle pose can help relieve lower back pain by releasing the lower *chakras* and allowing *prana* to flow through this area. Or to warm the extremities by spreading the heat from the heart *chakra* to the hands and feet, try Downward Facing Dog.

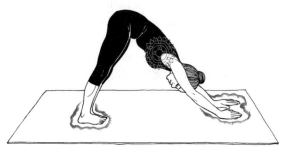

Downward Facing Dog directs heat from the heart *chakra* to the extremities.

Sometimes the power of two is greater than the power of one. If you have an interested partner, try meditating together, facing each other, legs crossed, knees touching, and holding hands. Focus on each of the *chakras* one at a time (perhaps take turns naming each *chakra*, from the Saturn *chakra* all the way up to the Thousand Petalled Lotus *chakra*), or stay silent and meditate individually while connecting physically, emotionally, and energetically through the *chakras* (see the following figure).

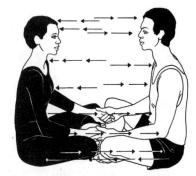

Connecting your *chakras* with a meditation partner.

Mudra Magic

Mudra means "seal," and technically, *mudras* refer to a variety of yoga practices that aren't poses exactly, but various techniques for sealing life-force energy inside the body to preserve it rather than let it escape. These techniques get pretty esoteric and can involve complex rituals, chanting, meditation, and some practices we Westerners might find a little odd.

The word *mudra*, however, is more commonly used today to refer to specific hand gestures used during meditation and *pranayama* to seal the fingers. *Prana* can escape out of the fingertips as it circulates through the body during meditation and *pranayama* exercises, and hand *mudras* bring the fingertips together in various ways for different, subtle effects. Hand *mudras*, in essence, create a *prana* circuit. The energy moves back around and into the body again.

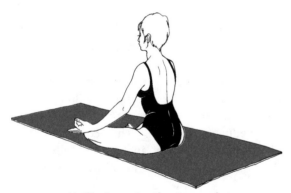

Meditating using the *Om mudra.*

Namaste Mudra: A Little Respect

Namaste (pronounced *nah-MAH-stay*) *mudra*, or the respect gesture, puts the palms together in prayerlike fashion to honor the inner light. Place your palms together and extend your fingers upward, as if you are praying. Hold your hands to your heart. Honor and respect the light within you and the light within all.

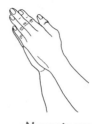

Namaste mudra.

Om Mudra: Simply Divine

Om (pronounced *AUM*) *mudra*, or the divinity gesture, invokes divine balance. Open your palms, and with each hand, bring the tip of your thumb to the tip of your index finger to form a complete circle, which represents the complete cycle and ultimate harmony of divinity. *Om.*

Om mudra.

Jnana Mudra: Be a Wise Soul

Jnana (pronounced *GAH-nah*) *mudra*, or the wisdom gesture, produces wisdom. Rest your hands, palms up, on your knees, and touch each index finger to the middle of each thumb. The wisdom gesture promotes harmonious inward expression and openness to life's beauty. This *mudra* produces wisdom and encourages the ego to realize that relinquishment brings wisdom. This *mudra* is often practiced during meditation.

Jnana mudra.

Buddhi Mudra: **How Enlightening!**

Buddhi mudra, or enlightenment gesture, is often associated with the Buddha and is ideal for centering and calming. Bring your thumb and index finger together, tip to tip, as in the *Om mudra*. Then bring the back of your hands together, knuckles touching, and rest your hands against your lower abdomen at your Jupiter *chakra*. This *mudra* represents divinity and the oneness of self and also the joining of all energies. It quiets the mind, stills action, and enlightens the self to its inner divinity. Try this *mudra* when you are feeling tense or rushed.

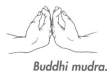

Buddhi mudra.

Mantras: **Beyond *Om***

"I'll do yoga," you say, "but I draw the line at chanting." Okay, so you've been put off by a few *om* stereotypes on television and in movies. But bear with us for just a little bit—chanting probably isn't at all what you assume, and once you understand what chanting is all about, you might just want to give it a try.

A *mantra* is a sound or sounds that resonate in the body and evoke certain energies. *Mantras* help stimulate the *chakras* by soothing your mind and awakening your senses. Herbert Benson, M.D., president and founder of the Mind/Body Medical Institute at Harvard Medical School, conducted many studies that showed how simple meditation including the repetition of a *mantra* (any word, sound, even a short prayer) induced a profound relaxation effect on the body. In his landmark book *The Relaxation Response* (Avon Books, 1976), Dr. Benson revealed the remarkable healing effects of this relaxation that seemed most effectively induced by *mantra* meditation.

Know Your Sanskrit

A *mantra* is a sacred sound used in meditation as the object of focus, meant to resonate within the body and awaken the *chakras*. The word *mantra* is a composite of two Sanskrit root words. The first word, *man*, means "continual or constant thinking." The second word, *tra*, means "to be free." *Mantra* is a process by which you free yourself from worries or doubts, but not from consciousness.

Although the *mantra* you try could be any meaningful word, phrase, or sound, *om* is a common *mantra* because it's designed to invoke a universal perspective: You see your bodymind in relation to its place in the big picture. In Sanskrit, *om* is spelled in three symbols that approximate the letter A-U-M, meant to invoke the resonating sound of this *mantra*.

Each letter is a sacred symbol:

◆ **A** represents the self in the material world.

◆ **U** represents the psychic realm.

◆ **M** represents indwelling spiritual light.

Chanting *aum* (*om*) unifies your perceptions so you can sense yourself as an integral part of the universe. Gradually, the chant helps you shed everything that separates you from the universe—all your negativity, illusions, and misperceptions of yourself and the world. *Aum* is a great *mantra* for anyone. Don't be embarrassed! Give it a try!

Many Sanskrit word combinations serve as common *mantras*, but any sequence of words meaningful to you can become a *mantra*. You might find something that works for you in the following list:

- Light (*inhalation*), love (*exhalation*). Love (*inhalation*), light (*exhalation*).

- One is all, all is one.

- *Om namah sivaya* (pronounced *OHM NAH-mah SHE-vah-yah*). (*Note: Siva* destroys and recreates. The energy that destroys the lower self builds the higher self.)

- Amen.

- Hallelujah.

- *Om Shanti Shanti Shanti* (pronounced *OHM SHAHN-tee*, meaning "all peace, peace, peace").

- *Hari Om* (pronounced *HA-ree OHM*, meaning "removing fear, uncovering bliss").

- *Hong Sau* (pronounced *HONG SAW*, meaning "the holy breath"; inhale *hong*, exhale *sau*).

Wise Yogi Tells Us

Om Shanti Shanti Shanti (pronounced *OHM SHAHN-tee SHAHN-tee SHAHN-tee*) is a great beginning *mantra* to try. *Shanti* means "peace," and when repeated three times, it balances the bodymindspirit. It's easy to use and to remember.

Mandalas: Goin' 'Round in Circles

While a *mantra* is meant to soothe the body and mind through sound, a *mandala* is meant to center the mind through sight. *Mandalas* are beautiful, usually circular, geometric designs that draw your eye to the center. *Mandala* means "circle" or "center," and the designs suggest the circular patterns that exist in so many levels of life, from atoms to solar systems.

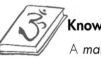

Know Your Sanskrit

A *mandala* is a circular geometric design used as a center of focus in meditation and meant to suggest the universe's circular motif (from atoms to solar systems) and the spirit's journey. *Mandala* means "circle" or "center."

Mandalas represent a pilgrimage to enlightenment. As you focus on the center of the *mandala*, you'll notice the outer parts shifting and changing in your peripheral vision; eventually, your focus will become clear, and the center will be all that you see.

Mandalas can also come in the form of a labyrinth, a *mandala* shape meant for walking. The most famous instance of this kind of labyrinth is in the Chartres Cathedral in France. This *mandala*-like pattern is different than a maze because there is only one way to the center and one way back out again, just like a *mandala*. However, a labyrinth is specifically designed to be physically traveled through, while a *mandala* is any pattern with these qualities in any form, from a painting on the wall to a complex Tibetan sand mosaic to a figure you draw in your journal.

Slow, meditative walking through the labyrinth *mandala* is symbolic of traveling the spiritual path into the mindbody and back out to the world again. These "walking *mandalas*" make possible a physical expression of meditation through movement.

Some religious institutions have "traveling labyrinths" available on a periodic basis. These *mandalas* are painted or printed on large mats of canvas. Unrolled, they provide a walking path for anyone who wants to come and try them. We've tried it, and the simple experience of walking on a painted canvas to the center of a *mandala* and back out is beautiful, profound, and enlightening.

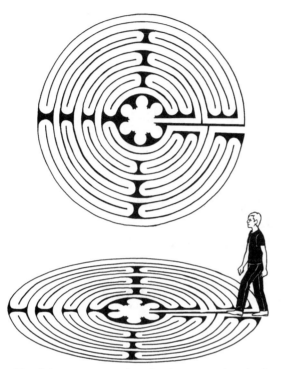

Mandalas are a metaphor for the spiritual path of the mind and body. This well-known *mandala* or labyrinth is built into the floor of Chartres Cathedral in France. Spiritual pilgrims literally walked through the labyrinth to attain spiritual insight. Get a pencil and try walking the Chartres *mandala* by tracing the path you would take to reach the center and then return from the center to the world again.

Using *mandalas* and *mantras* together is a wonderful way to meditate, because the combination of oral and visual stimulation awakens and clarifies your mindbodyspirit in multiple ways. Adding color to your *mandala* goes even further toward stimulating the senses. (And you thought meditation would be boring!)

The Least You Need to Know

◆ *Chakras* are energy centers in your body that govern different areas of your physical, emotional, and spiritual self.

◆ Unblocking and releasing *chakras* through meditation and targeted yoga poses can improve your physical, emotional, and spiritual health.

◆ *Mantras* are words or groups of words meant to resonate within the body for certain effects and are often used as an oral focus in meditation. The most well-known *mantra* is the Sanskrit word *om* (*aum*).

◆ *Mandalas* are circular patterns meant to focus the vision and, by extension, the consciousness during meditation. Labyrinths are "walking *mandalas*" through which the meditator follows a path to the center and back out again, symbolizing the spiritual path into the self and back to the world.

◆ Combining *mantras* and *mandalas* in meditation results in an even more powerful centering effect.

In This Chapter

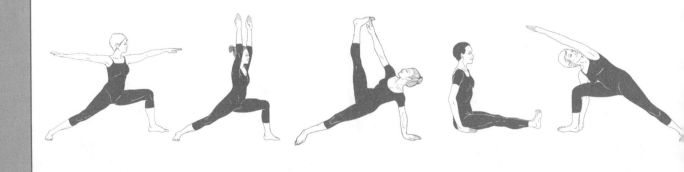

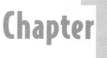

Chapter 17

Take the Forward Path

Forward bends are important for several reasons. They're wonderful for helping you focus inward and quiet your mind. As your body bends forward, it folds your heart into its center. Forward bends are also important to balance backbends, so include a few of each in your yoga practice.

Forward-Bending Basics

In forward bends, always bend from the hips, not the waist. Bend forward slightly and place your hands on your hip joints at the top of your thighs to feel the movement there.

Forward bends are great for stretching out and loosening the lower back muscles and also for lengthening the hamstrings. Believe it or not, the leg muscles, especially the *gluteus maximus* (the muscles of the derrière) often hold more stress than any other muscle group in the body! Forward bends help you reach that inner place where you can allow your lower back and hamstrings to relax and become fluid. Okay ... one, two, three, bend!

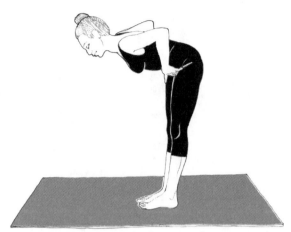

When bending forward, place your fingertips at the hip joints, the part where your thighs and legs meet. Bend forward and gently press in to more closely feel the movement forward from this point.

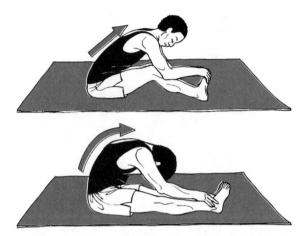

If your hamstrings are tight, let your knees bend and focus on keeping your back straight. Avoid the hunched, curved back that comes from trying to keep the legs straight by bending at the waist instead of the hips.

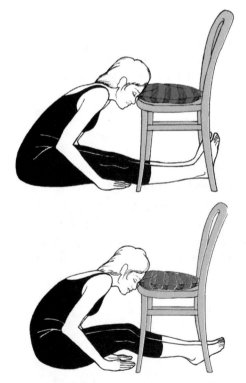

Modify forward bends using a chair and pillows for support. Bend from the hips and feel the slow, consistent release in the hip joints. Bend knees if the back is tight, and slowly the spine will lengthen.

Mudhasana: Child's Pose

Child's pose makes you feel safe and nurtured, as if you were still in the womb. *Mudhasana* (pronounced *moo-DAH-sah-nah*) activates your Venus and moon *chakras* (located behind your heart and at the base of your skull, respectively), relieves lower back pain, and improves your complexion. It also stimulates respiration because it compresses your diaphragm.

When practicing Child's pose, put some pillows or a blanket under your head to help lengthen your back if you find it hard to bend forward, or place a pillow or blanket between your knees and calves if your knees feel strained.

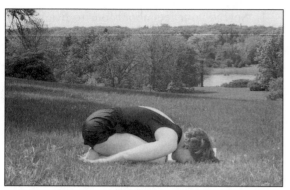

Child's pose.

1. Sit back on your heels, then bring your forehead to the floor.

2. Rest your arms alongside your body with your palms facing upward. The pose should feel completely relaxing.

3. Breathe deeply. Feel your diaphragm rising and sinking with each breath, like a baby's tummy. A baby hasn't yet learned shallow chest breathing.

4. **Yoga Adventure:** You can also modify this pose by stretching your arms out in front of you. Feel your spine lengthen as you relax into this elongated version of Child's pose.

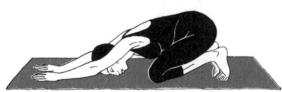

Child's pose variation with outstretched arms.

Uttanasana: Standing Head to Knees Pose

Uttanasana (pronounced *OOH-tah-NAH-sah-nah*) stretches the entire back of your body. It also tones your abdomen, decreases bloating, refreshes your mind, and clears your head. Forward bends are also conducive to relaxation

and sleep, so a few forward bends followed by Corpse pose in the evenings is a great way to wind down before sleep.

In forward bend, you might have to bend your knees, and that's fine! Your body's flexibility doesn't determine the benefits of this pose; the bend from the hips does the trick. As you become more flexible, you'll be able to grasp your big toes with your index fingers. For those who can fold in half, give yourselves a hug!

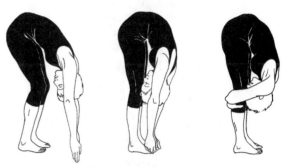

Standing Head to Knees pose.

1. Stand with your feet together. Inhale and raise your arms overhead.

2. Exhale and bend forward at your hips. Bending at the waist will curve your back. Try to bend at your hip joints to keep your heart open as you move forward. Work toward touching your chest to your knees. Keep your knees straight unless your back hurts, in which case you can bend your knees.

3. Be careful not to rock your weight back to your heels. Keep your weight evenly distributed over your feet. Don't round your back or turn your feet out; instead, bend forward from your hips, lengthening through your lower back. Don't force your head toward your knees—let gravity do the work as your head and neck stay relaxed. Don't be concerned with how far you bend. Focus on how open you can become as you "lift" forward.

4. **Getting Started:** If Standing Head to Knees is too intense for you, try relaxing into this pose using books, foam, and/or wooden blocks as props. Yoga blocks are available in many stores that sell fitness equipment. Wise yogis that we are, we use books! Rest each hand on a book, and rest your head on a stack of books reaching to a comfortable height for your flexibility.

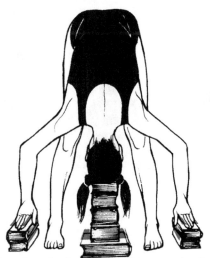

Standing Head to Knees with support books.

Forward Bend with V-Legs Pose

We love this forward bend because it feels so good! It gives a deep stretch to the hamstrings and muscles of the inner thighs.

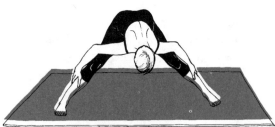

Forward Bend with V-Legs pose.

1. Spread your feet about four to five feet apart, toes pointed forward or slightly inward.

2. Exhale and bend slowly forward, dropping your head between your legs as you run your hands down each leg for support.

3. Go as far as you can to feel the stretch, but not so far as to cause pain.

4. As you bend down in this pose, grasp your thighs, calves, or ankles with your hands. Or rest your hands or forearms on the ground under your head. Clasp your elbows with your hands to stabilize your upper body on the ground if you can reach that far. If you have very flexible hamstrings, you might even be able to rest your head on your forearms or the floor. Once this pose is comfortable, it is very relaxing and stabilizing because you are forming a tripod with your two feet and your joined forearms and head.

5. **Yoga Adventure:** You can check your quadriceps tone in this pose. While holding Forward Bend with V-Legs, tense your thigh (quadriceps) muscles, lifting your kneecaps with the contraction. See how long you can hold this tension in your thigh muscles. If you can only hold it for a few seconds, you would probably benefit from more thigh-strengthening yoga poses. If your quadriceps muscles are rock-hard but you have trouble *releasing* the contraction, stretching and lengthening, yoga poses that target the thigh muscles are probably perfect for you.

Parshvottanasana: Feet Apart Side Angle Pose

In *parshvottanasana* (pronounced *PARSH-voh-tah-NAH-sah-nah*), you will tone your abdomen; straighten drooping shoulders; and make your hips, spine, and wrists more flexible.

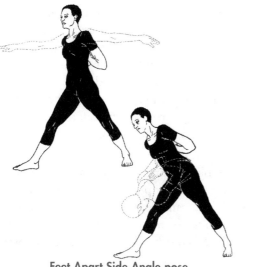

Feet Apart Side Angle pose.

means "head." You might guess that this pose, then, involves bringing the head and knees together. You're right! Sitting One Leg pose tones your abdomen, liver, spleen, and kidneys. It quiets your mind and aids digestion, as well as stretching and strengthening your lower back and chest. Men suffering from an enlarged prostate will benefit from this pose as well.

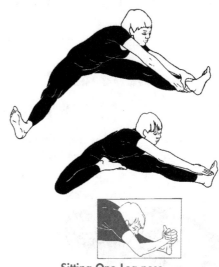

Sitting One Leg pose.

1. Stand with your feet three to four feet apart. Turn one foot out so it is perpendicular with the other foot, the heel of your turned foot lining up with the arch of your straight foot. Turn your body to face your turned-out foot.

2. Bring your hands into the *namaste* or prayer position behind your back with your fingers pointing up. If this is too difficult, simply clasp your hands behind your back or keep your hands at your sides as you move forward.

3. Inhale, lengthen your spine upward, then exhale, bringing your head toward your front knee.

4. Imagine your chest, rather than your head, moving toward your knees to help lengthen your spine and prevent rounding your back. Keep breathing throughout this pose.

Janu Shirshasana: Sitting One Leg Pose

In *janu shirshasana* (pronounced *JAH-noo shur-SHAH-sah-nah*), *janu* means "knee," and *shirsha*

1. Sit on the floor with your left leg straight in front of you, toes pointed upward. Your right leg should be bent in toward the straight leg.

2. Raise your hands over your head, exhale, and slowly bend forward over your straight leg.

3. Hold the stretch, then inhale as you rise back up. Repeat on the other side.

4. **Yoga Adventure:** It's alright to bend your knee! As you become more flexible, you'll be able to straighten your leg and actually grasp your foot with your hands. Sound impossible? Maybe not today, but that's okay!

Wise Yogi Tells Us

If you feel stress on your back doing the Sitting One Leg pose, bend the knee you are reaching toward. Angle your body directly over this knee. Release any competitive thoughts. Forget your goals and open your heart. Bend at your hips, not your waist. Don't hurry, be patient with yourself. Slowly your leg and hip will open. Have fun with the process.

Paschimothanasana: Sitting Forward Bend Pose

Sitting Forward Bend helps the spine be more flexible as it stretches the entire back of your body from your neck to your calf.

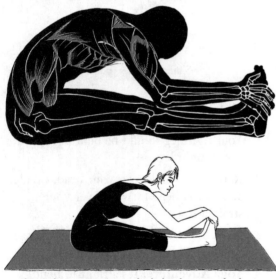

This is how your musculoskeletal system looks in Sitting Forward Bend.

1. Sit with your legs stretched out in front of you, feet together and relaxed.

2. Inhale and bend forward, folding your torso over your thighs and reaching your hands toward your feet. Don't strain your head toward your knees. Instead, keep your head up and gently ease your chest toward your thighs. When you have pulled yourself down as far as you can, relax your head down.

3. If you can reach your feet, flex them and hook your index fingers around your big toes. Gently pull to increase the stretch. If you can't reach that far, just ease your hands down your legs as far as you can. Keep your head in line with your spine.

Ardha Baddha Padma Pashchimottanasana: Bound Half Lotus Pose

Ardha baddha padma pashchimottanasana (pronounced *AHR-dah BAH-dah PAHD-mah PAH-shih-moh-tah-NAH-sah-nah*) is identical to Sitting One Leg pose, except that the foot of your bent leg is in a Half Lotus position, with one foot placed on the opposite thigh.

Ouch!

Not every pose is for every body. Be patient and kind with your body, and your body will respond accordingly. You will be amazed at the power of TLC (tender loving care!).

1. Sit on the floor with one leg in front of you (as in Sitting One Leg pose) and the other leg bent, foot placed on your opposite thigh in Half Lotus.

2. Bring your arm around your back and connect your hand to this foot.

3. Face your upper torso directly over your extended leg. Open your chest, exhale, and slowly bend forward. Repeat on the other side. If this pose seems impossible, be patient and the pose will come.

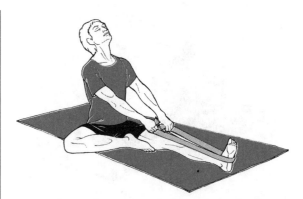

Stretch your hamstrings using a strap and pulling gently as you keep your back straight and neck in line with your spine.

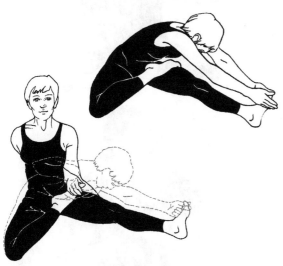

Bound Half Lotus pose.

4. **Getting Started:** Ease into Bound Half Lotus by sitting with one leg tucked into a Half Easy pose. Stretch your hamstring by looping a towel or strap around your foot and pulling gently rather than bending your body forward. Keep your back straight and your neck in line with your spine.

5. **Yoga Adventure:** For an extra challenge that not only adds a nice hamstring and inner thigh stretch but also helps make your hip joints more mobile, try Archer pose (*akarna dhanurasana*). From Bound Half Lotus, pick up the foot of your folded leg with the hand on the same side of your body and lift it gently by the ball of the foot toward your ear. Keep your elbow lifted. With your other hand, reach straight out toward the toe of your straight leg, grasping it if you can. Your body becomes bow, arrow, archer—bodymindspirit. Enjoy the lovely stretch!

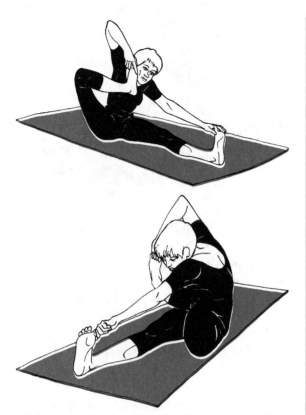

Adjust your feet from Bound Half Lotus into Archer pose for a great hamstring stretch that adds mobility to your hip joints.

6. **Yoga Adventure 2:** From Archer, you can give your hips an even greater stretch with Foot-to-Head pose (*eka pada sirasana*), but don't push this until you are flexible enough. From Archer pose, bend your outstretched knee and tuck your foot close to your body as in Easy pose, but take the foot you have in your raised hand and gently ease it behind your head so your heel rests on the opposite shoulder, toes pointed upward. Now both hands are free to rest in prayer pose (*namaste*). Breathe and hold for several moments, then gently raise your foot and place it back down into Full Easy pose.

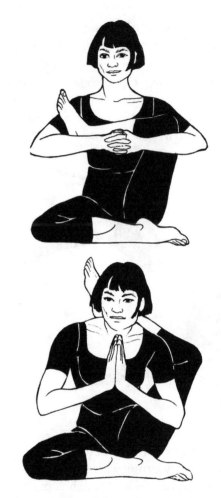

Foot-to-Head pose (*eka pada sirasana*) is an advanced pose for those with great hip flexibility.

Yoga *Mudra:* Ego Be Gone!

Yoga *Mudra* (pronounced *YOH-gah MOO-drah*) is a symbol of unity. This important pose inspires feelings of devotion and humility. It also stretches your legs and hips, opens your shoulders, and aids the gastrointestinal tract.

Wise Yogi Tells Us

Just a friendly reminder to your ego: Take a hike! When performing any yoga pose, especially more difficult poses, don't allow your ego to take over. If you find yourself thinking *Look at me touching the floor!* or *Wow, I'm so good at this!* re-adjust your thoughts. The aim of yoga is to eliminate ego, not to encourage it. Feel how the posture you're holding helps your mind become clear and see the truth: that you are one with the true world.

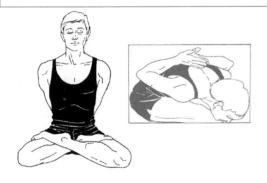

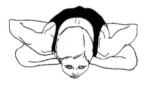

The Yoga *Mudra* pose.

1. Sit cross-legged or in Kneeling pose.
2. Move your arms behind your back, clasp your hands, and lower your head to the floor.
3. Keeping your arms straight, lift your clasped hands up over your head until your arms are perpendicular to the floor.
4. **Yoga Adventure:** Bring your hands into *namaste* behind your back.

Naukasana: Boat Pose

A yogi holding *naukasana* (pronounced *now-KAH-sah-nah*) looks like a boat bobbing on the waves, and *nauka* literally means "ship." Boat pose tones your stomach and intestines, strengthens your back, and activates your Mars *chakra* (located behind your navel).

In Boat pose, don't hold your breath, even as you are concentrating on balancing. Your feet may fall to the floor at first. Whether you are doing Full Boat pose or Half Boat pose (see the following description), keep your leg position steady and your knees together.

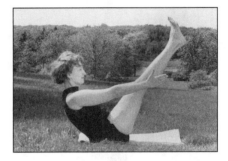

Boat pose.

1. For Full Boat pose, sit on the floor with your knees bent in front of you and your arms holding your knees.
2. Lean back to about a 45-degree angle, bring your feet off the floor, and balance on your tailbone.
3. Raise your feet straight up in the air so your body forms a V shape. For balance, extend your arms straight out, parallel to the floor at about knee level.
4. Imagine you are bobbing on top of the water like a little buoy.
5. **Getting Started:** If balancing in Full Boat pose is too difficult at first, start with Half Boat pose. Keep your knees bent, but instead of raising your feet all the way up, raise them to a right angle to the floor. Keep your knees together. Bring your hands alongside your feet with your palms facing in.

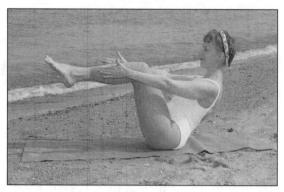

Half Boat pose.

Santulangasana: Balancing Chalice Pose

This challenging balance pose is great for improving concentration and also strengthens the abdomen and hips.

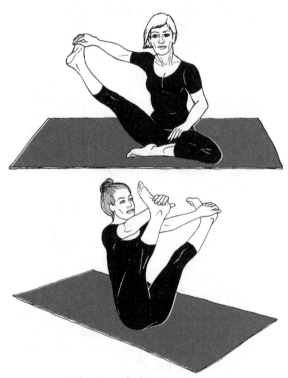

Balancing Chalice pose improves concentration and abdominal strength.

1. Begin in Easy pose with your back straight and your head lifted.

2. Grasp one ankle with your hand and inhale as you straighten your leg to the side. Exhale as you slowly bring the leg in front of you.

3. Grasp the other ankle with your other hand and inhale as you straighten the second leg to the side, then exhale as you slowly bring it forward. Your legs should form a V, your arms are straight and strong, and your back stays straight with head lifted.

4. Focus on a single point in front of you to help you balance, and hold as long as your abdominal strength allows or for a few controlled breaths.

5. Release your legs back down into Easy pose and breathe, resting for a moment to feel the difference between balanced sitting and stable sitting.

Kurmasana: Tortoise Pose

You'll look like a tortoise when you practice *kurmasana* (pronounced *koohr-MAH-sah-nah*). This pose keeps your lumbar limber! (In other words, it makes your lower spine more flexible.) It also strengthens your neck, massages your thyroid, aids digestion, and rejuvenates your nervous system. Take it slowly—just like a tortoise!

 A Yoga Minute

Hypothyroidism, the underproduction of the thyroid hormone, is a common condition and might be the underlying cause of many recurring illnesses and chronic fatigue. Symptoms of an underactive thyroid include fatigue, weight gain, weakness, dry skin, hair loss, recurrent infections, depression, and intolerance to cold. For a nice thyroid massage, try Turtle pose.

Does Tortoise pose seem impossible? Simply lower yourself as far as you can, let the corners of your mouth turn upward like a cute little turtle, and enjoy the journey to the floor, even if it takes many, many yoga practices to extend as big as a tortoise. Tortoises are not in a hurry. They live loooong lives!

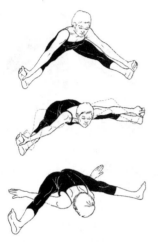

Tortoise pose.

1. Sit with your legs extended in front of you in a V shape. Bend your knees just slightly, and slide your arms under your knees with your palms on the floor.

2. Slowly straighten your legs again to hold your arms against the floor and bring your chest forward. Your chin will eventually reach the floor.

Adho Mukha Shvanasana: Downward Facing Dog Pose

Another pose named after the esteemed canine. Downward Facing Dog, *adho mukha shvanasana* (pronounced *AH-doh MOO-kah shvah-NAH-sah-nah*), brings heat to your body, strengthens and stretches your spine, and gives your heart a rest.

This is one of the better-known yoga poses—maybe because it feels so great to do it! Downward Facing Dog is easily adjustable for any flexibility level. You can reach down to the floor—or even to the seat of a firmly anchored chair—if you can't quite make it all the way down. Or if you are very flexible, you can press all the way down to the floor with your palms and your heels while pushing your hips up. *Ahh*, doesn't that feel great?

If you have trouble with this pose because of tight hamstrings, spend extra yoga time on Sitting Forward Bend to loosen the back of your legs. If Downward Facing Dog hurts your wrists, you might not be balancing your weight evenly. Try placing a rolled-up towel or blanket under the heel of each hand. This will take some of the pressure off your wrists. Then try to shift your weight back onto the heels of your feet. (All these heels! We definitely are talking about dogs!) Hold the pose only as long as you are comfortable. Little by little, your balance will shift, and this pose will eventually become quite soothing.

> **Ouch!**
>
> If your back is sore or tight, definitely keep your knees bent. Focus on spine lengthening, instead of legs straightening.

It might also help to concentrate on stretching out your lower back. Instead of rounding it, lengthen it. Remember the way your back is stretched out in Child's pose? Think about lifting your tailbone to the sky. If necessary, keep your knees slightly bent to return a natural curve to your lower back. When you are flexible and strong enough to perform Downward Facing Dog fully and peacefully, you will place as much weight on your feet as you do on your hands. To get this feeling of the full pose, have a partner lift your hips up and shift your weight back to center, as shown in the following illustration.

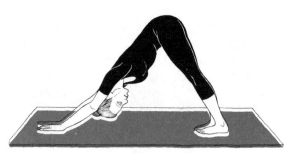

Downward Facing Dog.

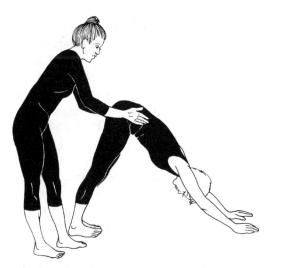

Checking hip alignment in Downward Facing Dog.

1. Get down on your hands and knees. Lift your tailbone up, bringing your knees off the floor so your body forms an upside-down V, with your palms and the balls of your feet touching the floor.

2. Bring your head down and your hips up. Keep your knees bent at first, then slowly bring your heels to the floor and straighten your legs. No rush to straighten those legs. With dedicated practice, they will open in their own time. Breathe and hold for as long as it feels good.

3. Have a partner check your hips to make sure they are straight rather than listing to one side, and weight is evenly distributed between your legs and arms.

4. **Yoga Adventure:** For an extra foot and calf stretch in Downward Facing Dog, alternately bend one leg and push into the other leg, feeling your heel powering into the ground and pushing up with your hips for a deep, one-leg isolation stretch. Repeat on the other side.

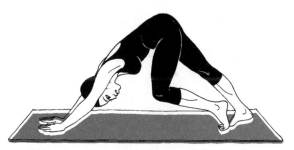
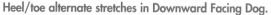

Heel/toe alternate stretches in Downward Facing Dog.

5. **Yoga Adventure 2:** To strengthen your leg muscles and improve your balance, try a heel lift in Downward Facing Dog. Exhale and bend your knees slightly and lift your heels off the ground. Feel your spine lengthen. Hold for a few seconds, then inhale and lower your heels back to the ground, keeping the spine elongated. Repeat several times.

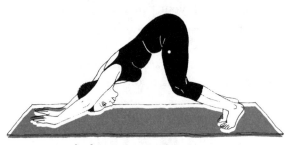

Heel Lift in Downward Facing Dog.

6. **Yoga Adventure 3:** To make Downward Facing Dog even more challenging, combine it with Elbow Dog, which deepens the leg stretch as it strengthens your shoulders and upper arms. From Downward Facing Dog pose, slowly lower yourself down onto your forearms, bringing your elbows to the ground. The more you do this pose, the more flexibility you will gain in your calves and hamstrings.

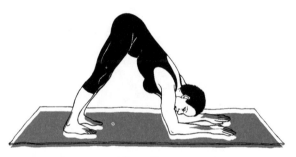

Elbow Dog.

Feeling worn out yet? The next chapter will give you a chance to let your body really relax so all that work can take effect. Corpse pose is, paradoxically, the easiest and most challenging yoga pose of all. Read on to learn more, and prepare to get really, really relaxed.

The Least You Need to Know

◆ Forward-bending postures—such as Standing Head to Knees, Feet Apart Side Angle, Sitting One Leg, Bound Half Lotus, Yoga *Mudra*, Boat, Half Boat, Tortoise, and Downward Facing Dog— help you internalize and quiet your mind.

◆ Forward bends are great for loosening your lower back and stretching out your hamstrings.

◆ Forward bends and backbends balance each other and should be practiced together.

In This Chapter

◆ Why Corpse pose is so named, and why it's the most important of all the poses

◆ More on *Om*

◆ How to relax and stop thinking

◆ Finding peace at last!

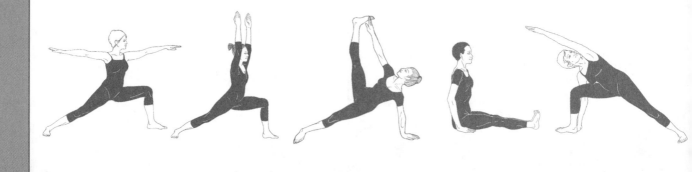

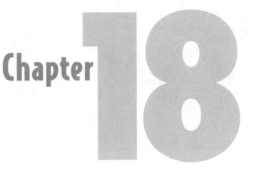

Chapter 18

Dead to the World

Of all the yoga poses, *shavasana* (pronounced *shah-VAH-sah-nah*), also known as *Corpse pose*, is the most important. *Shava* means "corpse," and just as it sounds, Corpse pose consists of lying on the floor in complete relaxation, still, peaceful, and corpselike. "How can lying on the floor be important?" you might ask. Or better yet, "How can imitating a corpse be important?"

Both good questions! Here's a good answer: The essence of peace comes from within, not from without. *Shavasana*'s goal is to relax the body so completely that the body becomes irrelevant, as if it were deceased. With the body "gone," the mind is set free to blossom. *Shavasana* sinks into that space between life and the beyond.

"But a corpse is dead!" you might continue to argue. "Isn't yoga about life?" Yes! But life and death are inseparable—they are all part of a bigger reality. By learning Corpse pose, you learn to live. By focusing inward, which means focusing beyond your body, your ego, and your superficial trappings of the "you" who walks around every day (clothes, habits, personality), you'll ultimately connect with the beauty of the universe. The surface "you" can finally fall away, and the inner "you," the Real You, can emerge. Imagine the resounding cosmic question: Will the Real You please stand up? If you've mastered *shavasana*, you'll know just who the Real You is! As your body lies corpselike, the Real You can stand.

How to Be a Corpse

Shavasana involves more than collapsing onto the floor in a crumpled heap after a long, hard day and *wishing* you were dead.

Let's practice Corpse pose with a little more focus!

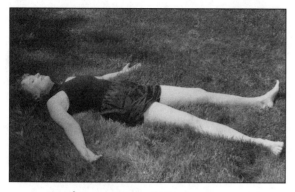

Shavasana: yoga's Corpse pose.

1. Lie comfortably on your back on the floor, and separate your legs so your feet are two to three feet apart. Let your toes fall out to the sides. Close your eyes.

2. Separate your arms so each hand is two to three feet from your body, with each palm facing upward.

3. Roll your head from side to side, releasing tension in your neck.

4. Roll your shoulders down and away from your ears.

5. Allow your attention to travel up and down your body, scanning for tight spots or contracted muscles. When you find a tight spot, gently tell the area to relax (out loud, if it helps). For example, "Chill out, right shoulder!" You might have to say it twice. Place a pillow under your knees or head if this helps you relax.

6. Repeat your body scan until your body is completely relaxed.

7. Now bring your attention to your breath. Listen to your breath. Don't try to control it. Simply observe it. Feel it flowing in and out of you. Make the sound and feel of your breath the sole focus of your attention.

8. If part of your body starts to tense up, redirect your mind to the tense area and focus on relaxing it again. Then return to the breath.

9. As thoughts pop into your mind (*If my computer crashes again today, I'm gonna throw it out the window. That new guy at the office sure is cute!*), let them pass back out of your mind. Imagine they are soap bubbles—allow your breath to blow them away softly, up into the sky.

10. Come back to the breath. Back to the breath. To the breath. The breath. Breath. *Om.*

11. **Getting Started:** For some people, lying on a firm floor and/or lying flat on their backs is uncomfortable, even painful. If this sounds like you, try Supported Corpse pose. Lie on the floor with a blanket or small pillow under your head and neck. Keep your arms at your sides, palms up, but rest your knees, lower legs, and feet on a chair so your legs are bent at a right angle. Rest, breathe, and relax.

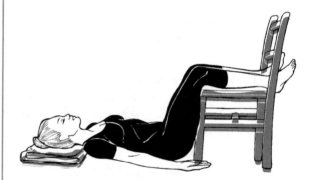

Supported Corpse Pose.

One for All, and All for *Om!*

Maybe lying on the floor is no problem for you, but everything after that is a real challenge. It isn't easy to relax, let alone clear the mind. *Om* to the rescue!

Om is the sound frequently chanted by yogis, because it is an all-encompassing sound. According to yogic thought, if all of life were translated into a single sound, the sound of the universe, that sound would be *Om.*

Try saying the sound now, right where you are sitting (or standing, or lying down, or wherever you happen to be at the moment). Take a deep breath, breathing from your diaphragm, and sing out the *o* sound as long as you can without your voice faltering. Don't be afraid to put some sound and strength behind it. If you're worried about keeping your volume down too much, you might not give the sound the breath support it requires. Stay strong and sing out the sound, which is pronounced like *oh*, then slowly let the *o* sound come to a close in a resonating, vibrating *mmmmm* sound.

Now take a breath, close your eyes, and try it again. Let the sound stretch out for as long as you can with the support of a deep breath. Use up all your breath, but don't strain yourself. Doesn't that feel good? Do it again if you'd like to. Notice how, when your entire body is vibrating with that sound, it's easier to concentrate on your breath and the sound than whether to have dessert with dinner tonight or whether you can convince someone else to do the dishes.

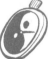 **A Yoga Minute**

According to an eyewitness account, Gandhi's last words to his assailant as he fell to the ground on, January 30, 1948, from a gunshot wound, were "Rama, Rama," which means "Praise God." This is the essence of yoga: to have one's thoughts continuously uplifted, even (especially!) in the transition from one existence to another.

Also notice how much *Om* sounds like "amen." If you've been to or go to church, you've probably heard the "amen" sung at the end of every hymn. Have you ever noticed that when a chorus of voices sings "amen," the voices often bloom from a single note into a harmony, like a multi-petalled flower opening in sound? Think how nicely this concept fits into the yoga way of thinking. Many voices harmonize to form a single, beautiful sound that is more complete than one voice alone, just as the universe is a beautiful blending of each soul into a single vibration of love.

In a nutshell, the point of chanting *Om* is to let the incredible power of sound and vibration work for you, pushing away worldly concerns and physical discomforts to bring your mind to a singular (yet universal) focus. Try it the next time you try Corpse pose. You'll be blissfully surprised!

When the Easiest Is the Hardest

Some of you might still be stuck on the idea that *shavasana* is the most important of all the postures. *How hard can it be?* you might wonder. *How hard can it be to lie on the floor and relax?* Actually, *shavasana* is the most challenging pose, even though it seems, at first, to be the easiest. Unlike some poses, where you first need to spend a lot of time developing strong ankles or upper arms or balance, Corpse pose can be assumed by anyone who can lie on the floor.

On the other hand, not only is relaxation a true challenge for many, but *shavasana* has a strong mental component, without which you aren't truly practicing *shavasana*. Just as you can hold Lotus pose perfectly without truly practicing yoga, you can certainly lie in what appears to be a perfect *shavasana* without coming close to a yogic state of mind. Ideally, *shavasana* could be practiced in the midst of total chaos, because the yogi in *shavasana* has utterly released him- or herself from the body. The body is merely a shell or a vessel, while the soul is directly connected with the universe. Certainly it takes a long while to reach this point, and Corpse pose can be practiced quite productively before this state is reached, but this is the ideal destination—and a challenging journey it is!

Wise Yogi Tells Us

Even though *shavasana* isn't meant to put you to sleep, practicing it in bed at night—particularly the steps for relaxing the body—can help lure even the most hardcore insomniac toward dreamland.

Let *shavasana* become a part of your workout, and take it just as seriously as any other posture—even *more* seriously. Your body will learn how to release all its tensions and will benefit even more from the other postures because of its time spent in *shavasana*. Your spirit, too, will learn how to soar beyond the limits of its "container." Now *that's* a powerful skill!

Open Up and Let Go: The Body

Your body is a complex organism with thousands of parts, all connected and related yet separate, too. It's no easy task to relax the whole thing, let alone transcend it completely. When practicing *shavasana*, it can help to have a plan for releasing each part of your body a little at a time. Read over the following steps for releasing and relaxing your lower body, upper body, and face. Enough times through, and you'll have the steps memorized.

The Lower Body: Going Nowhere

Once you are in Corpse pose and have followed all the steps mentioned earlier, but before you focus on your breath, relax your lower body:

1. Tighten one foot, curling your toes and contracting your foot muscles for a few seconds. Then release and feel the tension flowing from your foot.

2. Flex your ankle and tighten your calf, then relax both.

3. Lift your entire leg two inches off the ground. Tense your leg, especially your large thigh muscle. Squeeze! Then let your leg fall to the ground. With the release, imagine all the tension falling away.

4. Repeat these steps with your other foot and leg.

5. Lift your hips two inches off the floor and squeeze your buttocks as tightly as you can for several seconds. Then release the contraction and drop your hips back down. Feel all the tight areas releasing and relaxing. Your hip joints should feel loose and your buttocks muscles completely relaxed.

Ouch!

If lying flat on the floor is uncomfortable for your back, put pillows or blankets under your knees. This protects your lower back from undue strain. If your head or neck is uncomfortable, rest your head or neck on a small pillow, but make sure your throat feels open. Too many pillows could block the flow of energy through your neck; too few pillows could cause your neck to overstrain backward. If you have low blood pressure and your feet get cold, wear socks. Strive for a feeling of openness in all parts of your body.

The Upper Body: Still Rhythms

Continuing upward:

1. Contract your stomach muscles as tightly as you can, then release them.

2. Lift one arm about two inches off the floor. Squeeze your hand into a fist and hold it tightly. Flex your arm muscles for several seconds, then relax your entire arm and let it fall. Feel stress and tightness flowing down your arm and out the ends of your fingers. Repeat with your other arm.

3. Tighten your chest muscles, then release them. As you release them, try to feel your heartbeat. Gently tell your heart to relax, slow down, and rest.

4. Bring your shoulders up to your ears, tensing your shoulders for several seconds. Release them and feel all the stress dropping away. Many people carry tension in their shoulders. You might want to do this several times until your shoulders feel truly loose.

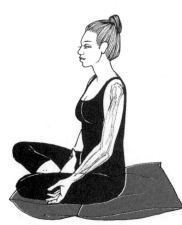

If lying down is uncomfortable, Corpse pose can be done seated. Try tensing muscles, then relaxing them to begin the seated *shavasana* journey.

The Ultimate Facial: Losing Your Senses

And now for the rest of you:

1. Lift your head two inches off the ground. Tense all your neck and facial muscles, scrunching up your face like a prune. Purse your lips and imagine you are trying to bring every part of your face to your nose. Release and lower your head.

2. Raise your head again, and open your eyes and mouth as wide as you possibly can. Stick your tongue out as far as you can. Really stretch that face for several seconds, then relax and lower your head to the ground.

3. Roll your head slowly and gently from one side to the other.

4. One at a time, scan your senses. First, notice what you can taste, then let it go. Take your mind away from your taste buds. Next, notice what you can smell, then release your sense of smell. Notice everything your body is touching, then imagine you are floating and can't feel anything. What can you hear? Let it go. Focus inward. Last, let go of your sight (even though your eyes should already be closed) by releasing all tension around your eyes. If you see light through your eyelids, gently release your awareness of it.

5. Now go back over each body part again, but this time, instead of physically tensing and releasing your muscles, mentally tell each part to relax. Really focus on each area, one at a time, and coax it to release all pain and tension. Consider this the start of a wonderful relationship between your mind and your body. Why shouldn't they converse?

6. After you've completed all these steps, you should feel very, very relaxed and internalized. Mentally scan your body a few more times, seeking out pockets of stress and releasing them. If any sensations try to creep back in, gently ignore them.

Now you're ready to leave your body behind and ride your breath.

Open Up and Let Go: The Mind

You've moved past your body and are now immersed in your mind. But that has to go, too. Yes, the mind is as distracting as the body when it comes to true relaxation—maybe more so! Even as you lie in Corpse pose, feeling proud that you've managed to transcend your body—at least to some extent—your mind is holding you back from true awareness. How? By making you feel proud, for one thing! Pride belongs to the ego, and in true awareness, there is no ego. So what's an active-minded person to do? Simple: Stop thinking.

Me? Stop Thinking? Forget About It!

To many, the prospect of not thinking seems far more of an effort than the most complicated yoga posture. We *are* our minds—aren't we? Not according to yogic philosophy. In fact, wise yogis tell us that we aren't our bodies or our minds at all. These are merely tools to help free our souls and bring them into fuller and more unifying consciousness.

As you rest in *shavasana*, attempting to keep your mind at bay, think about your mind merely as a tool to help you in your task. When used at the wrong time or for the wrong job, a tool can be a hindrance, but when used correctly, it will make any job easier. During *shavasana*, it's time to put the tools down. Put away your thoughts. Let them go. You can always pick them up again later.

Dream a Little Dream

Imagine waking up one morning with the memory of a beautiful dream. In the dream, you are walking through your home, and everything is familiar until you come upon a door you've never noticed before. You open the door and step through it into a new universe. Pure beauty surrounds you, and you are filled with a sense of bliss. You realize that you are perfect. You have no faults, no sins, no shortcomings, no guilt. You are a being of pure light, and the whimsically lovely universe that encompasses you is also you. Love radiates from you and into you. You vaguely remember the comparatively ponderous and painful life of

striving on the other side of the door through which you came, but as you look behind you, the door is gone, and you realize that other life was just a dream.

And then you wake up. Which was real and which was the dream? Yogic philosophy says that this life we lead in these earthbound bodies and minds is the dream, and that pure bliss is the reality. Yoga helps us wake from this dream. But even dreams exist for a reason, and we all move through this dream of our lives to learn about our souls. This dream is a lesson, albeit a very vivid one, but it's still only a dream.

Of course, we don't mean that right now you are really asleep and dreaming all this. (Or do we?) Life isn't a dream in the sense that we are used to thinking of dreams. But according to wise yogis, our interpretation of life is an illusion. Anything that isn't eternal and blissful is an illusion. Yoga, and especially *shavasana*, helps us work past our bodies and dig through our thoughts until we unearth the jewel that is cosmic consciousness. How extraordinary to awake to such a reality!

Give Your Mind a Breather

But let's get back to this "dream" we're all living and striving through called life. We have to live in the world, and we can't lie in Corpse pose all day long. We have to eat, sleep, make money, do our daily chores, and care for those who depend on us. What good is *shavasana* during the rest of the day?

Have you ever left all your worries behind and taken off for a vacation, even if just for the night? Maybe you found a last-minute babysitter and whisked your spouse off for a romantic evening alone. Maybe you took a personal day off from work, got in your car, and drove somewhere you'd never been before. If you've never done such a thing, you should try it. It's rejuvenating and gives you a new perspective on your everyday life. But even if you aren't at liberty to leave your regular life for a while, you can still practice *shavasana*—a mini-vacation for your mind.

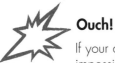

Ouch!

If your daily obligations make it impossible for you to get away for a restorative vacation, don't be discouraged. Practicing *shavasana* can give you the mental break you need … as good as a refreshing ocean breeze.

If you had a job where you had to work the same hours your mind has to work, you'd probably collapse in less than a week. Of course, our brains are made to be busy, but even the most efficient brain needs a break now and then. *Shavasana* turns everything off: the senses, the emotions, the thoughts. Only breath and pure consciousness exist. If you've ever uttered the words, "At last, I can just sit here and do nothing!" you know how your brain feels when you practice *shavasana*.

Wise Yogi Tells Us

"Do not take life's experiences too seriously. Above all, do not let them hurt you, for in reality, they are nothing but dream experiences. … If circumstances are bad and you have to bear them, do not make them a part of yourself. Play your part in life, but never forget that it is only a role."

—Paramahansa Yogananda

Quest for Peace

Perhaps the most compelling reason for us Westerners to practice *shavasana* is that it simply brings more peace into our lives. Imagine yourself calmer and more clear-headed, able to take any situation in stride and handle any emergency with unruffled confidence. The regular practice of *shavasana* can give you this gift. We can all use more peace in our lives, and this needn't be a futile wish. Take an active role in bringing peace to your life through *shavasana*, because even the most hectic and chaotic external life is miraculous and wonderful when peace lives inside you.

The Least You Need to Know

- If you practice only one yoga pose, practice *shavasana*.
- Mastering *shavasana* can be more strenuous and requires more discipline than the most physically demanding yoga postures!
- In *shavasana*, first you consciously relax your body, then you consciously relax your mind, then you let your consciousness go, too, living only in the breath and pure awareness.
- Learning to quiet your mind and remove scattered thinking will bring you peace.

In This Part

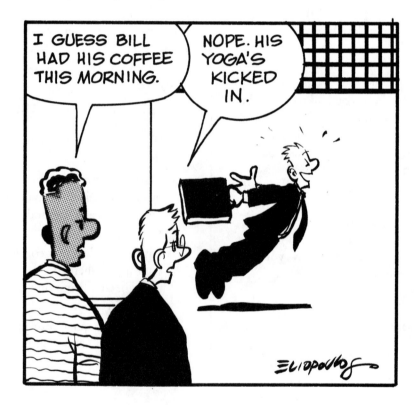

Yoga Sessions: Energy Flow

In this part, we'll really get you moving. First you'll learn about *vinyasana*, a method of yoga that strings postures together in a sequence with deep breathing to create an active, flowing routine full of movement and energy. Depending on which postures you include in your *vinyasana*, you'll experience a mild to strenuous cardiovascular workout. We give you some energizing *vinyasanas* to try, including the well-known and popular Sun Salutation, then set you free to create your own *vinyasana* routines. Have fun!

Next, we'll give you some targeted and fully illustrated sessions to fit into your day. Whether you have 5 minutes, 15 minutes, half an hour, or a full hour for yoga, we've got a sequence of poses that will fit into your life.

In This Chapter

◆ Yoga's Sun Salutation

◆ Yoga's Moon Salutation

◆ Combining postures in a sequence of motion

◆ How to create your own flow—move and groove!

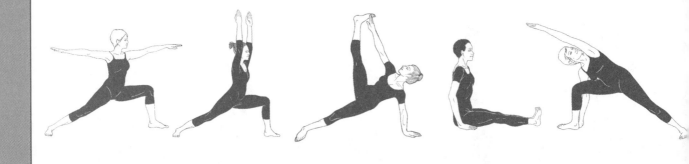

Chapter 19

Vinyasana: Moving with the Sun and the Moon

You're probably convinced by now that yoga can be tough and challenging to your strength and flexibility. But what about working up a *real* sweat? That's where *vinyasana* (pronounced *vin-YAH-sah-nah*) comes in! *Vinyasana* combines a series of yoga postures into a long, fluid, unified movement. Poses are held within a *vinyasana*, but the difference is that when you come out of one posture, you flow immediately into another posture. The right flow will give you a great workout, in addition to improving your balance, grace, speed, strength, and agility.

Sweat with the Rhythm

Continuous-flow sequences of yoga postures can be an invigorating cardiovascular workout. Repeating a series of postures in quick succession takes stamina and good lung capacity. A more slowly executed series of poses is also challenging, allowing you to enter each pose fully and deliberately while still engaging in continuous movement, a *vinyasana* flows in a moving meditation. Let the rhythm of your body and your breath move you to new levels of mindbody awareness.

Breathe to the Beat

Breath is extremely important in a *vinyasana*. Connecting posture to posture and movement to movement is more than just moving muscles. Every movement and every position of a *vinyasana* has an equivalent breath: an inhale, an exhale, or a hold. A good general guideline is to exhale when going into forward bends and inhale when going into backward bends.

The right breathwork in a *vinyasana* can make or break the flow of a series. Before you begin your *vinyasana*, determine your pace and your intention. For instance, maybe you decide to do the Sun Salutation in a slow and languid way this morning to warm you up. Let your breathing reflect this intention. Inhale and exhale deeply with each movement of this *vinyasana*. Perhaps you do it again this afternoon, but this time at a quicker, more energized pace. Again, let your breathing reflect your intention. Breathe to the rhythm of your movements so your breath and your body work together.

Let your mind work with your body, as they become one, using your breath as a monitor. If you can't breathe slowly enough, deepen your breath or allow for more than one breath in a position. If you can't keep up, slow the pace. Let your breath work for you. It will tell you when you are pushing yourself too hard.

Wise Yogi Tells Us

When you set your intention ahead of time, you'll be in a better frame of mind to notice and monitor your progress as you go. Are you revving up too much, when you had intended to go slow? Are you lagging behind when you had intended to keep an upbeat pace?

Always remember to breathe with your entire body during a *vinyasana*. Inhale fully, and exhale completely. Let the movements, the contractions and expansions, the bends and arches, twists and stretches, help your lungs and the muscles in your thoracic cavity draw breath in and push it out. Feel the breath traveling from your toes to your fingertips, your heels to your head. Let the breath be as integral to the movement as your physical body.

Bodymind in Motion

Just as your breath works for you during a *vinyasana*, so does your mind. More than your muscles are moving here! Your mind is to be equally engaged in the movement from pose to pose.

Making a purposeful effort to concentrate on the way your body feels and moves during a *vinyasana* is an excellent way to cultivate mindfulness. The *vinyasana* becomes a sort of meditation when practiced with this kind of intense focus. Let your moving body and flowing breath be the center of your meditation. Observe yourself from the inside out. Let your mind become the movement, let the movement become your body, let your body connect back to your mind in a complete circle.

You are one fully integrated, fully functioning yogi—so let's go with the flow!

Uttanatavasan: Leg Lifts

Uttanatavasan (pronounced *ooh-TAHN-ah-tah-VAH-sahn*), or Leg Lifts, involve a steady movement. They prepare the body to make the more fluid movements of a full *vinyasana*. Leg Lifts strengthen your stomach, which in turn supports your lower back. The deeper your breathing during this movement, the easier and smoother your *vinyasana* will become. Leg Lifts also help prepare your body for a Headstand.

Be careful not to use momentum to swing your legs up during Leg Lifts. Keep your movements slow and complete to build your strength, touching the ground and pausing before each lift. Don't separate your feet or bend your knees when you come down. If your back hurts, keep one knee bent, foot on the floor, but keep the other leg straight.

A Yoga Minute

Continuous practice of Leg Lifts can help alleviate lower back pain. A majority of Americans over age 40 suffer from it.

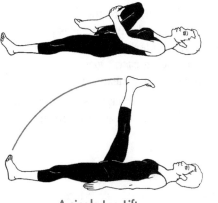

A single Leg Lift.

If you have a sensitive back, bend the knee you are not lifting and keep that foot firmly on the ground. This will protect your lower back as you continue to strengthen it with Leg Lifts. Leg Lifts build stomach and back muscles.

1. Lie on your back. Bend your left leg a little and press your lower back toward the floor slightly to avoid lower-back strain.

2. Inhale as you straighten your right leg and lift it straight up to the sky. When your leg is perpendicular to the floor, push your heel out.

3. Exhale and slowly lower your leg back down.

4. Repeat this movement on the same side, connecting each repetition with breath: Inhale as your leg goes up, exhale as your leg goes down.

5. After a satisfying number of repetitions (three or four—or more if you're up for it), switch to your left leg.

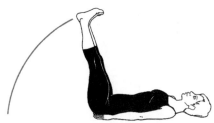

And now for the Double Leg Lift.

1. Begin the Double Leg Lift with your palms facing downward and tucked under your tailbone to keep your lower back from rising off the floor. Straighten your arms out under you. If you have long arms, they might go past your tailbone, which is fine.

2. Slowly inhale as you bring both legs straight up while you contract your abdominal muscles, pulling them in toward the floor to further support your lower back.

Wise Yogi Tells Us

While flowing through a Leg Lift, cup your hands over your ears and listen intently to your breath as it connects movement to movement. Is it smooth? Rocky? Does it sound like the ocean? The wind in the trees? Link the rhythm of your breath to the movements of your muscles. Notice everything. Be mindful. Close your eyes. Internalize.

3. Exhale as you bring both legs straight down, keeping your abdominals firmly contracted.

4. Do as many lifts as you can, inhaling as your legs go up, exhaling as your legs come down. Then rest.

Banarasana: Lunge Pose

We're soon going to introduce you to Sun Salutation, yoga's most well-known and beloved *vinyasana,* but be patient—we're still preparing you. Lunge pose is a pose that is used within Sun Salutation, and it is one of the movements some people find challenging, so practicing it on its own first can help make Sun Salutation easier and more enjoyable.

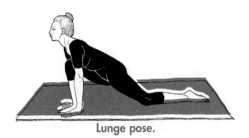

Lunge pose.

1. Stand in Mountain pose with your feet together, hands hanging down. Breathe.

2. Exhale and bend forward into Standing Head to Knees pose. Bend your knees if necessary to put your palms on the floor on both sides of your feet.

3. Inhale, and as you exhale, step one foot back behind you into what is commonly called a runner's lunge. Keep your chest forward and your head lifted.

4. Release your foot so the top of your foot is flat on the floor and drop your hips to try to make the line from your neck to your knee a straight line, diagonal with the floor. (It helps to do this in front of a mirror to check for the proper alignment.) Keep your palms flat on the floor so your fingers line up with your toes.

5. Hold for several moments, then draw your back foot back next to your other foot as you raise your hips, coming back into Standing Forward Bend.

6. Roll back up into Mountain pose.

7. Repeat with the other leg.

Surya Namaskara: Sun Salutation

The sun is the center of our solar system, and without its energy and warmth, we wouldn't be able to exist on this planet. This *vinyasana* is a devotional (not to mention great exercise). *Surya namaskara* (SOOR-yah nah-mahs-KAH-rah) offers

thanks and greetings to the sun, and although it can be performed any time, it is particularly appropriate and wonderful when performed outdoors at sunrise, facing east. *Surya* means "sun," and *namaskara* literally means "taking a bow."

Sun Salutation energizes, strengthens, and tones all the major muscles and organs in your body.

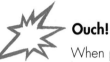 **Ouch!**

When performing Sun Salutation, keep your awareness focused. If you go too fast, your mind might stray from attending to the body, breath, and devotion to the sun. You should go fast enough to keep the movements flowing and get your body warm, but not so fast that you don't feel in control of your movements or breath.

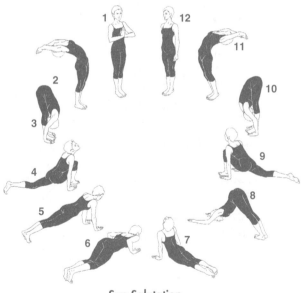

Sun Salutation.

1. Begin in Mountain pose with your hands in *namaste*, or prayer position. Center yourself and concentrate on a devotional attitude.

2. Inhale. Raise your arms up over your head and tilt them slightly back, as if you were encompassing the sun with love.

3. Exhale. Bring your hands straight down to the floor. Bend your knees to protect your lower back. Eventually, you may straighten your legs. Bring your palms alongside your feet. This position is a symbol of thanking the earth, where our feet are firmly planted.

4. Keeping your hands down, inhale and step your left foot back behind you. Stay low to the ground and look up. This represents that we are on the earth through the strength of the sun.

5. Exhale. Bring both legs back behind you and balance in Plank pose, as if you were about to lower yourself into a pushup. Push out at your heels for strength. This represents finding a balance between the sun and the earth. Pause.

6. Exhale further. Bring your knees, chest, and chin to the floor. Keep your tailbone up off the ground. You are thanking the earth.

7. Inhale into Upward Facing Dog pose and look up. Let the sun's warmth strengthen you.

8. Exhale and push up into Downward Facing Dog pose, lengthening your spine. Let the strength of the sun enter your spine.

9. Inhale as you bring your left foot forward. Look up and thank the sun as you proceed on your journey.

10. Exhale and bring both legs together. With your palms alongside your feet, humbly devote yourself to the sun. Open your moon *chakra* (located at the back of your head) to the sun's kind and steady energy.

11. Inhale as you bring your arms and body up, tilting into a slight backbend, again embracing the sun with love.

12. Exhale as you bring your hands back into the prayer position, standing in *tadasana*, Mountain pose.

13. Repeat the entire sequence again for a complete round. For the second half-round, bring your right leg back first to create a balance.

14. **Yoga Adventure:** Many different yoga teachers alter the Sun Salutation in many different ways, so if your teacher does Sun Salutation differently than the way we describe it in this book, that's fine! For example, some people add an extra step after step 3. After Standing Head to Knees pose, you can inhale and, keeping your back straight and your hands on the floor or on your ankles or lower legs, look up, separating your torso from your thighs. Then, exhale and bend back down before moving on to step 4.

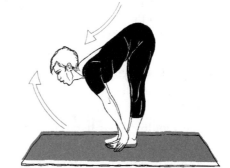

For variety, you can add this movement between steps 3 and 4 of the Sun Salutation as we've described it.

15. **Getting Started:** For some people, Sun Salutation is simply too difficult, strenuous, or not physically possible. If this sounds like you, try seated Sun Salutation, a gentler and less-strenuous version but a *vinyasana* nevertheless. Follow the following figures for this Sun Salutation adaptation. Don't forget to move through this *vinyasana* twice so you have a chance to use both legs. All the yoga postures can be adapted for use with chairs. It just takes some creativity and knowledge on the part of your teacher.

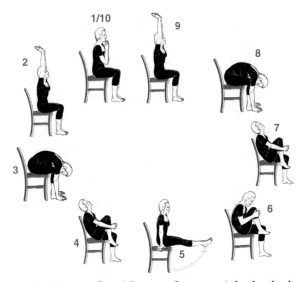

1. Sit comfortably on a firm, straight-backed chair with your feet planted on the ground, your palms together in front of your chest in prayer position (*namaste*). Concentrate and breathe, preparing yourself for the Seated Sun Salutation.

2. Inhale and raise your arms straight up, stretching your shoulders, arms, and upper back.

3. Exhale and drop your hands toward the floor, folding your body over your thighs. Relax and breathe for a moment, feeling the change in position.

4. Inhale and return to an upright seated position as you raise your right knee off the ground and hold it gently with your hands, tipping your head back just slightly.

5. Exhale and extend your bent leg forward and grasp the sides of the chair with your hands. If possible, lift your body slightly off the chair as you hold your legs out straight. One leg may remain planted on the floor for support.

6. Inhale and lower yourself back to the chair, then exhale and bend your extended leg, bringing your knee into your chest again, but this time keeping your head tilted forward toward your knee.

7. Inhale and continue to hold your bent knee, but lean your head back again in a controlled way, looking up.

8. Exhale and gently lower your leg to the floor, bringing your entire body back down over your thighs and dropping your hands to the floor beside your feet.

9. Inhale and raise your torso up again as you extend your arms overhead.

10. Exhale and return your hands to prayer position in front of your chest. Then, repeat the Sun Salutation with the opposite leg.

Chandra Namaskara: Moon Salutation

This Moon Salutation *vinyasana* restores vitality, strength, and flexibility to the entire body. It also improves digestion through the continual compression of the intestinal tract. *Chandra* means "moon," and just as the Sun Salutation greets and honors the sun, so *chandra namaskara* (pronounced *SHAHN-drah-nah MAHS-kah-rah*) greets and honors the moon. Try practicing this *vinyasana* outside on a clear evening when the moon is in full view. Serenity!

1. Stand in Mountain pose with your hands in *namaste*, or prayer position. Inhale and bring your arms over your head in a slight backbend, keeping your palms together. You are greeting the moon.

2. Exhale and bring your palms to the floor. You are thanking the earth for allowing you to stand on it.

3. Inhale and step your left foot back. Touch the side of your ankle to the floor. Your right leg is lunged forward with the weight of your body on your toes.

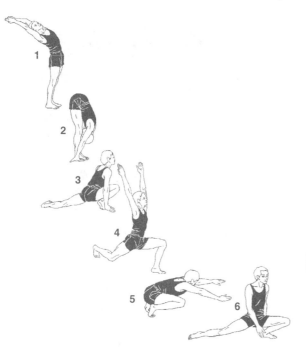

4. Exhale and switch the position of your feet. Keep your left knee at a right angle to the floor with your right knee touching the floor. Your weight is now supported by your left foot and right knee. Inhale and lift your arms straight up overhead toward the moon.

5. Then exhale into Child's pose (see Chapter 17), a symbol of turning inward.

6. Now inhale and step your right foot back with the side of your ankle touching the floor. Your left leg is lunged forward with the weight of your body on your toes. Exhale and switch the position of your feet as before. Your right knee is at a right angle to the floor, and your left knee is touching the floor. Your weight is now supported by your right foot and left knee.

7. Inhale and lift your arms straight up overhead. Thank you, moon!

8. Exhale and bring your hands back to the floor. Inhale into Upward Facing Dog. Strong and steady, the moon circles us.

9. Exhale into Child's pose again—the moon *chakra* at the back of your head will open for healing energy.

10. Inhale, bring your hands straight up overhead, and look up.

11. Exhale and bring your hands back to the floor. Inhale, push your hands against the floor, and stand up into Mountain pose.

12. *Namaste.*

Quite an energetic sequence of poses! The moon is a lunar/emotional/yin symbol. The strong physical movements in a Moon Salutation help balance your emotional side with your physical side.

Create Your Own Flow

The Sun and Moon Salutations are popular *vinyasanas* because they combine a series of poses that so nicely balance each other (a backbend, then a forward bend, and so on). But you, too, can create your own series of postures. Just keep them balanced—forward with backward, exhale with inhale, upright with inverted, one side with the other side, an expansion with a contraction, and so on. This will become easier as you familiarize yourself with the postures in this book.

Here are a few suggestions to get you started. All poses mentioned here are described elsewhere in this book or are explained here.

Warm Wonder *Vinyasana*

This *vinyasana* is quick, invigorating, and incredibly warming. We love to do this on a chilly winter evening before bed, or to warm up in the morning on a crisp fall day.

1. Start in Downward Facing Dog pose.

2. Inhale and flow into Plank pose.

3. Exhale, bend your elbows, and lower your body straight to the floor.

4. Inhale and push yourself up into Upward Facing Dog.

5. Exhale and push back into Downward Facing Dog.

6. Inhale, push one leg forward, turn to the side, and straighten up into Triangle pose.

7. Turn your chest back toward your bent knee and place your hands down alongside your feet. Exhale as you step back into Downward Facing Dog.

8. Step the other foot between your hands, and come up into Triangle pose on the other side.

9. Turn your torso over your bent knee, bring your hands alongside your feet, and push back into Downward Facing Dog. Hold for as long as comfortable.

10. Exhale into Child's pose, then rest. Hey, did somebody turn up the heat?

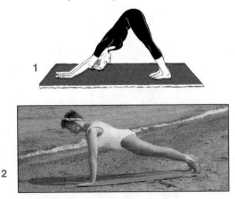

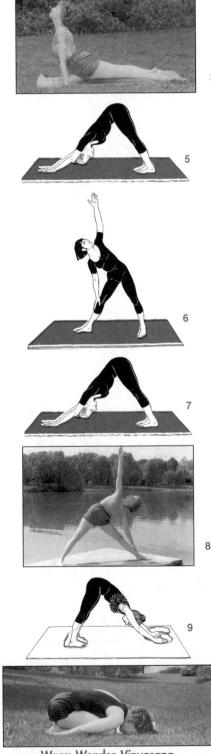

Warm Wonder *Vinyasana.*

Solar Flare *Vinyasana*

This is a super-powered *vinyasana* that strengthens the body as it brings strength, confidence, and a feeling of self-possession to the bodymind. It's great before you have to give a speech or go on a first date or otherwise radiate confidence!

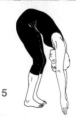

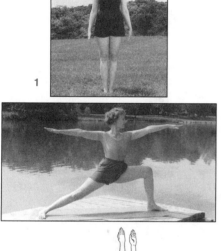

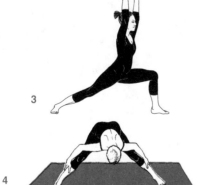

Solar Flare *Vinyasana.*

1. Start in Mountain pose.
2. Jump your feet three to four feet apart and assume Warrior 2 pose.
3. Hold for a few breaths, then change your body position to face forward with your arms overhead in Warrior 1 pose. Hold for a few breaths.

   Switch to the other side, doing Warrior 1 and 2 in the other direction.
4. Now, keeping your feet separated, turn your entire body to face forward and bend straight over with your knees straight. Bring your hands toward the floor and hold for a few breaths.
5. Come back up, jump your feet together, bend your knees, and place your palms flat on the floor. Slowly straighten your legs to further stretch the hamstrings. Breathe deeply. Rest.

Mild and Mindful *Vinyasana*

This is a calming and meditative *vinyasana* that helps you focus your mind as you relax your body.

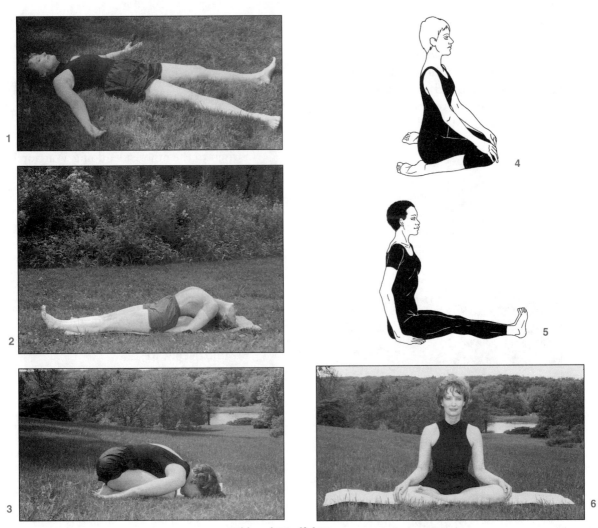

Mild and Mindful *Vinyasana.*

1. Start in *shavasana*.
2. Inhale and bring your hands under your tailbone, lifting up into Half Fish pose.
3. Hold for a few breaths, then come out of the pose, exhaling and rolling over into Child's pose.

4. Stay in Child's pose for a few breaths, inhale, sit up, exhale, and move into Hero pose.
5. Inhale as you move up, then exhale into Staff pose.
6. Inhale into any meditation pose such as Easy pose or Lotus pose, and—you guessed it!—meditate.

Moving with the Universe

While many yoga poses imitate animals or structures in nature (mountains, trees, and so on), a *vinyasana* imitates the rhythm and movement of the natural world, the universe, and the cosmos. The human body is like a universe in microcosm, with its own internal rhythms and movements. At the atomic level, the very atoms that make up everything are like tiny universes. Beyond our bodies, the world is full of cycles: the seasons, the years, the moons spinning around the planets, the planets spinning around the sun, the entire galaxy revolving.

A vinyasana helps us feel like a part of this magnificent, intricate, ultimately large, yet ultimately small cycle. The sun, moon, and earth all move in concert, and through a *vinyasana,* we move in concert, too. Everything is moving to a sacred rhythm, ancient and eternal, and the rhythm wouldn't be the same if any one thing did not move with it. We are all part of a wave in the ocean of the universe, and when we move with the tide, we are doing what comes naturally, what makes us a part of the whole.

Now if that's not a good reason to do a *vinyasana* every day, we don't know what is!

The Least You Need to Know

◆ A *vinyasana*, such as the Sun or Moon Salutation, is a sequence of postures strung together and performed in a series of flowing movements.

◆ A *vinyasana* is coordinated with the breath and the mind so that body, breath, and mind are integrated.

◆ The Sun Salutation is the most well-known *vinyasana*, but many others exist, and you can even create your own by doing sequences of poses that balance each other.

◆ *Vinyasanas* are great exercise for body and soul!

In This Chapter

- ◆ Why a little yoga goes a long way
- ◆ Three five-minute yoga sessions
- ◆ Three 15-minute yoga sessions

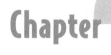

Yoga in Five Minutes or Fifteen Minutes

Will five minutes of yoga really do you any good? You bet your hurried self it will! Some yoga poses and pose sequences can make a big difference when you are stressed, tense, or need a quick energy boost. Try peppering these five-minute yoga sessions throughout your day to bring you serenity and balance.

For more detailed instructions on how to do any of these poses, see their original descriptions from previous chapters. Each pose is listed in the table of contents and the index for easy reference.

Yoga in Five Minutes

Here are three quick five-minute yoga sessions to use whenever you have five spare minutes—and who doesn't have five spare minutes at least once a day? You'll be glad you used the time for yoga instead of for a cup of coffee or a run to vendo-land for stale candy.

Session 1: Butterfly Take Flight

Let this movement help keep your seated meditation practice a wakeful one. Hold each pose for three breaths, then move into the next pose. Go back and forth and feel your energy soar, then return to your meditative pose. Repeat if you begin to feel sleepy again.

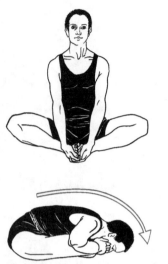

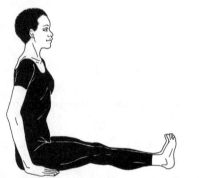

Relax into Butterfly pose, bringing your heels in toward your body only as far as you can still keep your spine straight, and bow forward. Hold for several breaths.

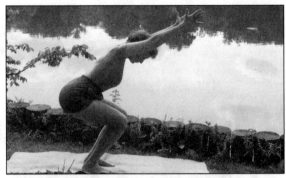

Session 2: Triple Stretch

Feel the full stretch of bodymindspirit in the powerful relationships inherent in this strength-producing sequence. Move slowly from one pose to the other, then repeat on the other side. Don't forget to breathe fully throughout this sequence.

Move into Lightning Bolt pose, breathing deeply, and arms straight up over your head, palms facing inward.

Straighten your legs and bring your hands to the floor directly under your shoulders, keeping your arms straight and fingers pointing forward. Hold Staff pose for several breaths.

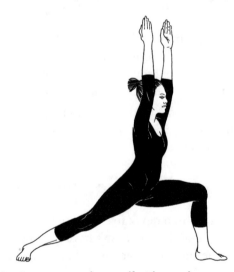

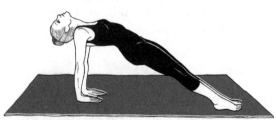

Flow into Upward Facing Plank pose, holding for several breaths with strong arms and a straight body.

Continue to ground yourself with your legs as you move into Warrior 1, lifting with your torso.

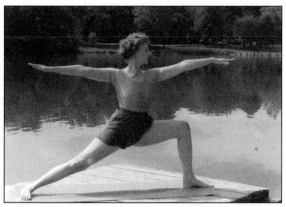

Bring the arms down parallel with the shoulders, Warrior 2. Breathe in strength and confidence. Exhale as you change sides.

Lengthen and Balance

This pose balances, lengthens, and strengthens the body for an infusion of serenity, grace, and confidence for whenever you need it. When you've completed this sequence, repeat, and then end with a few moments in Mountain pose.

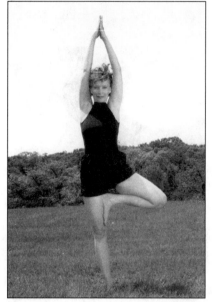

Move into Tree pose, balancing first on one side and then on the other.

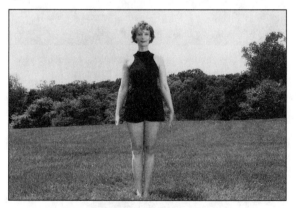

Begin by finding the strength of Mountain pose.

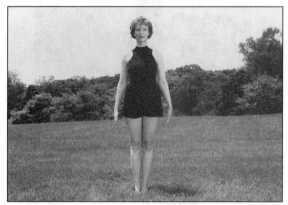

Come back to Mountain and rest for several breaths as you feel your body re-centering.

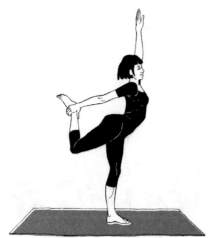

Move into Dancer pose, opening the chest and fully expanding the front of your body. Repeat with the other leg.

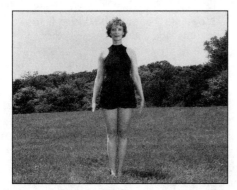

Again, return to Mountain pose, feeling your body re-centering as you breathe.

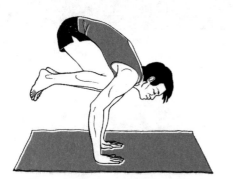

Squat down into Crow pose and feel the front of your body contracting for balance.

Return to Mountain pose.

Yoga in Fifteen Minutes

When you've got a little more time but still not a lot, try any of these three 15-minute yoga sessions. The first will help relax and center you. The second will energize your bodymind and help you gain perspective. The third will pump you up!

Session 1: Calm and Collected

This 15-minute sequence is perfect for relaxing after a long and stressful day or when you've been going too fast for too long and just need to put on the breaks for a precious quarter of an hour.

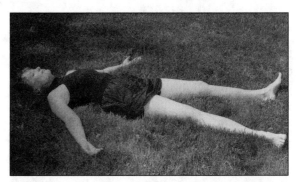

Spend a few minutes in total relaxation, releasing your thoughts and physical tensions.

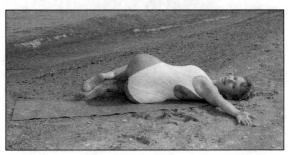

Loosen your spine by drawing your knees straight up and twisting slowly, first one way, then the other. Hold and relax into each side for at least several breaths.

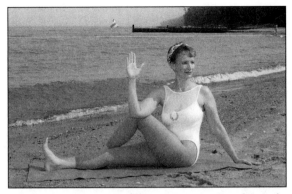

Further lengthen and twist your spine in Seated Spinal Twist, slowly rotating from one side, taking a few breaths there, and then from the other side. Breathe deeply.

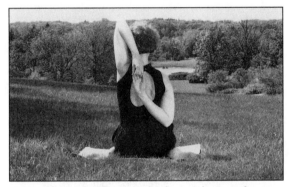

Open your shoulders, expand your chest, and open your hips by doing Cow pose in a cross-legged position.

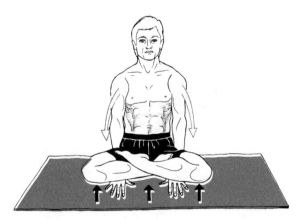

Release your arms to the floor and use your strength to raise your body and crossed legs in *tolasana* or Scales pose.

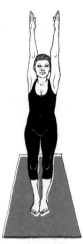

Come to standing and stretch your body out with several deep breaths in Mountain pose with your arms extended.

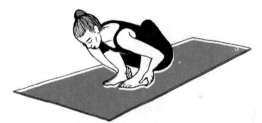

Squat down into Crouching pose and hold your ankles. Breathe!

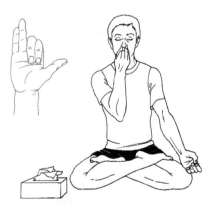

Crossing your legs into a seated meditative pose such as Easy pose or Lotus pose, center yourself through the calming effects of the *pranayama* technique called *nadi shodhana,* or Alternate Nostril Breathing, to bring the emotional and physical aspects of your body into balance.

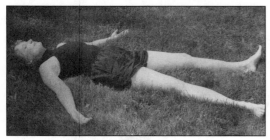

Return to *shavasana* to rest, release, and renew once more.

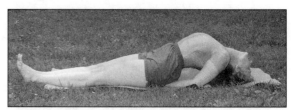

Roll over again and stretch into Half Fish pose, opening your chest, expanding your heart so recently nourished by the inversion against the wall, and stretching those legs so recently folded into Child's pose.

Session 2: Inversion Interest

Take a load off your feet and give yourself a whole new perspective with this 15-minute inversion sequence.

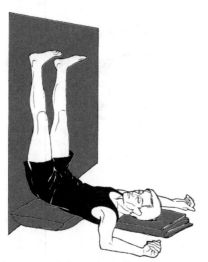

Begin by resting in this position for a few minutes with your legs and feet supported by a wall.

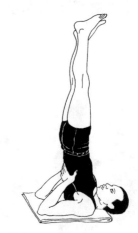

Balance Fish by coming up into Shoulderstand, elevating your legs, relaxing your heart, and nourishing your thyroid.

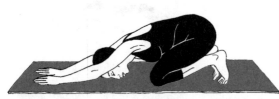

Slowly push yourself away from the wall, roll over, and come into extended Child's pose to balance the stretch of the hamstrings with a gentle contraction of the hamstrings.

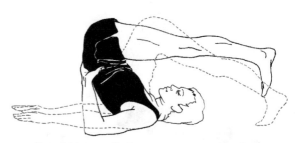

Roll with a controlled movement into Plough pose or *halasana*. Bring your feet back only as far as comfortable so as not to hurt your spine.

Chapter 20: Yoga in Five Minutes or Fifteen Minutes

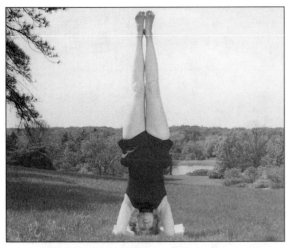

Roll back down from Plough and spend some time in Headstand, the king of all poses. Your mind and heart deserve it!

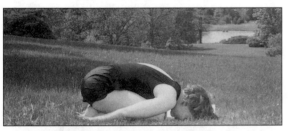

Relax back into Child's pose.

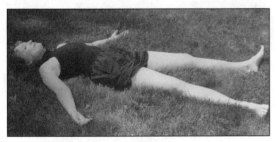

Finally, end with a full relaxation in *shavasana*.

Session 3: Move and Groove

Let this 15-minute session rock your world! It's great for getting geared up before you need to approach a task or project with lots of positive energy, whether it's an office party, a speech in front of your class, or dinner with the in-laws.

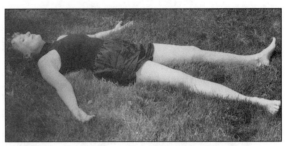

Prepare for this energizing sequence by releasing tensions in order to approach your practice of *vinyasana* calmly.

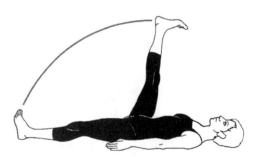

Let your breath guide you in these lifts as you inhale up and exhale down, repeating 12 on each side.

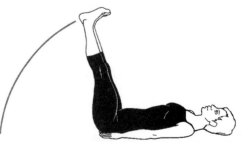

Place your arms under your spine for additional back support if needed and switch to Double Leg Lifts, inhaling up and exhaling down.

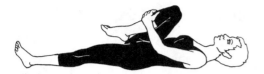

Bend your knees and hold each knee to your chest for several breaths to relax your back.

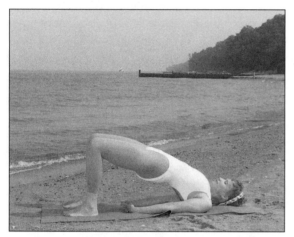

Expand the front part of your body and open your shoulders by lifting your body up into Bridge pose.

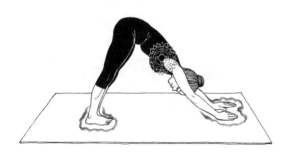

Lower from Bridge, roll over, and go into Downward Facing Dog.

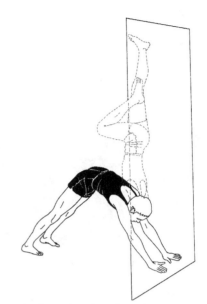

Lift your body up into Handstand. Give your arms a workout in this strength-building balance pose, extending your spine and balancingthe effects of Bridge pose.

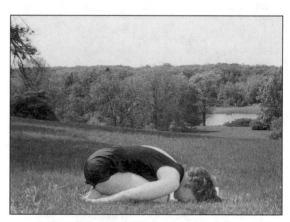

Relax and be nurtured, resting in the universal womb of Child's pose.

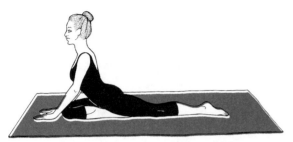

Come back up and stretch one leg straight back into Pigeon pose to open your hips and balance the stretches of this sequence.

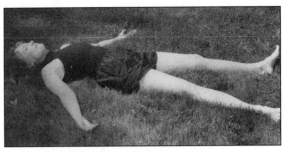

Ahhhh ... relax, release ....

The Least You Need to Know

◆ You don't have to have a lot of time to experience a lot of yoga.

◆ Five-minute yoga sessions can bring you practically instant calm or a burst of energy, and they are easy to fit into any schedule.

◆ Fifteen-minute yoga sessions don't take long, either, but you can accomplish significant stretching, strengthening, and relaxation with these brief yoga sequences.

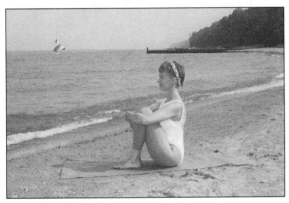

In a final reflection, sit and hold your knees to your chest. Breathe slowly and deeply.

In This Chapter

◆ Spending more time on your yoga sessions allows you to spend more time in poses and relax into total yoga mode

◆ A sample 30-minute yoga session

◆ A sample 60-minute yoga session

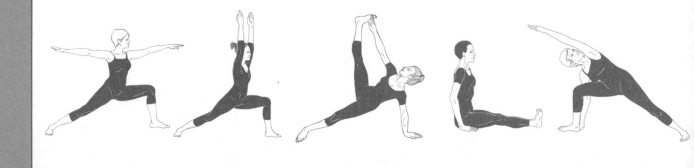

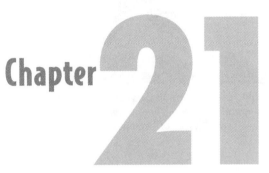

Chapter 21

Yoga in Thirty Minutes or an Hour

Sometimes it's nice to stop hurrying and spend a more dedicated chunk of time on yoga at least once or twice a week. You might enjoy it so much that you'll decide that a daily 30 minutes or an hour are just what you need. These sessions give you time to really sink into your yoga, spend as much time as you need to spend in each pose, and feel supremely and luxuriously *not* rushed.

Thirty-Minute Session: Downward Facing Dog Dig It

We think a 30-minute daily yoga session is the perfect foundation to combine with an hourly yoga class. This amount of time spent in daily practice helps you to maintain your practice and your yoga mindbody balance all week long.

Following is a sample 30-minute session we've put together. The more familiar you become with different yoga poses, the more you will enjoy creating your own 30-minute sessions. You can also ask your yoga teacher for some alternative ideas.

The following is a great all-over balancing series of vigorous yoga postures. It's both relaxing and really feels like exercise (because, of course, it *is* exercise!). We love to do this sequence to wake up in the morning or to counter that late-afternoon sag time.

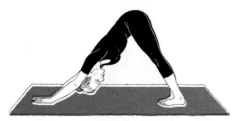

Begin your session with Downward Facing Dog, a great strength-building, spine-lengthening, overall-good-for-beginning stretch.

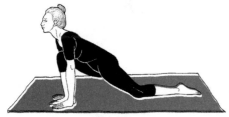

As you exhale, step one leg forward into a Lunge and hold for several breaths.

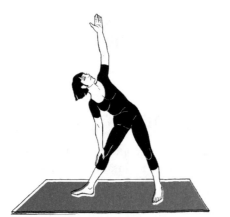

Expand Lunge by twisting to one side and straightening up into Triangle pose.

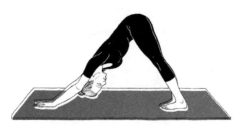

Relax back into Downward Facing Dog, evening the stretch of the spine, then repeat this series of steps on the other side.

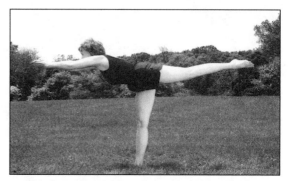

This time, come out of Downward Facing Dog by lunging one foot forward and straightening up into Warrior 3. Hold for several long, deep, expansive breaths.

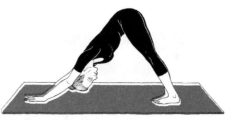

Relax back into the ever-wonderful Downward Facing Dog, then repeat the Warrior 3 sequence on the other side. After completing the sequence on the other side, and from Downward Facing Dog, jump both feet up between your hands on the floor.

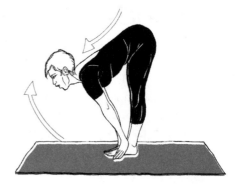

Straighten your torso up into Standing Forward Bend, keeping your head lifted and looking up. Feel the long stretch in your spine and breathe deeply.

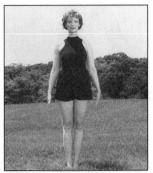

Rise up into Mountain pose and hold, firmly rooted, for a few breaths.

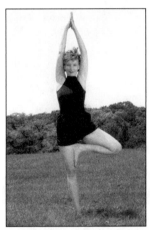

Lift one leg and both arms up to balance in Tree pose, remaining rooted but growing and breathing.

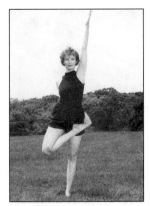

Lower your arms and grasp your foot, moving into Standing Half Bound Lotus. Hold strong and steady, breathing deeply. Repeat Tree and Standing Half Bound Lotus on the other side.

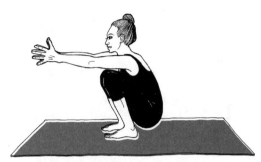

Sink down into Extended Lightning Bolt, radiating energy into all your limbs.

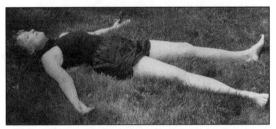

Relax into this final relaxation pose.

Yoga in an Hour: Strength-Building Oasis of Peace

This extended yoga session is similar to what you might encounter in an hour-long yoga class. It builds strength as it builds inner peace. Take your time between poses. Spend as much time as you need to spend in each pose and enjoy the lotus flower opening inside you.

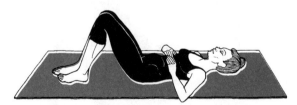

Relax into Corpse pose and pay attention as your lungs expand fully. Feel this expansion by placing your hands over your lower ribs, and try gradually to deepen your breaths.

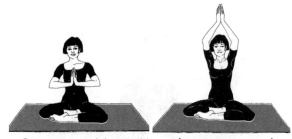

Come up to a sitting position such as Easy pose and work with slow deep breaths, raising and lowering your arms in *namaste mudra*, further opening your chest.

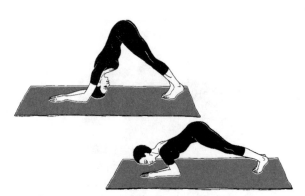

This exercise strengthens your upper arms and shoulders. Coming up into Elbow Dog, alternate your chin coming toward your hands and then back toward your feet. Exhale forward, inhale back in the movement of a Dolphin.

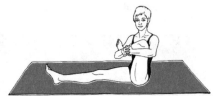

Open the lower part of your body by rocking your lower legs, one at a time, rockin' and rollin' those hips.

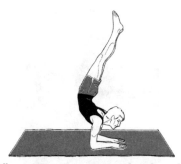

From Elbow Dog, separate your hands, palms flat, bend your knees, walk your legs in close to your hands, and lift your torso and head into Scorpion. If this is too difficult, hold Elbow Dog for several long breaths instead.

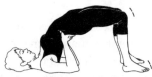

Open your spine through this Expanded Spinal Twist, twisting on both sides.

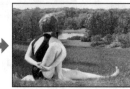

Relax back and let your inhale guide you into Bridge pose. Breathe deeply.

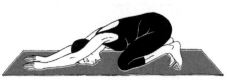

Relax back into Child's pose with your arms stretched out in front of you to lengthen your spine.

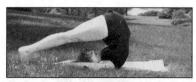

Lower back to the floor and roll your legs over your head, lengthening and stretching your spine fully into Plough pose. Extend your arms to touch your feet. Breathe, hold for at least several breaths, then roll back up onto your heels.

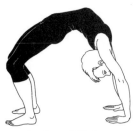

Roll over onto your back and lift the center of your body. Imagine a string connected to your navel, lifting you up into the shape of a wheel.

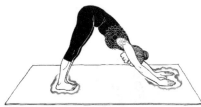

Lower your body to the ground, roll over again, and come up into Downward Facing Dog. Feel the heat in your body as you balance the energizing effects of Downward Facing Dog by further lengthening your spine.

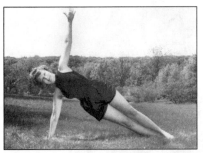

Turn your body to the side and balance on your strong arms, lengthening and straightening your body so it makes an angle with the floor. Repeat on the opposite side, coming into Downward Facing Dog in between sides.

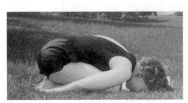

Come back down again into Child's pose, this time with your arms alongside your body. Relax.

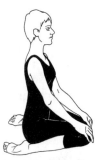

Sit up into Hero pose. If your tailbone can touch the ground, try relaxing back into it for a fuller quadriceps stretch.

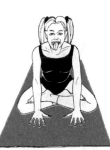

Come back up into a release of your body in Lion's pose, either in Lotus or remaining on your knees in Hero, and roar.

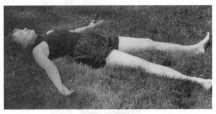

Purrr back down to the floor, and relax into *shavasana*.

The Least You Need to Know

◆ A daily 30- or 60-minute yoga session will keep you centered and your mindbodyspirit in balance.

◆ A 30-minute yoga session is a good way to support a weekly hour-long yoga class.

◆ Have to miss yoga class this week? Do one or two hour-long sessions for an almost-as-good-as-class mindbody workout.

In This Part

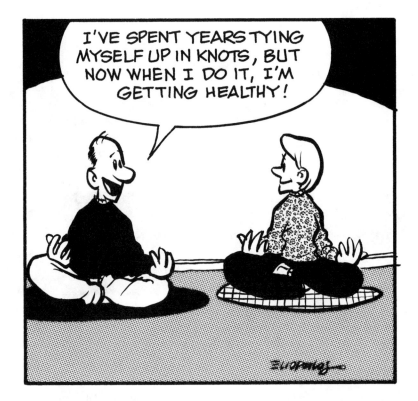

Part 7

Living Your Yoga

Yoga doesn't exist in a vacuum, and neither do you. Yoga is designed not for a single, isolated practice, but as a way of life, and this part will show you how to incorporate the yoga way into your daily existence with partner yoga or yoga with your family and children. We'll devote a section to the unique needs, strengths, and challenges of women (from PMS to postpartum depression to menopause and beyond) and the yoga poses to accompany those issues.

Next, we discuss diet and how what you eat can affect who you are. Yoga divides foods into three categories: *sattvic*, *rajasic*, and *tamasic*. Find out which category your favorite foods belong to and how they might be helping or hindering your physical and mental well-being.

Last, you'll read about how different postures and other yoga lifestyle changes can help you with various minor complaints, such as headaches or stomachaches, and even how you can help your body help itself when you suffer from more serious health conditions such as arthritis or heart disease. Make yoga a part of your health and vitality. You'll be glad you did!

In This Chapter

- How yoga is different when practiced in pairs

- Great postures for partners

- How yoga can make all your relationships—even the sexual ones—more spiritual

- Meditation for two

- Yoga for kids and families

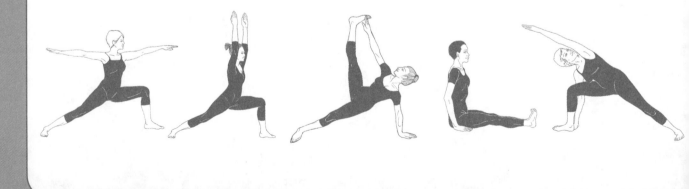

Chapter 22

Partner Yoga: For Two—or More!

Why practice yoga with anyone else? Isn't yoga a solitary and self-reflective pursuit? Yes, it is. But the journey can also involve spiritual communion between two bodies and two souls. Also, postures you can perform alone can be modified or performed more deeply or intensely when someone else helps you. Plus, practicing yoga with a friend, partner, or spouse can deepen your relationship, because you'll be undertaking at least certain paths of your yoga journey hand in hand.

Double Your Insight

Finding wholeness and balance within yourself is important. However, because you probably aren't a hermit living alone in a cave or on a mountaintop, it's also important to find wholeness and balance in your relationships. Practicing yoga with a fellow yogi can expand your sense of balance and improve your relationship, not only with your yoga partner but with all your fellow earthlings.

Double yoga helps unfold your awareness, so it blankets your entire household, community, country, and planet. It gives you insight into the journeys, desires, suffering, and joy of others. It helps you understand that every human being is as complex, interesting, and beautiful as you are. It is also an excellent way to bond together, physically and spiritually, in a partnership. Try yoga with the man or woman you love and add a whole new dimension to your practice.

Postures for Partners: Part 1

So let's try a few! Grab (nonviolently, of course!) your spouse, partner, child, or friend, and try this set of postures for partners.

Be a Mountain Range

A first and easy posture to try is Mountain pose, but because there are two of you, let's make it a mountain range. This is also a nice pose to do with the whole family! The more people involved, the longer your mountain range!

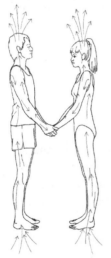

Be a mountain range.

1. Face your partner, standing about two feet apart, and close your eyes. This distance is close enough to allow you to sense each other and to hold hands without arm strain, but far enough away to allow you to maintain a sense of your own space.

2. After you're both centered, hold hands. Take some time to become aware of your partner across from you (keep your eyes closed). Feel your partner's form and energy, then feel the energy flow between you as it traverses the bridge made from your joined hands.

3. Next, connect with the grounding energy of the earth. Feel how it pulls you toward its center. Feel your feet and legs connecting and becoming one with the earth.

4. Let the earth's energy move through your body, from toe to head and beyond, and through your joined hands so you and your partner are joined with the earthlike mountains.

5. **Yoga Adventure:** For more than two people, stand side by side in Mountain pose, holding hands, and feet lined up. You can also stand with your legs about two feet apart so the sides of each person's foot stands firmly against the side of the next person's foot.

Warrior 2 Pose for Two

This pose will help you find balance with a partner. In the process, you'll both become stronger.

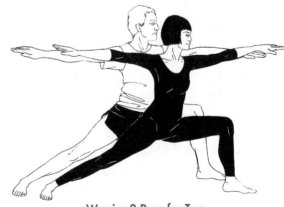

Warrior 2 Pose for Two.

1. Stand with one of you in front (Partner A) and one behind (Partner B). Both perform the Warrior 2 pose (Chapter 11). Once you are both in position, Partner A balances the extended arms and hands on top of the back of Partner B's extended arms, forming a chain of energy.

2. Partner B keeps Partner A's arms and hands at shoulder height. Partner B will expend more effort, but Partner A should keep the arms energized and strong rather than let them sag limply on Partner B's. Partner B should be supporting an energy flow, not a limp noodle.

3. Switch sides. Now Partner A holds Partner B's arms up. Breathe. Try to increase the length of time holding the pose. Encourage each other to hang in there. This pose is difficult and builds arm strength in addition to doubling the warrior energy.

Stretch and Pull

Both partners receive a nice spine stretch in this pose for two.

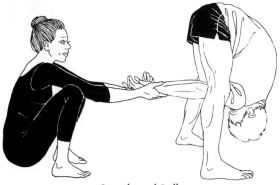

Stretch and Pull.

1. Again, stand with one partner in front (Partner A) and one behind (Partner B). Partner B squats with heels on the floor. Partner A performs a forward bend, keeping the knees straight or slightly bending them and folding the torso forward at the hips. Partner A should be able to see Partner B between his or her legs. (Peek-a-boo!)

2. Partner A reaches both hands between the legs, and Partner B grasps Partner A's wrists, pulling slightly to help Partner A stretch.

3. At the same time, Partner B bends down into a full squat, stretching the back.

4. Hold and take some breaths.

5. Switch places and do it again.

Lengthen Your Spines Together

Continue to lengthen the spine—maybe even grow an inch with this one!

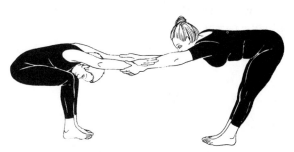

Lengthen Your Spines Together.

1. Face each other, hold hands, then take a big step away from each other.

2. Bend at your hips, but don't clunk heads! Be sure to step far enough away from each other that you don't collide.

3. Bring your tailbones up and out. Take turns pulling gently on each other to lengthen your spines.

4. Then find a balance—pull—and both of you come down into a squat. Keep your heels on the ground. Stretch those spines.

5. Slowly come back up, balancing and stretching all the way back to standing.

Ouch! _____

When you're helping someone else stretch (or he or she is helping you), keep the lines of communication open. You can't feel when someone else is starting to hurt (unless you're extremely attuned), so let each other know when you're being pushed or pulled just far enough.

The "S" in Sex Stands for "Spirituality"

Practicing yoga with your partner can deepen all aspects of your relationship, even your physical relationship. When practicing "couples yoga" with your partner or spouse, don't simply hold the positions. Take full advantage of your partner's proximity. Feel your partner's energy, body shape, and movement.

A Yoga Minute _____

Mae West once said, "Sex is an emotion in motion." How true! One of the benefits of the fourth _yama_, _brahmacharya_ (see Chapter 6), is that it teaches you to separate lust from a purer, spiritual connection. When you're fraught with emotional desire for the physical, you cannot perceive a deeper reality. Transcending intense emotions permits the spirit to manifest itself.

Truly connecting with your partner on a spiritual level is a much more blissful experience than physical connection void of any emotional or spiritual bond. It can even be a bit alarming if you aren't used to really knowing someone on this level, because souls are much more sensitive than bodies. This is a goal you can work toward when practicing yoga with your partner. Physical intimacy may seem mighty intimate, but it can also lack intimacy without a deeper bond.

Problems in your relationship might surface, too, as you work together in different postures. You should be prepared for this possibility. Your bodies can reflect your minds, so when you have difficulty with a double posture, look into what's wrong and see if you can't find what's happening on a deeper level. Working through the barriers in your physical partnership can reveal the barriers in your spiritual partnership. Take the lessons you learn about each other into your hearts and memorize them. They're lessons in true love!

Postures for Partners: Part 2

Double yoga is a fun way to exercise your relationships. Let's try a few more poses for two.

Massage Your Spines Together

This pose will help your partner connect to the muscles along the spine. A flexible spine equals a youthful body. Help your partner loosen up his or her spine.

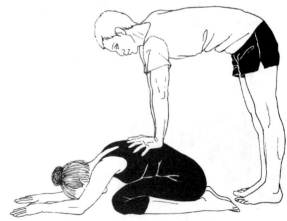

Massage Your Spines Together.

1. Partner A sits in Child's pose (see Chapter 17).

2. Partner B stands behind Partner A and places a palm on either side of Partner A's spine at the lower back. Partner B

gradually walks the hands up to the neck and back down to the lower back. Partner B keeps as much of the palm on Partner A's back as possible at all times, pressing gently. Don't press directly on the spine; stay on either side.

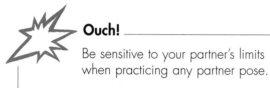

Ouch!

Be sensitive to your partner's limits when practicing any partner pose.

Forward Bend Together

This pose starts to look complicated, but it really isn't. It's only two poses in one. Partner B helps Partner A lengthen the spine by pushing down on Partner A's hipbone. Conversely, Partner A helps Partner B lengthen the hamstrings by pushing down on Partner B's heels.

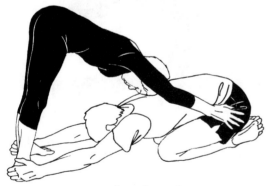

Forward Bend Together.

1. Partner A gets into Child's pose with arms outstretched in front (Chapter 17).

2. Partner B stands in front of Partner A. Partner A holds Partner B's ankles as Partner B assumes Downward Facing Dog (Chapter 17) over the top of Partner A, placing the hands on either side of Partner A's hips, palms facing in.

3. Partner B helps Partner A lengthen the spine, while Partner A helps Partner B lengthen the hamstrings.

4. Hold as long as is comfortable, then switch positions.

Forward Bend and Backbend Together

Try this one with a partner who is about the same size as you are. If one of you is much larger, he or she should be Partner A, and the positions shouldn't be reversed.

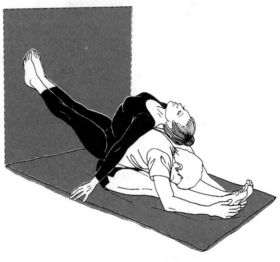

Forward Bend and Backbend Together.

1. Partner A sits on the floor a few feet from a wall with the back to the wall and the feet in front and together. Bending at the waist, Partner A brings the chest toward the thighs. Bend your knees if needed.

2. Partner B lies on Partner A's back, facing up, and props the feet against the wall so that the feet are slightly higher than the head. Partner B's fingers can rest lightly on the ground on either side of Partner A's hips.

3. Hold for a while, then switch.

Hero Pose for Two

Who says heroes can't come in pairs? This pose retains the tall, proud posture of Hero pose but lets two in on the fun.

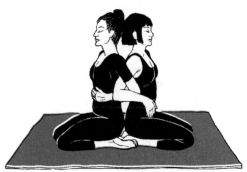

Hero Pose for Two with locked arms.

1. Sit in Hero pose, back to back.
2. Link arms and pull gently to further expand the chest and breathing area.
3. As you both breathe, feel your spine and head stretching upward, and feel your partner doing the same thing.
4. Notice how deeply you are able to breathe together.

Boat Pose for Two

Boat Pose for Two helps calm the rocky waters and strengthens tummies, too (or two!).

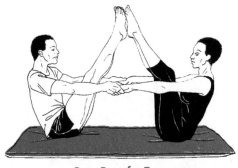

Boat Pose for Two.

1. Face each other so your hips are three to four feet apart. Both partners assume Boat pose (Chapter 17).
2. Place your feet sole to sole, and grasp hands on the outsides of your legs. Now you look like a schooner!

Modified Shoulderstand for Two

This energizing and supportive inversion brings two energies together in a vibrant flow. You'll feel great after this pose, and more energetically linked to your partner. You can also do this pose in a triad or in a group of four. Just put your heads together and touch toes.

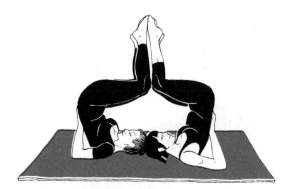

Modified Shoulderstand for Two.

1. Lie down so the crowns of your heads are barely touching.
2. Gently raise your legs and hips, supporting your hips with your arms.
3. Bend your knees over your head and tilt back until you feel your partner's legs. Rest your lower legs against each other.
4. Hold until one or both of you are ready to come back down.

Wise Yogi Tells Us

Try double heart gazing to connect your heart *chakras*. Sit facing each other in any meditative pose with your knees touching. Look into each other's eyes. Really look, past the surface. Place your right hand on your partner's heart, and have your partner place his or her right hand on your heart. Then each partner covers his or her own heart (and the partner's right hand) with the left hand. Feel the energy flowing between your heart *chakras*, connecting you to each other. Close your eyes and continue to feel the energy.

Partner Tree

Balance the inverted Shoulderstand for two with this upright standing pose. This pose is a balance pose, yet the partnership makes it incredibly stable and grounding.

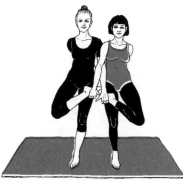

Partner Tree.

1. Stand side by side, shoulders touching or a couple inches apart.
2. Each partner bends outside knees and brings feet up.
3. Clasp each other's feet and bring opposite hands behind you. Hold opposite hands together.

Don't miss out on the great physical, emotional, and spiritual benefits of yoga for two. This type of workout is an enriching complement to your solo yoga practice and can be very fulfilling. Vary your solitary communion with one of fellowship. Partner yoga will increase your joy.

Yokids

Kids take naturally to yoga because it's so much fun. Getting the whole family involved in a yoga routine is a great way to keep you motivated. When your whole family practices yoga together, the family bond is strengthened. Everyone learns more about the other family members—what they can and can't do, what they like and dislike, and how they like to play. Love is built on intimacy like this, and yoga offers the perfect environment to cultivate and nurture family intimacy.

Turn Off the TV and Play!

Kids today watch a lot of television and play a lot of video games. Sure, some television is stimulating and offers children valuable information. But healthy kids are built from exercise, nutritious food, and imaginative play. Encourage your kids to turn off the tube and get moving, using both their bodies and their minds more actively. Interacting with you and with each other (other siblings or friends) builds children's social skills and teaches them much more about the world than any half-hour sitcom or 60-minute talk show.

The Lessons Yoga Teaches Kids

Yoga teaches kids valuable lessons about life. You'll probably teach your children all the following in one way or another, but yoga can deepen and reinforce all these healthy and life-affirming ideas:

- Exercise is fun!
- Exercise equals active play.
- When the body and the mind combine into imagination, there are no limits.

- Things that are good for you don't have to be unpleasant—they can actually be the highlights of your day!

- "Feeling" like different animals and objects such as trees makes children more sensitive, not only to their own bodies, but to all our fellow inhabitants of the earth.

- Families who play well together, grow well together.

- The earth and all its creatures have a lot to teach us about how to move and how to live.

- Sometimes it's fun to be quiet, still, and reflective.

- Kids can learn to be patient, too.

- Your body is your friend, ally, and instrument.

Yoga for All Ages and Stages

Yoga is both fun and beneficial for kids of any age. You can do yoga with your newborn infant, your toddler, your preschooler, your kindergartner, your fourth-grader, your eighth-grader, your high school sophomore, or your high school graduate. Older kids often enjoy establishing and growing in an individual yoga practice, too. If you've set them on the yoga path, chances are they'll continue it on their own. What a great gift to give your child!

But yoga is a little different, depending on the age of your child. Infant yoga is, naturally, a completely different kind of practice than yoga for teens. In general, encourage younger kids to talk, respond, and flex their imaginations while practicing yoga. Teens might appreciate a more internalized practice, or maybe not, if they are practicing yoga with a group of friends.

Let's look briefly at some yoga approaches for kids of all ages. Also feel free to adapt any of the basic poses in this book in ways that are fun (and safe) for your child's developmental level.

Wise Yogi Tells Us

Let your children's yoga workout be fun and full of communication when they need it so they can get the most out of each pose, and you'll have a better idea of how they're doing, what they do and don't understand, and how you can best progress with them. When yoga is a family affair, everyone stays in better touch.

Baby Love

Babies are great for cuddling, but they make great yogis, too! Babies do some yoga poses all on their own—like Cobra pose, when they look up from a prone position to find the source of a noise. Babies naturally push and test their bodies so they can develop their muscles, mobility, coordination, and dexterity. And you can help your infant optimize this development with some simple moves that can help get her accustomed to the idea of touch, play, and movement. Have fun; listen to your baby; and keep the attitude loving, gentle, and responsive.

Put your daughter on her back on a blanket, smile, tell her you are going to move together with nature, then gently take one of her feet in your hand. Wiggle each toe, flex and point her foot, rotate her ankle, flex and straighten her knee, flex and straighten her hip. Move her leg ever so gently around and around. Her leg is moving like butterfly wings, gently and softly. Tell her all about it! Have fun! Then do the same thing on the other leg and each arm. Let your imagination suggest ideas for what your baby's arms and legs could be as you move each limb through its range of motion—a slithery snake, a regal flamingo. Through your words and kind movements, your baby will be introduced to the glory of nature.

Turn your baby gently onto her stomach and, using a rattle or your voice, make a noise above her head until she moves her eyes or head, or (if developmentally appropriate) she pushes herself up to see what all the commotion is about. Let her see you or the rattle, and smile. Cobra pose!

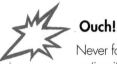

Ouch!

Never force your baby's body in a direction it doesn't want to go. Also pay attention to your baby's response to movement. If he or she isn't in the mood, try again later.

Babies can even do *shavasana!* Place your child on her back and give a gentle massage, starting at her feet and working your way around her limbs, then gently rubbing her delicate chest, tummy, and head. Ah, now that's one relaxed baby! (*Shh*—lights out!)

Toddler Time!

Toddlers are finally able to explore nature on their own, although occasionally they will need help from you to figure out how move. Toddlers love to move, make noise, and expend that immense toddler energy. Who knows—if you set an example in your movements, you might end up with fewer tantrums on your hands (for you and your baby)!

Here are a few fun toddler poses to try:

◆ **A Roar, and More!** Everyone get on your hands and knees, sit back on your heels, stick our your tongue as far as possible, and look up. You're all lions, so everybody roar!

◆ **Hop to It!** Everyone squat down on the floor and hop around like frogs. A few "ribbits" offered up to the heavens never hurt anyone.

◆ **Flower Power.** Everyone curl up on the ground like seeds, then imagine being watered and the sun shining. Slowly expand, then rise up out of the ground. Slowly, now! Gradually get taller and taller until head, face, and arms open up into a beautiful bloom.

Peppy Preschoolers

Preschoolers have super-powered imaginations and are developing the coordination, flexibility, and balance to accomplish even more yoga poses. Although preschoolers would also enjoy the toddler poses in the preceding section, the following poses are great fun for preschoolers, too, and use preschool skills toddlers haven't quite mastered.

◆ **Mountain's Majesty.** Stand as in the classic Mountain pose. Ask your kids what it feels like to be a mountain. What kind of mountain are they? Rocky and imposing? Rounded, green foothills? Volcano? Is anybody about to explode?

◆ **Be the Tree.** Everyone stand firmly rooted with both feet on the ground (unlike the classic Tree pose on one foot). Now let your kids feel how the weather is gradually changing: from sunny and still, to windy, to blustery, to an all-out thunderstorm. How do all the trees shift and move with the weather? Have everyone make appropriate wind and leaf-rustling sounds. Is that a tornado? *Woahhhhh!* (Don't be surprised if a few trees fall over!)

◆ **Leg Lifts at Sea.** Everyone lies on their backs. Have each child raise one leg up and breathe in. Then, have each child lower the leg down as they breathe out. As they continue doing this, have them imagine they are at the beach. When they breathe, you hear the waves coming in and going out. Close your eyes, and soon you will all be at the beach. What a beautiful time together you're all having as the sounds of their breaths become stronger and the waves become fuller.

◆ **Dogs and Cats.** Have a group of children form a circle in Downward Dog pose. Choose one or two children to crawl under the children in Downward Dog pose and pretend they are kitties. Meow! See if the dogs can stay up and strong as the little kitties travel underneath the doggies. Tell the doggies to say "Ruff" when the kitty comes underneath them. This will make the kitty move faster! The kitty can relax and do a Cat stretch between each dog.

Yoga K-6

Kids in grade school are learning machines, so you can take advantage of those burgeoning minds to really expand the possibilities of a yoga practice. As kids progress through grade school, they become increasingly independent, but try to continue practicing with them. A family who practices yoga together is making memories to last a lifetime!

Try these next two poses with younger grade-school kids. Kindergartners enjoy them.

- **For the Birds.** Each person choose a type of bird, then practice standing, hopping, and flying like that bird. Notice how a sparrow is different from a great blue heron, a mockingbird different from a vulture, a hummingbird different from an eagle. (And remind your kids—birds don't bump into each other!)
- **Circle of Peace.** Sitting cross-legged in a circle, cross your arms in front of you, and hold hands with the person next to you. Close your eyes. Inhale love and exhale peace. Do this several times, then begin to bend your body forward on peace. Inhale up love, exhale down peace. This is similar to yoga *mudra* pose—the pose of yoga, a pose to help your family connect more deeply to each other and to the world around them.
- **Boats on Waves of Wonder.** Start out on your backs, with your knees bent in, holding on to your knees. Rock back and forth, massaging your spine. As you rock steadily, you are able to rock fuller. Gradually, you come up into Boat pose and hold. When you are ready to let go, roll back down and rock again, then come

up again. Watch the family of boats move along the rocky waters, every so often coming into the strong calm of Boat pose, then going back to ride the waves again.

- **Fly Like an Eagle.** Standing straight in Mountain, bend your knees and bring your arms out to shoulder height. Fly the way an eagle does with his strong wings. Pull your arms (wings) in to your body and wrap them around each other. As you do this, simultaneously wrap one leg around the other. Now you are standing as an eagle stands when its relaxed—strong and majestically balanced. When you loosen your footing, bring your wings out and try again.

Invent your own nature poses. The possibilities are endless.

> **Ouch!**
>
> Kids taking the significant step of starting grade school might be under pressures adults aren't aware of. No longer under our watchful eyes, they can suffer from peer pressure, pressure to succeed, and learning problems—even in kindergarten! Let yoga be a bridge between you and your grade-schooler. It will help your child handle stress and keep the lines of communication open between you.

Kids can also learn breathing exercises, but keep them simple. Have kids rest their hands on your stomach to feel how your stomach moves gently when you bring your breath lower. Then have them try this on each other. Ask them if they remember when they were sleeping in the crib and their tummies moved up and down. Ask them to pretend they are in the crib now.

Kids can even meditate! Have kids sit quietly and focus on a pleasant part of nature, like a flower, a butterfly, a tree. At first, rather than stress the absence of thought, suggest that your kids focus on one single beautiful feeling, such as love, happiness, or peacefulness. When thoughts arise, refocus on how the feeling *feels* instead. Imagine a happy tree, a sensitive butterfly, or an open flower. Tell the children to join in the beautiful feelings of nature. Afterward, discuss what they came up with. Children are master yogis. You might learn a lot from them.

Teen Yogis

Teenagers can gain great benefits from a regular yoga practice, which will help keep them physically fit, strong, flexible, and confident. The self-esteem teens can gain from yoga might be the most important benefit of all. Yoga can also help kids develop self-discipline and gain control over their bodies, which are subject to intense hormonal fluctuations and strong emotions during these years.

Teens can do any of the yoga poses adults can do and often more of them, because teens still have a degree of flexibility adults have allowed to slip away. Encourage your teens to read this book and work through it—with you, on their own, or both. Let yoga be a connection between the two of you and an avenue for communication. Even if they don't always show it, your teens want to connect with you and need to maintain that bond as they move toward becoming adults themselves.

Family Yoga

Lots of yoga poses can be adapted to become group poses. The gentleness and focus you bring to your practice will be seen by your children. You are the best example. Let your peace radiate within you. Let your acceptance of yourself transfer into a nonjudgmental, open vessel and a beacon of peace for your children. There are so many stresses in our lives in this modern world. Let yoga be an opportunity for you and your family to come together without expectations. Come together in peace, and let the movement of your breath together guide you all into ever-deepening understandings and expressions of love between you.

As you travel through poses, together or alone, end your family yoga session together as one. Sitting cross-legged together, each person brings their hands together in front of their chest in *namaste* (prayer) *mudra*. Close your eyes and inhale deeply together. As you exhale, sing "*Shanti, shanti, shanti*" together as a family, then slowly open your eyes and say "*Namaste*. The light within me honors the light within you." Say it with deep meaning and an appreciation for its truth. Whatever difficult roads we might travel as a family, yoga brings us all together with reverence, as one.

> **Ouch!**
>
> Fun yoga now could mean a lifetime love of yoga. Yoga that is boring or authoritarian might turn kids off for good. Never push a child into a pose or into doing yoga. Let your love and joy for your own practice be the motivation for your children to want to discover this on their own. Kids love to play. Poses can be playful. You might want to try more playfulness with your own yoga practice, too! Have fun!

The Least You Need to Know

◆ Practicing yoga with a partner is fun and can deepen your relationship, making all aspects of your partnership—physical, emotional, and intellectual—more spiritual.

◆ Practicing yoga with a partner can help you stretch farther than you could alone.

◆ Kids of all ages can experience yoga and learn to love it for a lifetime.

◆ Practice yoga as a family to build memories that will last a lifetime.

In This Chapter

- ◆ What is beauty?
- ◆ How yoga can help you through PMS and menstruation
- ◆ Yoga for pregnant and new mothers
- ◆ Yoga for menopause

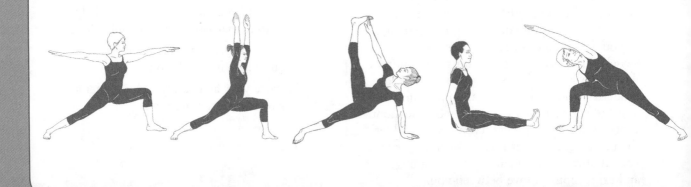

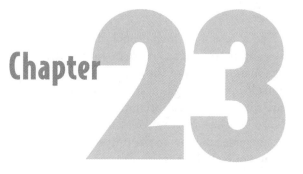

Chapter

For Women Only

This chapter is for all you female yoginis out there! Being a woman means certain things biologically and certain things culturally, too. We experience menstruation as our first rite of passage into womanhood, many of us experience childbirth, and eventually we all experience menopause. We're also raised in a culture obsessed with beauty, youth, and the female body. Women have many unique challenges, and yoga can help with all of them by helping keep us fit, strong, clear-thinking, and joyful.

The Truth About Beauty

Beauty really isn't skin-deep. In fact, it has nothing to do with your skin—not really. Beauty begins much deeper, so it's no wonder that many beautiful women don't believe they're beautiful. If you haven't found your inner self and aren't in touch with who you are, you won't be able to perceive your true beauty, even if you just signed a modeling contract. Your inner beauty has nothing to do with your hair color or facial wrinkles or cellulite or breast size. These are transitory features of your soul's container. These aren't you.

The most important first step any woman can take in dealing with the issue of beauty is to practice *ahimsa*, or nonviolence. Nonviolent acceptance of yourself, not only physically but mentally and spiritually, is yoga's dictum. Don't commit violence to your body, either physically, by trying to force it to conform to some cultural ideal, or mentally, by hating it or obsessing over it. Remember that your body is a tool. Keep it well maintained so it doesn't interfere with the real you. Keep it clean, strong, and flexible, but also keep it in its place.

The true you is much deeper, more complex, and more spectacular than your body. You are a manifestation of the universe. Finding yourself through yoga means finding the beautiful, spiritual you and bringing it out for everyone to see. Loving yourself means loving the universe, and loving the universe means loving yourself, because you're one and the same: You're both exquisitely radiant.

Managing PMS with Yoga

When you're suffering from PMS, you probably don't feel very radiant. PMS, or premenstrual syndrome, is a condition that affects a lot of women before the onset of their menstrual periods. Symptoms are as diverse as overall discomfort, bloating, backache, headache, irritability, food cravings, depression, exaggerated emotions or sudden lack of emotion, acne, painful or swollen breasts, insomnia, fatigue, even uncharacteristically violent or suicidal behavior. Some women get emotional, uncomfortable, or hungrier, yet everyone is different, and each woman may experience different symptoms from month to month. Many women experience no symptoms at all.

Wise Yogi Tells Us

Most women need extra calcium all month long, but many of us don't get the 1,000 mg per day we really need. Recent studies show that increased calcium intake can dramatically relieve some of the uncomfortable symptoms of PMS, so make sure that when it's that time of the month, you've "got milk" (or at least, calcium supplements!).

PMS commonly occurs during the week or two before the start of your period and can last until menstruation starts. You might notice a dramatic disappearance of symptoms, which can signal when menstruation is just about to begin (handy for the irregularly cycled among us). Symptoms are generally attributed to the production of hormones related to the menstrual cycle. You might not care about the cause so much as a good remedy when you're in the throes.

How can yoga help? Be dedicated to your regular yoga routine during PMS. Your hormone-wracked body will appreciate the familiar routine and the exercise. Triangle pose, sitting poses to open the hips, and twisting poses for lower back stiffness are all excellent for PMS. Although all the *asanas* activate the body, poses that stimulate the glandular and reproductive systems such as Cobra, Bow, and Bridge poses are good to practice during PMS.

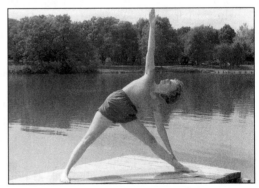

Triangle pose can help relieve lower back and hip pain associated with PMS.

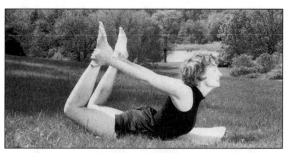

Bow pose can help relieve abdominal cramps associated with menstruation.

Wise Yogi Tells Us

When you're feeling particularly PMS-y, lie on your back with your buttocks against a wall. Put your legs up against the wall, separate them a bit, and lie there for a while—very relaxing.

Also, step up your *pranayama* practice. As your body sheds its uterine lining, support it by cleansing the rest of your body through *pranayama* (deep-breathing exercises). *Pranayama* also eases irritability, depression, and moodiness. *Mantra* work, too, can be of great benefit when your emotions are changing rapidly. The steady flow and vibration of a *mantra* soothes your nervous system and can help transform negative outbursts into outbursts of pure inspiration!

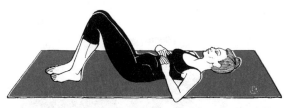

Stressed from PMS? Relax. Breathe deeply. Go with the flow (so to speak!).

Wise Yogi Tells Us

Evening primrose oil, dong quai, blessed thistle, cayenne, raspberry leaves, sarsaparilla, and Siberian ginseng are herbs known to help relieve symptoms of PMS such as bloating, pain, and depression. Look for these herbs in your local health food store, and take as directed.

And no matter how bad PMS is, stress only makes it worse—just one more reason to keep practicing yoga! All the stress-reduction benefits of yoga can also help lessen the effects of PMS. Don't forget *shavasana* (the relaxation pose in Chapter 18)—do it as often as you can. When you are feeling physically or emotionally uncomfortable, you'll welcome *shavasana*'s utterly relaxed state, especially when you get so relaxed that you don't even feel your body anymore!

Meditation, too, can be helpful when you are uncomfortable but in a good frame of mind. Meditation, including *shavasana*, can help you move beyond your physical body for a while and give you a break from your body's aches and pains.

Going Full Cycle: Celebrating Menstruation

Some women are pleased by the arrival of their menstrual period each month—or so we hear. Most of us are a little miffed. *This again?* we think. *Why do I have to go through this every month?!* Do you really want to know?

Technically speaking, menstruation is part of your body's fertility cycle. About every month, from puberty to menopause, your womb first builds up nourishment for a potential embryo and, after ovulation, if pregnancy has not occurred, sheds this tissue in a self-cleansing process before beginning to prepare anew for next month's cycle. All of this happens because of the work of your hormones, which fluctuate throughout the month but seem to cause the most trouble in terms of discomfort during the premenstrual period.

Ouch!

PMS can literally be a big pain, and eating certain foods just before you expect PMS symptoms can make it worse. Even if you crave them, try to avoid chocolate, anything with caffeine, alcohol, excess salt, red meat, sugar, and overly processed foods, which seem to aggravate PMS symptoms in some women. Focus on calcium and fiber instead. A fresh apple and a glass of milk, anyone?

But that's not really what you mean when you wonder why you have to go through menstruation—we know that. We're just trying to remind you what it's all about. Your menstrual cycle sets you apart as a woman. (Well, it isn't the *only* clue, but it's certainly an unmistakable one!) Menstruation is a monthly marker of fertility and one of the few biologically imposed rituals we, as women, have.

Women have often been compared to the moon, probably because we both operate in cycles. Study the moon for a few months, watching it nightly as its lighted section swells, then shrinks each month. Feel a kinship with the moon. See if you can notice its effect on you. Do you feel different during a full moon than during a new moon? How does your menstrual cycle synchronize with the moon's cycle? Pay attention to the beautiful regularity of the moon's waxing and waning, then carry that reverence over to your own body. Your cycle is similarly splendid—even if it doesn't always feel that way.

Wise Yogi Tells Us

Rather than fighting gravity, yoga makes a friend of gravity. So during those times when we want to encourage movement out of the body, such as during menstruation, it's counterproductive to work against gravity by practicing inversions like the Headstand or the Plough. Thank gravity for helping your body with its monthly "out with the old, in with the new" process and do not overly extend inversions during this time.

Incorporating yoga into your menstrual ritual is a nice way to make the experience even more positive. You can do most yoga postures you normally do (listen to your body especially well during this sensitive time, and enjoy a nice, relaxing rest on the floor with your legs and feet up against the wall), but you might enjoy creating a special yoga routine for the week of your menstrual period. Try the following variations of poses for your menstrual cycle sessions.

An extra-long *shavasana* is the perfect way to end your yoga practice during your menstrual cycle.

You might also want to experiment with Triangle, Cobra, Bow (great for cramps if you're up to it, and very energizing), Wheel (also great for cramps), Bridge, Butterfly, Lotus, and Moon Salutation. These are all just suggestions to help make this cycle a more comfortable one.

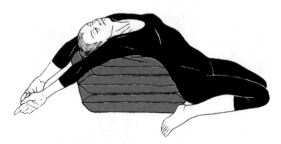

A modified Child's pose eases menstruation or brings comfort during pregnancy.

1. Sit in Hero, Butterfly, or Lotus pose. Place a few pillows stacked on top of each other directly behind you. Lie back on top of the pillows. Extend your arms over your head. This position opens the Venus *chakra* and is also a good variation to perform during pregnancy.

2. Sit with your feet in front of you, widely separated. Place a few pillows stacked on top of each other in front of your navel. Bend forward, bringing your hands toward your feet.

So You're Having a Baby!

Pregnancy yoga is slightly different than regular yoga, and perhaps even more wonderful. Yoga helps you develop a greater awareness of your body so you can respond better to your body's subtle signals (such as *You're doing too much today* or *You need to get up and move today* or *You could really use a hearty serving of broccoli today*).

Because yoga gets you moving, you'll be in better shape for the hard work of labor. Recovery and getting back to your prepregnancy shape will be easier, too. Taking a prenatal yoga class can be a lot of fun. You'll get to meet similarly minded pregnant women, you'll get qualified instruction on the safest and most beneficial yoga poses, and you might be more motivated to keep up your workout. Plus, in the last month or two when your baby is getting big, he or she may be able to move more freely as you open your body in a stretch.

A few caveats are in order first, however. Take these precautions when practicing pregnancy yoga:

◆ Tell your doctor you are practicing yoga, and get permission for all poses you plan on practicing. If your doctor isn't familiar with yoga, bring pictures of the poses you'd like to do.

◆ Avoid extreme stretching positions and any position that puts pressure on or contracts your uterus. Skull Shining Breath might be too jarring for your baby, and full forward bends will probably be uncomfortable for you and baby, too. Be careful also with spinal twists. Try to focus on the upper part of the spine and do not overtwist the mid- and lower parts of your spine.

◆ Avoid full backbends such as Wheel pose and full forward bends such as Standing Head to Knees—maintain that abdominal space. Give that little him or her inside you a little room!

◆ Keep standing poses to a minimum, and never jump into them.

◆ Remember that your center of balance is completely different than it was before you were pregnant. Be careful doing balance poses. If you fall, the baby is well cushioned in your uterus, but you could injure yourself.

◆ Don't lie on your stomach for any pose.

◆ After the twentieth week, don't lie on your back for any pose (which will probably start to become uncomfortable, anyway). The weight of the baby can hinder your blood flow.

The following are suggestions only. If any pose feels uncomfortable or strenuous, stop at once. If you experience dizziness, sudden swelling, extreme shortness of breath, or vaginal bleeding, see your doctor immediately. Your best approach to these postures is to listen to your body and to never take it where it doesn't want to go.

◆ *Tadasana,* **Mountain pose.** Focus on tilting your lower back in to prevent the weight of the baby from pressing against your lumbar. Bend your knees slightly and place your hands on top of your knees. Tighten your thigh muscles and watch your kneecaps lift upward. Straighten your legs and try to lift your kneecaps.

Wise Yogi Tells Us

After the twentieth week, practice *shavasana* with lots of pillows, lying on your left side instead of your back.

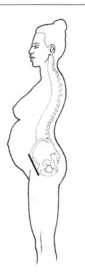

The added weight of pregnancy can create a condition called "lordosis," a swayback effect. Practice *tadasana*, Mountain pose, and concentrate on maintaining the proper spinal and pelvic alignment.

◆ *Shavasana*, **Corpse pose.** After your twentieth week, practice *shavasana* lying on your left side. A pillow for your head and pillows between your knees can take pressure of your neck, lower back, and hips, which might all be suffering from the change in your center of gravity.

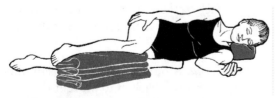

After the twentieth week of pregnancy, practice *shavasana* by lying on your left side.

◆ **Hero pose.** Sitting in Hero pose helps reduce swelling in your ankles, reduces fatigue, and improves circulation in your legs. Place a stack of pillows behind you and lean back. Bring your hands alongside your body to push yourself back up.

◆ **Child's pose.** Support your body with a stack of pillows placed between your knees, or stand on your knees and cross your arms over the back of a chair and lean forward. You might want a pillow or blanket under your knees as well, to protect and cushion them.

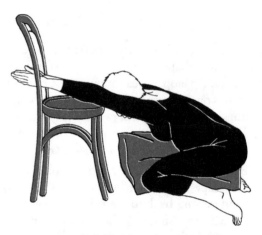

A variation of Child's pose during pregnancy.

◆ **Simple hamstring stretches.** Your hamstrings are the tendons at the back of your knees. Hamstring stretches relieve pressure on your lower back. Be gentle when you stretch.

◆ **Twisting poses should be performed gently.** When not pregnant, your focus should be on twisting your entire spine. During pregnancy, however, most of your twisting will be in your neck, shoulders, and head. Lift your spine as you inhale, and twist as you exhale.

Ouch!

At the first sign of leg cramps (common in pregnancy), draw your toes upward and push out your heel. Practice this movement so you can be ready to perform it in a split second when a leg cramp wakes you up in the middle of the night.

◆ **Use chairs for support whenever you can.** For example, try Warrior 2 pose or Side Angle Stretch seated on the center of a chair. It is more freeing and takes the weight off your legs.

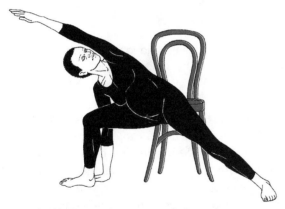

Side Angle Stretch variation during pregnancy.

◆ **Another way to use a chair is to try the Downward Facing Dog while standing and using the back of the chair for support.** What a wonderful stretch and release for your spine! Holding on to the chair takes some of the pressure off your legs in this pose. You'll feel freer, and so will your little passenger.

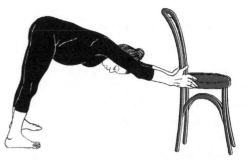

Downward Facing Dog variation during pregnancy. If you don't have a steady, firm chair to use, place your hands against a wall and stretch this way.

◆ **Learn some inspirational *mantras* to practice during childbirth.** They'll be much more productive than yelling and swearing at your partner, midwife, or doctor. Let your baby experience the transcendent vibrations of a *mantra*. If nothing else, transform your "*Aaaahhhhhhh!*" into "*Aaaauuuummmm!*"

◆ **Butterfly pose can help you relax, open your hips, and prepare for labor.** If your hip joints are tight, sit supported with a pillow under each knee. Hold the position only as long as it is comfortable. Move into an easy pose and rest if you need to.

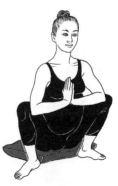

If Butterfly pose is comfortable for you, you might want to try this more advanced squatting pose. Stack the pillows as high on the floor as you need to, to reduce stress on your joints and muscles. When you are ready, return to a seated meditative position and breathe deeply and fully.

New Mama Yoga

Once you're home with your new little bundle, you might be a bit incredulous that you could have any time for yoga. You don't even have time to sleep! The first few weeks of transition are stressful but also joyful. You might feel alternately ecstatic and despairing, frustrated and overflowing with love.

Practicing yoga now is important because you need the energy. Filling your body with *prana* through breathing exercises and 10 minutes daily in *shavasana* will recharge you and make the little sleep you do get more productive. Your body also needs all its resources to heal itself after childbirth.

You probably need some mental maintenance, too. Your hormones might be making you extra emotional or a little depressed right after childbirth. Add to that the fact that your entire life has changed and will never be the same. Pile on top of that the fact that your jeans look hopelessly small, and even though you aren't pregnant anymore, all you might be able to wear are your old maternity clothes. Remember that it takes time to adjust to any major life change. It will also take your body time to readjust to a nonpregnant state. Be patient. Be kind to yourself. It took you nine months to get to childbirth, so give yourself nine months to get back. You have just accomplished something magnificent, and it has changed you. Accept the change lovingly and with joy.

Give yourself time to practice yoga each day, either when your baby is sleeping or when your partner, a family member, or a friend can play with the baby. Consider it pampering time and a well-deserved reward.

With your doctor's approval, you can usually start gentle yoga postures two weeks after delivery or a few weeks longer if you had a cesarean section. Hold off on inverted poses for at least six weeks.

All women have postnatal bleeding for a few weeks after pregnancy. Watch this flow for signs that you're going too fast. If the bleeding gets heavier or brighter red, you need to slow down and give your doctor a call. Start with just a few poses, and gradually work back to your regular routine as your body lets you know it's ready.

Wise Yogi Tells Us

A high-sugar diet will make you feel tired any time, but especially in the early weeks after childbirth. Sure, you deserve a treat now and then, but a diet based on whole-grain foods like whole-wheat bread and brown rice, sufficient iron (best sources are dark, leafy greens, wheat germ, and meat), and lots of vegetables is the best diet to combat fatigue.

The most beneficial pose for you right now is *shavasana*, which you can even do on the day you give birth. *Shavasana* can help ease labor pains, help you recoup your energy before all that pushing, and can also help you relax after the whole process is finished and you have a sleeping baby on your chest.

Any chance you get, take some deep breaths and practice these revitalizing poses. You'll handle all your new challenges with greater inner strength and energy. The following poses are also wonderful for a gentle postpregnancy routine:

- *Tadasana*, **Mountain pose.** Take some time to stand in Mountain pose, and notice how your center of gravity has shifted yet again. Let *tadasana* help you reacquaint yourself with your newly autonomous body.

- **Child's pose.** Let yourself be the child for a few minutes each day.

◆ **Lying Down Spinal Twist.** Let your body relax for long periods of time in this pose to make up for all the spinal twisting you needed to forego during pregnancy. Relax and enjoy!

Wise Yogi Tells Us

The postpartum (the period after childbirth) time is a good time to read the *Yoga Sutras* or other yoga texts. Keep them on a bedside or end table to read while nursing your baby or while baby is sleeping … or read them out loud to your baby to help quiet her with the sound of your voice and get her started on her yoga journey at the outset!

More important than any postures at this point is your attitude. Being a new mother isn't easy. If you're feeling frustrated or unhappy and think you must be a bad mother, give yourself a break! All new mothers feel like that sometimes. Remember *ahimsa*: Treat yourself nonviolently. Your feelings are completely normal. Don't be afraid to talk to your partner, your close friends, or a counselor about your feelings. Just remember that you're entering an exciting new leg of your life journey.

Easing Through Menopause

Menopause is the time of life when a woman stops ovulating. Although the age at which it occurs varies greatly, it commonly occurs around age 50. Yet menopause means much more to women than this simple biological definition. The thought of menopause is daunting to many, and it's no wonder! Our culture puts so much emphasis on youth and beauty, especially for women, that aging is difficult enough.

Because women are finally beginning to share their experiences of menopause and more information is available, this transition from fertility to the next stage of life is easier to prepare for. Far from being the end of life, menopause signals a period of life during which spiritual growth can soar. Women who have passed through menopause often feel stronger, more in charge of their lives, and more intimately acquainted with their souls than ever before. Age brings wisdom, and once a woman is no longer a childbearer, her body can focus on its own journey. Increasing numbers of strong, vibrant, amazing older women have become important figures in our culture. Look to these women as examples for your own life. This next stage of your journey may be the most thrilling yet. It's certainly full of possibilities.

But first, you have to get through the menopause, and that isn't always pleasant. A hot flash is still a hot flash (you could call it a recharge!), whether or not it signals an exhilarating life transition. Menopause comes with lots of other physical complaints beyond the often-cited hot flashes. Dizziness, depression, heart palpitations, decreased sex drive, and shortness of breath are all symptoms of decreased estrogen levels.

Yoga balances the endocrine system and can ease the difficult transition by stabilizing hormone levels. Inverted postures are particularly helpful for hot flashes, because they cool the body and fill it with *prana. Pranayama*, too, is cooling to the body.

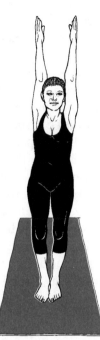

Practice breathing in Mountain pose. Inhale and lift your arms over your head. Exhale and bring your arms and hands down into Prayer pose. Return to Mountain and repeat. Yoga breathing helps lower blood pressure and reduce stress in mind and body.

Ouch!

When we hear the word *meno-pause*, most of us think of hot flashes, but you can experience a range of other physical symptoms. Considering menopause can last for five years, you'll probably want to do everything you can to minimize the unpleasantness.

As you work through menopause, incorporate these postures into your yoga routine:

- Headstand and other inversions, like Shoulderstand and Plough. If you've never mastered Headstand, now's the time to try. Headstand might reduce your hot flashes. All the inversions will make you feel more vital, too, because they replenish and rejuvenate your body. However, don't do inversions if you have high blood pressure.

- Downward Facing Dog and other forward-bending postures, such as Standing Head to Knees and Yoga *Mudra*. These forward-bending poses help you focus inwardly, an important process right now. Instead of shunning your body or feeling that it has betrayed you, embrace it, get to know it all over again, and let it work for you, leading you to a higher spiritual plane.

- Sun Salutation. Celebrate how your body has moved beyond moonlike cycles and catapulted like a rocket on toward the sun. Make the sun your newest ally. If you're up to it, start rising at dawn to practice yoga. Notice how, although the earth moves and turns and changes, the sun burns steadily and luminously in the center of our solar system. Meditate on how your body has become sunlike and strong, glowing with newfound steadiness and bliss.

◆ Any weight-bearing postures and activities. A drop in your estrogen level can cause you to lose bone mass, but you can easily counter this by exercising your bones. Postures that put stress on your bones such as inversions, standing postures, and Downward Facing Dog all increase bone mass. Light weightlifting is great for your bones and so is walking. Take a walk in the fresh air every day to keep your bones strong, your lungs full, and your heart light.

◆ Place a folded blanket or pillows about nine inches high against a wall. Support your lower and mid-back on the blanket, stretch your legs up the wall, and let your shoulder blades and head rest on the floor. Rest in this pose for 10 minutes with your eyes closed; focus on your breathing. This pose is cooling and therapeutic for any pelvic or abdominal problems.

◆ Start regular meditation. You're in an excellent time of life to begin meditation. You have a better sense of yourself than ever before. Take advantage of your wisdom and experience, and reap the benefits of meditation.

Most important, know that your life is far from over. You're a strong, vibrant woman with much to offer the world. Cultivate your soul like a garden and find your place in the universe.

The Least You Need to Know

◆ Beauty has nothing to do with your physical appearance. If you care for your body and radiate inner bliss, you'll be beautiful.

◆ Yoga can help reduce symptoms of PMS and menstruation.

◆ Yoga can be tailored to accommodate pregnancy and new motherhood.

◆ Yoga can ease the transition of menopause.

In This Chapter

◆ Three types of foods bring out three types of personal qualities

◆ Moderate eating is best

◆ The benefits of a lacto vegetarian diet

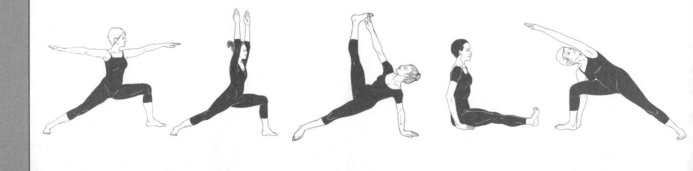

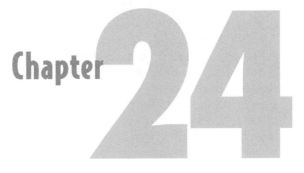

Chapter 24

Yogi Is What Yogi Eats

Now that you've got a handle on yoga's basic principles and are happily posturing away, let's consider another extremely important but often overlooked aspect of yoga: diet. It only makes sense that if your body, mind, and spirit are one, how you feed your body will influence the whole package. Western scientists have long recognized that a healthful diet is crucial to good health, although through the decades, the definition of *healthful* has certainly changed.

Gunas Gracious!

A fundamental principle is the yoga diet's primary influence. Yogis have traditionally divided food (and everything else, but we'll just talk about food in this chapter) into three categories, called *gunas*. The three *gunas* are *sattva*, *rajas*, and *tamas* (there's that triangle again!), and each represents a different type of energy. When applied to food, these energies go into our bodies and affect us in different ways, making us more balanced, or imbalanced, depending on our individual needs and the food we eat. *Sattvic* food promotes health, vitality, strength, and tranquillity; *rajasic* food promotes excessive energy, agitation, and discontentment; and *tamasic* food promotes lethargy, laziness, and inactivity.

Imagine a teeter-totter. The three *gunas* exist along the board of the teeter-totter, with *rajas* on one end, *tamas* on the other end, and *sattva* squarely in the middle. For example, if you tend to be a *rajasic* type of person, or you eat a lot of *rajasic* food (such as meat, hot peppers, double espressos, and other stimulating kinds of foods) and then you eat *tamasic* food (such as processed or preserved food or alcohol), you could achieve an uneasy balance, like two kids standing on either side of the teeter-totter. The slightest shift, and both kids will topple.

Know Your Sanskrit

Gunas are the three categories into which yoga divides all foods. The three *gunas* are **sattva, rajas,** and **tamas.** *Sattvic* foods like milk and organic produce promote balance, health, vitality, and strength; *rajasic* foods like caffeine and hot spices promote excessive energy, restlessness, and discontent; *tamasic* foods such as overly processed or high-sugar, high-fat foods promote lethargy, laziness, and inactivity.

But what if the two kids sit right over the teeter-totter's fulcrum? They'll be pretty stable, and that is what *sattvic* food—such as fresh, organic fruits, vegetables, and grains in or close to their natural state (and other *sattvic* influences like a regular schedule, plenty of sleep, and a steady routine)—does for your body. It balances you in a stable way. Your health will be much less likely to topple. You'll find the state of *samyama* much more accessible.

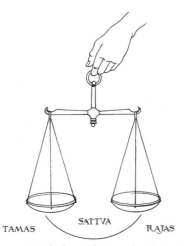

Achieve a *sattvic* balance for good yoga nutrition.

Samyama is what yogis strive for. It means holding your consciousness together through concentration, meditation, and contemplation in an attempt to understand everything about the object of your investigation, whether that is poetry, the study of medicine, or the study of yoga postures. *Samyama* is the final state that results from the active process of learning. In other words, it is total absorption in your activity and in your life itself.

On the other hand, *duhkha* is what often leads us astray. *Duhkha* is a feeling of discomfort or pain, suffering, sickness, or simply mental limitation. It is that deep-down feeling that something is wrong or out of place. *Duhkha* keeps you from achieving *samyama*. It makes you feel like you don't have the ability or are somehow inadequate—not healthy enough or strong enough or smart enough. *Duhkha* can arise out of excessive desire for something—even desire for enlightenment! It can be likened to a mental "virus" that infects your attitude and progress. *Duhkha* is like balancing on the end of the teeter-totter. You might be level at the moment, but it doesn't feel very good or secure. You are in fear of falling.

Know Your Sanskrit

Samyama (pronounced *SAHM-YAH-mah*) is a state that exists when concentration, meditation, and contemplation are all producing a perfectly balanced, concentrated meditational state. *Sam* means "together," and *yama* means "discipline."

Duhkha (*DOO-kah*) is pain, suffering, trouble, and discomfort. From *dur*, which means "bad," and *kha*, which means "axle hole" or "space" (hence, being in a bad space), *duhkha* is a mental state during which limitations and a profound sense of "wrongness" are perceived. *Duhkha* holds us back from self-actualization.

So how are *samyama* and *duhkha* related to the three *gunas?* Too many *rajasic* and/or *tamasic* foods produce *duhkha*, that's how! Balance is maintained with *sattvic* foods, and in fact, yoga itself can be seen as a process of "*sattvification.*" It helps keep you *duhkha*-free.

So we know we want to maintain a *sattvic* state of mind as often as possible. What better way than to eat a *sattvic* diet? Because feeding the body is akin to feeding the mind, *sattvic* food will encourage a *sattvic* mental state once we are balanced. However, *sattvic* foods won't necessarily be able to balance someone who is naturally very *rajasic* or *tamasic*. For instance, a very *tamasic* person—one who has very little energy and leads a sedentary life—might find that a little *rajasic* food like coffee or a nice hot salsa can help restore a balance. Then *sattvic* food makes a great "maintenance diet." A swinging pendulum isn't easy to stop. The way it best comes to rest is by a slow change in the intensity of its swing.

What's Your Nature?

As we mentioned, the *gunas* don't just apply to food. They are qualities that can be applied to the universe in general. The mind is made up of these three states. *Tamas* is lassitude, resistance to change, and also constancy. *Rajas* is activity and agitation. *Sattva* is clarity, tranquillity, and compassion. These three states also represent the three states of personal evolution: first the mind is dull, then it becomes active, and then, ideally, it finds true compassion. One aspect is usually dominant in each person's personality.

Yes, one of these qualities is probably dominant in you. Knowing which is your type can help you balance yourself. If you're a typical *rajas*-natured Westerner, for example, you can consciously minimize or eliminate *rajasic* food from your diet, replacing it with *sattvic* food. You'll probably notice a distinct difference in the way you feel—calmer, clearer, and less agitated.

Not sure which type you are? Take this mini-quiz to get a better picture of yourself:

1. If I'm feeling under a lot of stress, I'll be most likely to …
   a. Go take a nap. At least I'll be able to forget about it all for a while.
   b. Pace back and forth, worrying and wasting time.
   c. Analyze why I'm under stress and make a plan to deal with it.
2. I would describe my diet as …
   a. Centered around my food addictions: caffeine, sugar, or salt. Meals are really important to me because I have to have my food! It would be very difficult for me to give up any food I love.
   b. Very irregular. I grab a bite of whatever is handiest when I have the time. Sometimes I forget to eat or am so stressed out that I eat way too much without realizing it.
   c. Healthful, well-balanced, with lots of fruits and vegetables. Not a big fan of dead meat.
3. In my personal relationships, I tend to be …
   a. The passive one.
   b. The dominant one.
   c. Fairly equal with the others in my life.

If you had mostly A answers, you're probably *tamas*-natured. You'd rather lie on the couch than go for a jog; you tend to get addicted to pleasurable things like sugar, cigarettes, or coffee; and you have a hard time getting things done. You might have difficulty getting yourself into a habit of practicing yoga postures, but yoga will be of great benefit to you, revving up your system, increasing your energy level, and giving you the get-up-and-go you need to get through the day.

If you had mostly B answers, you're probably *rajas*-natured. You're typically overwrought, excited, anxious, or agitated. You get a lot done and fast, but you have a hard time relaxing and quieting your mind. For you, meditation is a real challenge, but you could really use the skill of being able to calm that overactive mind of yours. If you suffer from insomnia, regular yoga practice can help you sleep. In fact, regular practice of anything is good for the impetuous and routine-resistant *rajas*-natured.

If you had mostly C answers, you tend to be *sattvic*-natured. You adhere to the sensible notion of moderation in many aspects of your life, and the *yogic* lifestyle will probably be relatively easy for you to adopt. You find a sense of peace in yoga postures, you find meditation enjoyable, and you already follow the *yogic* diet without even intending to! In fact, you might wonder why you haven't discovered yoga before now.

Wise Yogi Tells Us

Feeling stressed out? Gently heat 1 cup low-fat milk on the stove or in the microwave. Pour it into a mug and add 1 tablespoon honey and a pinch of dried ginger. Stir, find a comfy seat, and relax. Sip slowly. *Ahhhhh!* Don't drink milk? Cut a two-inch slice of fresh gingerroot, peel it, and slice it into discs. Put it in the bottom of a mug or cup and pour boiling water over it. Let it steep for about five minutes, then remove the ginger. Add a squeeze of fresh lemon juice and a tablespoon of honey. *Mmmm!*

Yogi Food

So let's cut to the chase: What kind of food is *sattvic* food? *Sattvic* foods are pure foods. Most foods that are fresh, organically grown, additive- and preservative-free, unprocessed, and alkaline are considered *sattvic*. These include the following:

- Fresh fruits and juices
- Most fresh vegetables
- Whole-grain cereals
- Nuts and seeds, especially almonds and sesame seeds
- Pulses (dried peas, beans, and lentils)
- Milk and milk products (unfermented), including butter
- Honey

A Yoga Minute

Traditionally, milk has been an important part of the yogi's diet and has always been considered *sattvic*. However, milk today is not what it used to be. Choose organic milk rather than milk from factory farms when possible for the best possible sattvic energy, or if you choose to avoid dairy products, try organic soy milk for a lovely *sattvic* alternative.

Sattvic foods help you think more clearly, because your body is unclouded and unhindered by impurities, chemicals, and stimulants. *Sattvic* foods promote contemplative thought, vitality, energy, tranquillity, happiness, and overall health. Most serious yoga practitioners exist primarily on *sattvic* foods, although because food in and of itself is not an obsession for the healthy yogi, occasional tastes of other foods when these are offered aren't a problem. The wise yogi eats moderately, and moderation means *not* being obsessive about anything— even moderation!

If you're unable to drink milk or choose to avoid all dairy products (a truly nonviolent approach to eating), simply update our list of *sattvic* foods by eliminating milk. Stick with soy milk and other soy products, organic produce, and whole grains, the foods that remain *sattvic* even in our complicated world.

Wise Yogi Tells Us

If you aren't ready for all-out vegetarianism, try it for a day. Tell yourself you can have a cheeseburger tomorrow, but today you'll stick with hearty split-pea soup over rice or a steaming plate of pasta with sautéed mushrooms. Tomorrow, before your cheeseburger, notice how you feel. Lighter? Hungrier? No different? Calmer? Try it again next week.

Pungent, Spicy Westerners

As we've mentioned, Westerners tend to be *rajas*-natured because Western life is so *rajas*-oriented—high-speed and agitated! Our culture rewards high energy, overachievement, even anxiety and agitation if they help get the job done! *Rajasic* foods are generally the stimulating kind: spicy, sour, pungent, and bitter. The following are examples of *rajasic* food:

- All meat
- All fish
- Eggs
- Hot peppers
- Most strong spices, especially black and red pepper
- Coffee, tea, cola, and other stimulating, caffeine-laden beverages

Ancient cultures often fed their warriors meat before sending them off to battle, because it was known that meat increased aggression and agitation. After a good meat-fest, warriors could fight and kill better. Assuming you don't have the need to fight and kill anyone, however, why not try cutting down or even eliminating most *rajasic* foods from your diet? You might find a new sense of calm and a clearer head.

Of course, a little *rajasic* food now and then won't hurt anyone. It's what you do most of the time that counts. But if you exist on steak and eggs, or spicy beef burritos, or sausage-and-pepper sandwiches, or coffee and diet cola, even a nonyogi can tell you you're not going to be at your healthiest.

Stale Leftovers for Couch Potatoes

Tamasic food is considered impure and includes anything stale, old, aged, fermented, spoiled, overly processed, preservative-filled, or addictive. Here are some examples of *tamasic* food:

- Coffee, tea, cola, and other sources of caffeine (on this list, too, because they are both stimulating and addictive).
- Alcohol, including wine and beer.
- Aged cheese, yogurt, other fermented dairy products.
- Foods that are canned, pickled, or highly salted.
- Tobacco (we know, you smoke it, you don't eat it—but it still counts!).
- Any food that's been sitting around too long, even if it still looks good (for example, produce that has been heavily sprayed and waxed so it can last through a journey across country and long periods of storage).
- Anything processed, packaged, frozen, or preserved, from that "lite" microwavable dinner to that box of snack cakes that would last five years in your pantry.

Tamasic foods dull your mind. They make you feel tired and sap your ambition and strength (just what the preserving process—*tamasa*-fying!—does to fresh, or *sattvic*, food). Too much *tamasic* food will drain away your energy and your vitality, eventually bringing on a lack of joy in life, if not serious illness. No matter how much coloring and how many preservatives are added to make the food look good, when your body ingests it, the "makeup" comes right off and the food's true quality is revealed.

Unfortunately, many Westerners are addicted to *tamasic* food, especially sources of caffeine and alcohol. Also, we've been tricked into believing we don't have time for anything but preservative-laden "convenience" food. Our supermarkets are brimming with *tamasic* fare, but that doesn't mean you have to put it in your cart. A stock of tomato soup or commercial spaghetti sauce will keep longer than a stock of fresh tomatoes, but it certainly isn't better, or worth the price!

A Yoga Minute

Maybe you're wondering how caffeine can be both *rajasic* and *tamasic*. The stimulating quality of caffeine—that "buzz" that shifts you into high gear—is indeed *rajasic*, but there's more to caffeine than its stimulating nature. Coffee, tea, and cola are also addictive, and addictive substances are *tamasic*. The habit-forming nature of caffeine woos the *tamas*-natured; plus, the stimulating effect gets hard-to-move *tamas*-natured folks up on their feet and out the door to work. Yes, yes, we understand. You *love* your cup of coffee! (We love ours, too.) Fear not. Remember, it's what you do most of the time that counts. If the rest of your diet is basically *sattvic*, an occasional cup of coffee isn't going to hurt.

Moderation in All Things (as If You Didn't Know!)

But wait! Just because you now know which foods are best for you doesn't mean you should throw down this book, run to the kitchen, and start indulging. Calm down, you *rajas*-natured ones. Don't plan your indulgent feast just yet, you *tamas*-natured folk. Cultivating *sattva* means more than shoveling in massive quantities of the "right" foods. It also involves a few principles of eating:

◆ **Eat slowly.** Chew each bite 50 times (or if that's just too much to ask, start with 10 times and work your way up). Taste your food. Don't think about what you're going to eat next or what you need to do next. Give your meal some time. Give each bite some time.

◆ **Eat with full attention to eating.** That means no TV, no newspaper, and no trancelike gazing at the back of the cereal box, fascinating as it might be.

◆ **Enjoy your food, and savor the eating experience.** Live in the moment of your meal!

◆ **Don't eat too much.** Try to leave the table with a little room left in your stomach.

◆ **Don't eat too often.** That means avoiding between-meal snacking, late-night binges, and 3 A.M. Dagwood sandwiches.

If food is too important to you, it will control you. If you have a food addiction, you already know what it's like to be controlled. Food is meant to keep you alive and to enhance your existence; food isn't meant to fill emotional voids.

Overindulgence taxes your body, and it's been suggested that regular and consistent undereating (not undernourishment—an important distinction) increases longevity. That means more time on this earth for practicing yoga and more time to enjoy the improved you. Remember the old and familiar adage (did your parents ever tell you this?), "Moderation in all things"? This is a seriously important concept. Live moderately, and you'll live well.

Fasting

Sometimes the best way to let food work for you is to give your body a rest from food. Moderate eating is great, but sometimes even the moderate eater can benefit from a short juice fast. Occasional one-day juice fasts (nothing but fresh fruit and vegetable juice) are excellent system cleansers. However, fasting should not be overdone. Remember, moderation! For more information on fasting, check out *The Complete Idiot's Guide to Fasting* by Eve Adamson and Linda Horning, R.D.

Another great and easy way to fast is to eat a healthy breakfast, a hearty lunch, and an early, light supper, then not to eat anything but juice and water after 5 P.M. If you fast too often or for too long, or fast while only drinking water, you're committing violence on your own body (and that isn't following the *yama* of *ahimsa*, or nonviolence!). Before altering your diet or performing a fast, consult your physician or a licensed dietitian to come up with the best nutritional plan for your individual health and fitness needs.

Ouch! _____

If you are fasting and experience headaches, dizziness, or other discomfort beyond mild hunger, give yourself a break, practice nonviolence, and have something to eat. Fasting is not about hurting yourself. When breaking a fast, make sure you begin eating gradually again. Start with soup, bread, a salad, or something else natural (close to its natural state) and light in fat and calories.

Breaking the Addiction with Yoga

If you do suffer from food addictions, breaking them can be extremely difficult. Maybe you can't even imagine shelving your life-sustaining coffee mug. Maybe you binge on cookies every weekend or are seemingly incapable of passing a fast-food restaurant without driving through for a double cheeseburger and fries.

We have a nice little secret for you: You don't have to feel guilty. You don't have to deprive yourself. All you have to do is practice all the *other* aspects of yoga: the postures, the breathing, the meditation. Here's where yoga works its magic. Yoga is transformative. It changes you. If you diligently practice it, within a few weeks or months you'll be able to enjoy a cup of coffee without needing more or feeling addicted. Or maybe you won't want it at all. You won't feel the need for the caffeine. Fresh fruit will seem far more luscious than a bag of processed, store-bought cookies. And fast food will seem downright ... barbaric?

The point is, you don't really need to try to change your habits. You don't need to suffer and strive. If you're disciplined in the other areas of yoga, yoga will help you with the rest.

C'mon, Vegetarian?

Okay, we'll say it again: Here's where yoga works its magic. Yoga is transformative. It changes you.

Westerners are funny about vegetarianism. They seem to fall into two camps. There's the "Of *course* I'm a vegetarian. Aren't *you?*" camp, and the "You aren't *actually* one of those *vegetarians*, are you?" camp. Even if you're a vegetarian and don't judge meat-eaters, or a meat-eater who doesn't judge vegetarians, many who don't share your views about meat will assume you're in the "opposite camp" and will be on the defensive.

We aren't sure why this antagonistic scenario has developed in the West, but it has. If you're a vegetarian or have tried without success to quit eating meat, you have surely encountered "the attitude." Also, if you eat meat but know a lot of vegetarians, you may have felt similarly maligned. Similarly, you don't have to justify your meat-eating habits or your vegetarian habits to anyone but yourself.

So let's all try, just for a minute, to let go of all that. Let's be objective, as far as that's possible. Do you like meat? Could you do without it? Aside from what anyone else in the world might think, does the idea of a vegetarian diet appeal to you? Although some yogis are *vegans* and some are *fruitarians*, the most common yogi diet is a *lacto vegetarian* diet.

What exactly *is* a vegetarian, then, you ask? *Vegetarian* is a blanket term, and there are indeed several *kinds* of vegetarians. Check out this vegetarian primer, and you'll be an expert on the variety and range of vegetarian diets!

- **Lacto vegetarians** don't eat any meat, poultry, fish, or eggs. Their diets consist primarily of fruits, vegetables, whole grains (like rice, oats, and wheat), pasta, nuts, seeds, pulses (dried beans, peas, and lentils), milk, and milk products.

- **Lacto ovo vegetarians** are the same as lacto vegetarians but also eat eggs.

- **Vegans** eat no animal substance of any kind, including all dairy products. Diligent vegans even avoid eating things like gelatin and other products made with preservatives or other ingredients made from animal parts (like rennet), and wearing leather or other clothing made from animals.

- **Fruitarians** eat primarily fruit, but also some vegetables. The primary rule for fruitarians is that all food must be consumed raw. Yes, that means avoiding *all* cooked foods, and eating mostly raw fruits and seeds.

There are a lot of great reasons to practice a vegetarian diet:

- A vegetarian diet is in harmony with *ahimsa*, the *niyama* of nonviolence.

- A vegetarian diet is healthier for your heart, because it tends to be low in cholesterol and saturated fat.

- According to many wise yogis, when an animal is slaughtered, it is filled with intense fear and anxiety. Eating that meat transfers the terrible fear to you.

- A vegetarian diet makes many people feel lighter, more energetic, and healthier. Physical activity becomes less of an effort, and food becomes less of an obsession.

But what if your answer to the question of whether you could eat from the lacto vegetarian menu is a resounding "No way!"? As we said before, don't force yourself to do anything you aren't yet ready to do. You can certainly be committed to yoga without being committed to vegetarianism. In fact, many yoga teachers don't encourage vegetarianism or any dietary modification, especially to their Western students. These teachers know that yoga will do that job on its own, when the time is right.

Wise Yogi Tells Us

Some meat-eaters feel guilty eating meat in front of vegetarians, and some vegetarians feel guilty because they don't want their meat-eating friends to feel guilty. The true yogic way is to not judge others or yourself harshly. Yoga is a path of loving acceptance. No guilt, no condescension. PURE Joy.

Many yogis start out with no intention of becoming vegetarians, but the more yoga transforms them, the less interested they are in meat, until finally, one day … poof! … another vegetarian is born. Simply deciding to become a vegetarian will not magically grant you a kind heart. Plenty of mean-spirited vegetarians are walking around out there in the world! Vegetarianism doesn't make you a yogi; yoga leads you to nonviolence, which might eventually lead you to vegetarianism. Maybe this day is in your near future, and maybe it's a long, long way off. It's your journey. What's right for you is unique, and only you can truly determine your own course. So consider vegetarianism, be open to the idea, but if it just isn't "you" (or at least, the "you" you are today), let it go. Maybe it will come back to surprise you when you're ready for it.

Vegetarian or not, do try to eat a healthy, fresh, primarily *sattvic* diet. Everyone can agree that fresh, whole, unprocessed food is a delight to eat. A diet of *sattvic* food makes living so much nicer, yoga practice so much easier, and might even make this wonderful life of yours a little bit longer and a little bit more wonderful.

The Least You Need to Know

◆ Different types of foods—*sattvic, rajasic,* and *tamasic*—have different effects on you.

◆ Fresh, whole, unprocessed food helps you think more clearly. Stimulating food can agitate you, and stale or preservative-filled food can sap your energy.

◆ Moderation in all things is best!

◆ A lacto vegetarian diet has many health-related and spiritual benefits.

In This Chapter

- ◆ What makes you sick? Germs? Human failing? Can you prevent it?

- ◆ How yoga can help your nagging complaints

- ◆ How yoga can help when your condition is more serious

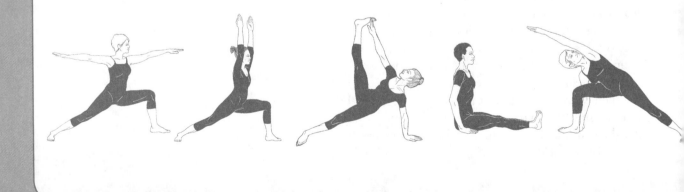

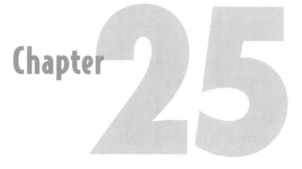

Chapter

Yoga and Healing

If you're human (which we assume you all are), chances are you've experienced illness and pain in your lifetime. Even if you've never been seriously ill, you've certainly had a cold, the flu, maybe insomnia, possibly indigestion, an occasional headache, or an aching back.

Our human bodies are far from perfectly functioning, especially considering how much and how vigorously we use them. But pain and discomfort aren't necessarily par for the course in the life of a yogi. The yogi has a few tricks, and you, as a novice yogi, are privy to this health-inspiring information. Read on for how to help prevent, relieve, and sometimes even heal your health problems.

What Makes You Sick?

Theories abound concerning the cause of illness and pain, but many yogis believe that although illness can be caused by physical factors such as viruses, bacteria, and accidents, illness can also be brought on or encouraged by …

◆ Insufficient *prana*, or life force, within the body, sometimes indicated by shallow breathing.

◆ An imbalance in the mindbody—for example, too much focus on the mental and not enough on the physical, or vice versa.

◆ Too much *rajasic* (causing agitation) and/or *tamasic* (causing lethargy) food or addictive substances like caffeine, tobacco, and/or alcohol.

◆ Lack of good personal hygiene.

◆ Unhappiness, pessimism, and/or negativity.

One of the characteristics of conventional, or *allopathic,* medicine is that it tends to pinpoint and isolate a problem or symptom and treat it, and it alone, which is sometimes just what the body needs. The body is like a machine that occasionally requires the repair of a specific part (a broken bone, a clogged heart, a ruptured appendix, etc.).

Holistic medicine tends to first look at the "big picture," or the whole person. What are you doing that could be causing your illness (*roga*), pain, or disease (*vyadhi*)? Who are you? How is your general health (*svasthya*)? What is your health history? How is your posture? What is your attitude? What is your view of life? Holistic medicine seeks the answers to all these questions in an effort to find the source of a problem, rather than merely treating the symptoms of a condition or illness.

Know Your Sanskrit

Svasthya (pronounced *SVAH-sthyah*) is the Sanskrit word for "health," from *sva-stha,* which means "one's own state." *Roga* (*ROH-gah*) means "sickness," and *vyadhi* (*VYAH-dee*) means "disease."

Yoga, too, takes this holistic approach to your health. Yoga treatments are great when used in conjunction with traditional health care, because such an approach results in an all-encompassing treatment. Yoga works on your body and your mind to free them of impurities and imbalances that could cause health problems for you later. Many specific yoga poses also compress and release internal organs and organ systems to help stimulate energy and healing.

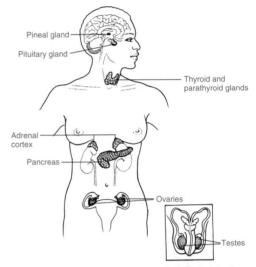

The endocrine system is a group of glands that manufacture hormones. Many yoga poses compress and stimulate these glands.

The problem with this kind of thinking is that it's easy to blame yourself for your illness. *If only I would have exercised more,* or *If only I would have eaten better.* Blame only generates more negativity. Instead, when you encounter a health problem, we encourage you to use yoga to help you focus on the positive, on healing, on relaxation, on letting your body do what it needs to do and letting your mind see the beauty and the joy in life, even in pain.

The "moderation in all things" adage comes into play in health as well as in diet, and this is a yoga concept you can actually control in your life. Anything you do to an extreme will cause an imbalance in your body and mind, or in your first three sheaths of existence. Remember *ahimsa,* or nonviolence? Practice it by refusing to commit violence to your body with obsessive actions. Also, observe *santosha,* or contentment, by practicing satisfaction, peace, and tranquillity. You'll have a much easier time staying obsession-free, positive, and balanced.

Physical Cleansing

One focus of ancient Indian yoga life science is cleanliness. Yoga includes several cleansing rituals or practices that were originally designed to keep the body clean, balanced, and in optimal health.

But you take showers. You wash your hair. You use deodorant. You don't smell bad. Isn't that enough? Not to the yogi! Of course, nothing should become an obsession, but according to yoga tradition, the body needs some hygienic upkeep to keep it from becoming a hindrance to the spirit and an impediment to *kundalini* energy, not to mention imbalanced and eventually vulnerable to disease.

This cleanliness is called *shodhana* and consists of cleansing rituals, or *shat kriyas*, for the body. Hatha Yoga also concerns strict observance of dental hygiene. Yogis not only brush their teeth, but also rinse their mouths, massage their gums, and scrape their tongues to keep them clean. And don't forget to visit your dentist every six months! (If you follow that yogi regimen, your dentist will be very impressed.)

Read on for more on some of the other *shat kriyas*.

Know Your Sanskrit

Shat kriyas (pronounced *SHOT kree-yahs*) are the purification rituals of Hatha Yoga. *Shodhana* (*sho-DAH-nah*) is purification of the body.

Sthala Basti (Ground Colon Cleansing): Elimination = Illumination!

Let's start at the bottom. This ritual helps relieve gas and keeps the bowels moving smoothly. It also improves digestion and gives your body a lighter feel.

Sit with your legs stretched out in front of you. Grab your big toes, right toe with your right hand, left toe with your left hand. Bend forward, bringing your head toward your knees just a little, so it feels comfortable. Relax your abdominal muscles, then churn them up and down. While churning your muscles, "lock" your anus (called the *mula bandha*). Be very careful not to push yourself too hard. This ritual should feel comfortable. Be sure to practice this ritual on an empty stomach.

Nauli Kriya (Rolling Cleansing): Tummy Toner

This kriya stokes the gastric fire and improves digestion. It helps keep the bowels healthy, cures constipation, and reduces belly fat.

Perform this ritual by bending your knees slightly from a standing position with your legs about one foot apart or slightly more. Let your hands rest on your thighs. Exhale fully, then lift your lower abdomen up and in. Hold your breath. Next, perform the muscle churning described in the Ground Colon Cleansing ritual, but with the abdominal muscles, moving them in more of a circular, side to side motion than an up-and-down motion. Rotate the muscles in this way as quickly as you can for as long as you can without discomfort. Don't push to the point where you become exhausted.

After the muscle churning, relax and let your breath flow in and out. This makes one round. Work up to several rounds, eventually reaching 100 or so churning rotations.

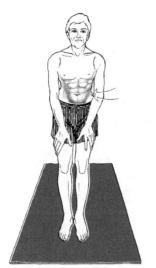

Isolate your abdominal muscles to cleanse and tone your colon.

Wise Yogi Tells Us

If all these cleansing rituals seem like a little too much to you, keep in mind that they stem from ancient Indian practices based in a culture that considers the body ultimately earthy.

Beyond Cleansing

Yoga health is about more than cleansing and moderation, although these are both extremely important for health maintenance. Also take care of yourself. Get regular massages. Meditate every day for at least a few minutes. Take time for yourself, and actively work to manage yourself. Practice Hatha Yoga every day, or at least every few days. Then, even if you do get sick, you'll know you are taking the best possible care of your body and allowing yourself to fully access your inner mindbody healing power.

Yoga for Those Nagging Complaints

Beyond cleanliness, yoga is also good therapy for the minor health problems that plague you. You'll probably find that with regular, consistent yoga practice, you'll suffer less often from minor complaints. If they do arise, however, try a few appropriate yoga *asanas* (postures) and stick with your yoga rules for living (*yamas* and *niyamas*) for effective relief.

A Yoga Minute

Back pain sufferers might need more calcium and magnesium. Great sources are milk, yogurt, cheese, dark leafy greens like collard greens and kale, calcium-fortified orange juice, almonds, calcium-fortified tofu, broccoli, wheat bran, wheat germ, whole-wheat flour, calcium-fortified cereal, dried beans, peanut butter, and dried apricots. If you have a spine-related injury, however, be sure to check with your doctor before trying any yoga postures. Once your doctor gives the go-ahead, practice under the supervision of an experienced teacher to be sure you perform the poses correctly and don't injure yourself further.

Oh, My Aching Back ...

Because we all walk around upright, our backs are bound to suffer. Our poor spines carry all that weight around and are continually jarred by the pounding of our feet, not to mention twisted and contorted by less-than-perfect postures. Weak stomach muscles are a common cause of back pain.

Injury to a disc or vertebrae can cause back pain. Yoga can help in these cases. If you suffer from back pain, include the following exercises, which strengthen the stomach and/or tone the spine, in your yoga routine:

- ◆ Cobra pose (Chapter 12)
- ◆ Single Leg Lifts (Chapter 13)
- ◆ Boat pose (Chapter 17)

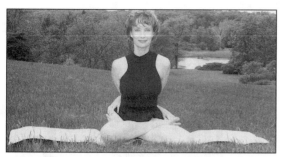

Practicing yoga can help you protect against bone and muscle loss, prevent the compression fractures common with osteoporosis, and encourage good posture as you age.

Oh, My Aching Head ...

It's the rare individual indeed who can say he or she has never suffered from a headache. Unfortunately, it's often difficult to find the source of a headache. Headaches can be caused by a negative reaction to a certain food, air pollution, allergies, sinus problems, eyestrain, stress, and any number of other factors.

Try eliminating suspected sources of regular headaches, such as caffeine, poor posture, or a particular food. If your headache is severe or your headache patterns change, see a doctor. For occasional, irregular headaches, however, your best bet might be to step up your yoga practice to put your body in the best possible condition for curing itself.

For headache relief, try the following:

◆ Try *pranayama* breathing techniques (Chapter 15).

◆ Gently rotate and flex your neck and toes.

◆ Practice inverted postures where your head is lowered briefly. These might help a headache, because inverted postures increase the flow of oxygen to the brain, but don't try these if you have high blood pressure.

◆ Make sure you maintain a balanced diet. Decrease or eliminate your intake of nuts, aged cheeses, chocolate, caffeine, and food containing nitrates (like luncheon meats

and hot dogs). These foods produce allergylike reactions in many people.

◆ Take a tip from reflexology, a healing art that uses targeted foot massage to reduce pain and induce healing. Pull on your big toe gently, straight from its socket, and hold the pull. Feel your headache melt away!

Why Am I So Tired?

Fatigue is a common problem in our overextended and fast-paced lives. Sometimes we simply wear ourselves out! Fatigue can also be caused by stress and extreme mental exertion, such as when you've been studying excessively, or when you're bothered by an emotional problem such as depression or anxiety. A good holistic health-care practitioner or therapist might be able to help you discover the underlying cause of your fatigue. If you notice unusual fatigue, however, even when you've gotten enough sleep, consult a physician.

Wise Yogi Tells Us

A few lifestyle modifications could be the answer to eliminating fatigue in your life. Try the following:

◆ Getting off caffeine ASAP!

◆ Not eating anything sweet before noon.

◆ Eating a low-fat diet. Too much fat slows you down and wears you out.

◆ Maintaining a positive attitude. Don't sweat the small stuff!

◆ Lifting your own weight in yoga postures ... and don't tell us your weight depresses you and that's why you don't lift it. We encourage you to lift it gradually!

For occasional bouts of fatigue during the day, a 20-minute power nap can work wonders. If you aren't in a position to take a nap, try the following:

- Practicing *shavasana*, or Corpse pose, for five minutes. (Chapter 10)
- Doing deep-breathing exercises to replenish your *prana*.
- Doing backbends to help energize you. (Chapter 14)

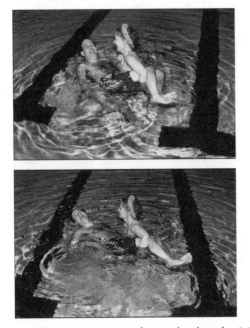

Yoga in the water is a great fatigue-battler, plus it is a nonimpact form of exercise. Here, Joan assists her friend Bob in a supported water spinal twist for a wonderful back release.

Why Can't I Sleep?

On the other hand we have the insomniacs. If you have trouble getting to sleep, common sense will probably tell you to lay off the caffeine, especially in the evening, and not to eat a whole pepperoni pizza at midnight. Stress is a common cause of insomnia, too. How can you sleep if your mind is abuzz with the worries of the day? Maybe you aren't purposefully sabotaging your body's ability to snooze, but if you nevertheless can't seem to catch even a few winks, try the following:

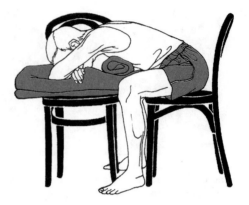

Forward bends are calming and can help induce sleep. This refreshing supported Child's pose stretch can help you relax.

- Meditate. Evening meditation can calm and still your mind, making sleep easier. Many wise yogis sit in Full Lotus in meditation so that if—or when—they fall asleep, they won't fall over!
- *Shavasana* is as good for insomnia as it is for fatigue. (Chapter 18)
- Forward bends quiet the body and mind. (Chapter 17)
- To help you get to sleep, take a warm bath before bed, and don't eat for at least six hours before bedtime.
- Dried lavender in your bath or stuffed in your pillowcase can help soothe you to sleep.

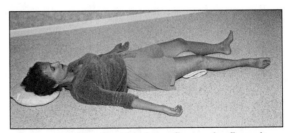

If you are uncomfortable lying flat on the floor due to lower back or joint pain, place a pillow or rolled blanket under your knees and another under your head and neck for support when practicing yoga's *shavasana* pose.

What's Up with My Digestion?

The digestive system is tricky. Maybe you've noticed you can eat chili dogs, cotton candy, and ice cream all day some days and feel fine, while on other days, a few bites of an enchilada are all it takes to give you heartburn all night long. Part of the reason is that much of your digestive success depends on the manner in which you eat. If you eat slowly, concentrate on your food, and enjoy the experience, you'll have a better chance of digesting without a hitch. Rushed, stressed eating or eating when you aren't hungry or aren't feeling well will lead you down a short path to indigestion.

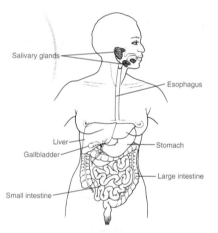

The organs of digestion are stimulated by forward-bending yoga poses, while back bends give the digestive system space to work.

Some people have chronic digestive problems, which could signal a number of possible health issues. If you suffer from frequent heartburn, indigestion, bloating, gas, or stomach cramps after eating, see your doctor. Occasional cases can be alleviated by a few good yoga poses.

- Try *shavasana*.
- Poses that move the digestive area through compression and opening are good for improving digestion. Try Fish pose (Chapter 14), which lengthens the abdomen,

followed by Child's pose (Chapter 18), which compresses the abdomen, or include Lightning Bolt pose in your routine (Chapter 11).

- The Sun Salutation (Chapter 16) is an excellent flowing series of poses to move and open the digestive system.

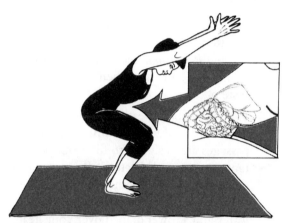

Lightning Bolt pose compresses the digestive system to help stimulate and balance the digestive organs.

This Cold Won't Go Away ...

Having a cold all winter long is frustrating as well as counterproductive to your happiness and well-being. If you can't get rid of your cold or keep getting colds back-to-back, consider where the virus is coming from. Are you washing your hands often enough? Do you frequently touch your face? Are you in contact with a lot of people all day long?

During the cold season, cold germs are everywhere, so be extra careful about hygiene. If you have kids, make sure they wash their hands before they eat and before they touch food others will eat. Remind them to wash their hands when they're away from home (at school or a friend's house) before eating and after touching anything that might not be sanitary, such as anything in a public bathroom.

Some colds have been known to turn into more serious problems, like sinus infections, bronchitis, or even pneumonia, so it's in your best interest to do everything you can to prevent them. Increase your intake of vitamin C, preferably through real food such as fresh citrus fruit, fresh-squeezed juice, strawberries, and broccoli. Also …

◆ Do lots of *pranayama* to keep your breathing passages clear. Keep a tissue nearby! *Pranayama* techniques also work to increase and strengthen the immune system.

◆ When possible, breathe through your nose instead of your mouth. Your nasal passages are designed to filter out pollutants, viruses, and bacteria. If you are too congested to breathe through your nose, sit with your head over a bowl of hot water and a towel draped over your head to clear that congestion.

◆ If your cold comes with a headache, try the previously mentioned headache relief suggestions.

◆ Poses that open the chest can feel great when you are congested. Try the Bow, Fish, and Cobra poses. (Chapter 12)

◆ Regular use of a neti pot will help to clear nasal sinuses and congestion.

Wise Yogi Tells Us

If you have nasal congestion, try using a *neti* pot. A *neti* pot is a pot specifically tailored to the nose! A mixture of saline solution is poured into one nostril and comes out the other nostril with the appropriate tilt of the head. *Neti* pots are traditionally used in the yoga practice of a cleansing ritual called *neti* (described in Chapter 15).

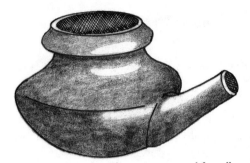

Neti pots are used to clear sinuses and for allergy sufferers.

Eyestrain Drain

Working at a computer or poring over paperwork all day can really strain your eyes. Yoga has many balancing exercises to help your eyes focus far away when they've been focused too close for too long, or to exercise and stretch the tiny muscles of your eye when they have been fixed in one place for too long (like that computer monitor). Try focusing on your thumb held at arm's length and following it up, down, right, left, and in clockwise and counterclockwise circles.

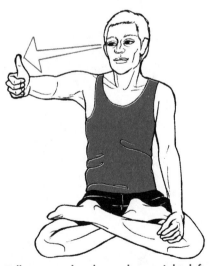

Follow your thumb up, down, right, left, and in circles to relieve eyestrain.

When It's More Serious

The one-on-one, personal attention to your specific needs can be a tremendous asset to your healing process.

> **Ouch!**
>
> This book is meant to complement, not replace, your doctor! If you are sick, injured, or suffer chronic pain, seek medical attention from a licensed medical professional. Tell your doctor you'd like to make yoga a part of your ongoing treatment plan.

AIDS

Because the AIDS virus attacks the immune system, yoga can be of great benefit in extending life expectancy by encouraging the immune system to rally. Practice your regular yoga routine diligently. The general and gentle nonviolent practice of Hatha Yoga will increase your overall circulation and the delivery of oxygen throughout your body. *Pranayama* techniques and relaxation techniques both boost the immune system.

Arthritis

Chronic joint pain—including such common joint problems as TMJ, tennis elbow, and carpal tunnel syndrome—can be seriously debilitating. If you suffer from arthritis in particular or joint pain in general, relaxation is key to easing your distress. Yoga can be a great help, but if you have arthritis, it's important not to push yourself beyond what your body can do. Don't exercise joints that are inflamed.

However, many people with arthritis drastically decrease activity due to pain. Your joints should periodically be mobilized to keep them limber and clean. Yoga encourages you to keep

moving, gently. As long as the following postures don't hurt, include them in your regular practice:

- ◆ *Vinyasana* routines (Chapter 13), such as a slow Sun Salutation, are excellent for maintaining your mobility.
- ◆ Try self-massage to bring warmth and circulation to painful areas.
- ◆ *Pranayama* increases your circulation and helps with pain.

Asthma, Allergies, and Respiratory Problems

When your breath is disturbed, your *prana* delivery system is disturbed, and that's a big deal. You don't want to mess with the life force! If you suffer from asthma, allergies, or other respiratory problems, you know how frustrating, let alone dangerous, breathing difficulties can be. Try the following to keep your breath flowing freely:

- ◆ Practice poses that open and stretch the chest: Tree, Warrior (Chapter 11), Fish, Bow, and Cobra poses (Chapter 12). Be careful not to hold your breath while holding these poses.
- ◆ Two deep breaths while holding a pose are better than 10 shallow breaths.
- ◆ Eat a healthy diet!

Cancer

In 1931, Dr. Otto Heinrich Warburg won the Nobel Prize in Medicine for his discovery that suboptimal oxygenation of tissues and cells is the underlying cause of cancer. Translation? Give your body oxygen! Yogis discovered thousands of years ago that the quality of one's breath has a direct and profound influence on the quality of one's life. *Pranayama*, therefore, is one of the best things you can do to keep your body filled with oxygen (and *prana!*).

In addition, evidence is building to support the claim that you can prevent many cancers by changing lifestyle habits like smoking, drinking, and high fat intake. However, knowing this doesn't help the person already afflicted with cancer, and might even make you feel worse. If you have cancer, don't blame yourself or waste time thinking about what you might have done differently. Instead, focus on your future and getting well.

Many cancers are curable, and even advanced cancers have been cured. Several studies have shown that cancer survivors tend to take charge of their illness by learning all they can about it and by having a positive attitude. Believe in yourself, the healing power of your body, and the healing power of your treatment regimen. Cultivate your own spirituality. Meditate, fill your lungs and body with *prana* through breathing exercises, and practice your Hatha Yoga routine slowly, steadily, and consistently to improve your circulation and overall strength. It is also important to eat a diet consisting of pure, whole foods. Bring meditation into your life. Meditation removes obstacles and illusions.

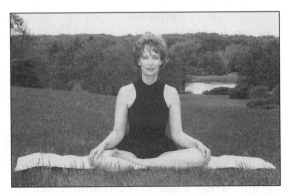

Meditating can bring positive energy to your mindbody, refreshing your immune system and your outlook.

Cardiovascular Disease

Your heart is the pump that keeps your body running. When your heart begins to lose efficiency or fails, your life is in immediate jeopardy. The best course of action is to prevent heart disease by eating a healthy, low-fat diet and by exercising regularly, but even perfectly healthy individuals are sometimes struck by cardiovascular disease. Maybe it's a matter of genetics. Sometimes the reason is a mystery. The treatment needn't be mysterious, however. In addition to your regular medical care, remember the following:

- Yoga can help you make the lifestyle changes you need for a better, happier heart. Yoga will decrease stress and increase circulation.

- The fastest way to reduce stress is to alter your breath. Deepen it. Inverted postures (Chapter 15) take pressure off your heart because it doesn't have to work as hard to pump blood to your extremities. More oxygen is pushed through the wall of your lungs, purifying your blood—but first get your doctor's permission to practice inversions.

- Yoga *asanas* in general stretch the major blood vessels, keeping them open and elastic.

Wise Yogi Tells Us

Even if you are unable to do a certain yoga pose because of illness, injury, or chronic pain, visualizing yourself going through a pose might increase the life force. First visualize the pose, then visualize flowing into the pose, becoming one with the pose, flowing out of the pose, and releasing. Like Pavlov's dog, we can ultimately think "Fish pose" and our body will benefit.

Diabetes

If you have diabetes, your blood has too much sugar and you might need to take insulin, which reduces blood sugar levels. Diabetes can be extremely serious if it isn't treated, but when treated, people with this condition can live virtually unencumbered by health problems.

For the diabetic, dietary control and weight control are crucial. Yoga is great for both and is, therefore, an excellent addition to the regular routine of anyone with diabetes. Yoga also helps with stress and improves the function of the pancreas, the organ that regulates blood sugar by producing insulin. Include the following in your routine:

◆ Obviously, you'll need a healthy diet. Yoga builds your confidence, concentration, and willpower, enabling you to want to stick with healthy eating habits.

◆ Because circulation in the extremities is important for those with diabetes, try resting your legs up against a wall as you lie back and relax. A slow, steady *vinyasana* routine will also help you maintain good circulation.

◆ Practice *pranayama* and meditation to help gain focus and control.

Illness, disease, and pain don't have to keep you from a fulfilling yoga practice. With your doctor's and yoga teacher's guidance, progress at a pace that is right for you and let yoga help your body help itself.

The Least You Need to Know

◆ Many things can cause or encourage illness or injury, from insufficient *prana* causing a depressed immune system to a lack of good hygiene to losing touch with your mindbody or becoming otherwise imbalanced.

◆ Don't blame yourself for getting sick or injured. Instead, focus on loving yourself and letting your body use its natural processes for healing.

◆ The regular practice of yoga *asanas* and *pranayama* exercises is a great way to prevent health problems and to help your body heal itself when health problems occur.

◆ Yoga can help with your minor health complaints, such as colds, minor back pain, and fatigue.

◆ With the approval of your doctor, yoga can also help more serious problems, such as diabetes, cancer, and migraine headaches.

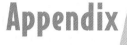

Glossary

Wondering about a yoga term? Here is your yoga terminology resource!

abhinivesha   Survival instinct.

adho mukha shavasana   Downward Facing Dog; a forward bend.

adho mukha vrksasana   The Handstand; an inversion.

adrenal glands   A pair of glands located just above the kidneys (in mammals); these glands secrete epinephrine (a stimulant) and certain steroids.

afferent nerves   The nerves that carry messages from the body to the brain.

ahimsa   One of the *yamas;* nonviolence.

allopathic medicine   The traditional medicine of Western culture, which focuses on a specific disease or problem and treats it.

Alzheimer's disease   A degenerative brain disease most common in the elderly.

ananda-maya-kosha   The bliss sheath and fifth sheath of existence.

anna-maya-kosha   The physical body and first sheath of existence.

apana   A type of *prana;* the vital energy of excretion that flows downward and out of the body, ridding it of impurities.

aparigraha   One of the *yamas;* nongreed.

ardha baddha padma pashchimottanasana   Bound Half Lotus pose; a seated forward-bending pose.

ardha baddha padmottanasana   Standing Half Bound Lotus pose; an advanced balancing pose.

asanas   The postures, or exercises, of yoga designed to help you master control of your body.

Ashtanga Yoga   Literally refers to the Eight Limbs of Yoga; in Western culture, this type of yoga has come to mean a Hatha Yoga practice that includes an intense *vinyasana* workout.

asmita   Ego or individuality.

asteya   One of the *yamas;* nonstealing.

astral body   The vehicle of the spirit, corresponding with the mind; higher than the physical body, but below the causal body.

aum   A sacred sound (also referred to as *om*) commonly used as a *mantra* during meditation and representative of the absolute or oneness of the universe; a rough approximation of the sound of the universe's vibration.

avidya   Incorrect comprehension.

baddha konasana   The Butterfly; a sitting posture.

baddha padmasana   The Bound Lotus; a meditative pose.

bandha   Literally "to bind" or "to lock," *bandhas* are muscular locks used during postures and breathing exercises to intensify the energy of *prana* so it can eliminate impurities from the body.

Bhagavad Gita   One of India's most beloved and famous sacred texts, this is the epic story of Arjuna, a warrior-prince who confronts moral dilemmas and is led to a better understanding of reality through the intercession of the god Krishna.

Bhakti Yoga   Sincere, heartfelt devotion to the divine is the primary focus of this type of yoga.

bhastrika   Literally "bellows," *bhastrika* is a breathing technique that imitates the action of a bellows.

bhramari   Also known as Bee Breath, this breathing technique imitates the sound of a bee.

bhujangasana   The Cobra; a backbend.

brahmacharya   One of the *yamas;* chastity or nonlust.

brahman   The absolute, or divinity itself.

buddhi   The intellect.

cakrasana   The Wheel; a backbend.

causal body   The subtlest body, it houses the spirit; higher than the physical and astral bodies.

chakras   Centers of energy that exist between the base of your spinal column and the crown of your head.

chandra namaskara   Moon salutation; a *vinyasana.*

circadian rhythms   The physiological rhythms people experience throughout the course of a 24-hour day.

dandasana   The Staff; a sitting posture.

deltoids   Muscles that lift and rotate the arms.

dhanurasana   The Bow; a backbend.

dharana   Orienting the mind toward a single point.

dhyana   Meditation, or the process of quieting the mind to free yourself from preconceptions and illusions.

diaphragm   A large, flat muscle at the base of the thoracic cavity that controls breathing.

duhkha   Pain, suffering, trouble, and discomfort; a mental state during which limitations and a profound sense of dissatisfaction are perceived.

dvesha   Refusal.

estrogen   Several hormones that produce sexual changes in female mammals.

fruitarian   A person who eats only raw fruits, "vegetable fruits" like tomatoes and cucumbers, nuts, and seeds, but nothing cooked or killed.

garudasana   The Eagle; a balance posture.

ghee   Clarified butter, or butter from which all solids have been removed, leaving only the oil; a traditional Indian food.

gomukhasana   The Cow; a sitting posture.

gunas   The three primary qualities existing in the universe—*sattva, rajas,* and *tamas*—can apply to the mind and to influences on the body, such as food.

guru   Literally "dispeller of darkness," a guru is a personal spiritual advisor who helps direct the yogi toward enlightenment.

halasana   The Plough; an inversion.

Hatha Yoga   A type of yoga primarily concerned with mastering control over the physical body as a path to enlightenment; Hatha Yoga combines opposing forces to achieve balance.

Hatha-Yoga-Pradipika   A fourteenth-century, comprehensive guide to Hatha Yoga.

holistic medicine   An approach to medicine in which the patient's entire lifestyle, environment, and personality are considered in the treatment of disease.

ida   A channel on the left side of the spine through which *prana* moves.

intercostals Muscles that expand the ribs.

ishvara-pranidhana One of the *niyamas;* centering on the divine.

jalandhara bandha A *bandha* that locks the throat.

janu shirshasana Sitting One Leg; a forward bend.

japa The process of repeating a *mantra* over and over for the purpose of clearing the mind.

Jnana Yoga This type of yoga emphasizes questioning, meditation, and contemplation as paths to enlightenment.

Jupiter *chakra* Located on the spine near the genitals, this energy center involves water, sexuality, passion, and the creation of life.

kali yuga The fourth of four ages (*yuga* means "age"), and the age in which we are now living; the shortest of all the ages, *kali yuga* is more than 432,000 years long.

kapalabhati A cleansing ritual for the respiratory tract, lungs, and sinuses; also called *skull shining.*

karma The law of cause and effect, or the movement toward balanced consciousness; everything you do, say, or even think has an immediate effect on the universe that will reverberate back to you in some way.

Karma Yoga Selfless action and service to others are emphasized in this type of yoga.

Kevali Kumbhaka A *pranayama* technique involving retaining the breath, it helps increase breath control and lung capacity.

koshas The five sheaths of existence that comprise the body.

Krishna A popular Hindu god.

Kriya Yoga The yoga of action and participation in life.

kundalini Literally "she who is coiled," *kundalini* is a psychospiritual energy force in the body that is often compared to a snake lying curled at the base of the spine, waiting to be awakened. When fully awakened, it is said to actually restructure the body, allowing the yogi to control previously involuntary bodily functions.

Kundalini Yoga This esoteric and mystical form of yoga is centered around awakening and employing *kundalini* energy.

kurmasana The Tortoise; a forward bend.

lacto vegetarianism A form of vegetarianism in which no meat, poultry, fish, or eggs are consumed; but milk and milk products are consumed.

lacto-ovo vegetarianism A form of vegetarianism in which no meat, poultry, or fish is consumed; but eggs, milk, and milk products are consumed.

larynx The area of the throat containing the vocal cords.

ligaments Bands of tissue connecting bones to bones or holding organs in place.

mandalas Beautiful, usually circular, geometric designs that draw your eye to the center and are used as a center of focus in meditation.

mano-maya-kosha The mind sheath and third sheath of existence.

mantra A sound or sounds that resonate in the body and evoke certain energies during meditation.

Mantra Yoga The chanting of *mantras* characterizes this type of yoga.

maricyasana The Half Spinal Twist; a twisting pose.

Mars *chakra* Located on the spine behind the navel, this energy center is associated with digestion or "gastric fire," your sense of self, and physical actions.

matsyasana The Fish; a backbend.

Matsyendra A Hindu sage and one of the first teachers of Hatha Yoga.

menopause The period in a woman's life, usually somewhere between her late 30s and her early 60s, when menstruation ceases.

Mercury *chakra* Located in the throat, this energy center governs communication.

moon *chakra* Located behind your head at the base of your skull, the moon *chakra* complements the sun *chakra*. Energy enters the moon *chakra*, travels down to the Saturn *chakra*, then rises up and exits the sun *chakra*.

mudhasana Child's pose; a forward bend.

mudras Hand gestures that direct the life current through the body.

mula bandha An anal lock.

murccha kumbkhaka A *pranayama* technique also known as third eye breathing, this exercise involves breathing with a focus on the third eye, or the area between and just above the eyebrows (the sixth *chakra*).

nadi shodhana A breathing exercise in which nostrils are alternated for inhalation and exhalation.

nadis Subtle vibratory passages of psychospiritual energy.

namaste mudra A *mudra* in which the hands are placed together in prayerlike fashion to honor the inner light.

naukasana The Full Boat; a balance pose.

nauli A cleansing ritual for the inner abdomen.

niyamas Five observances or personal disciplines, as defined by Patanjali in his *Yoga Sutras*; the *niyamas* are *saucha, santosha, tapas, svadhyaya,* and *ishvar-pranidhana*.

Occident The West (Europe and the Americas), as opposed to the Orient.

om A sacred sound (also referred to as *aum*) commonly used as a *mantra* during meditation and representative of the absolute or oneness of the universe; a rough approximation of the sound of the universe's vibration.

Orient The East (Asia), as opposed to the Occident.

padma shirshasana The Lotus Headstand; an inversion.

padmasana The Lotus pose, a meditative posture in which the legs are crossed and each foot is placed on the opposite thigh; the pose is said to resemble the perfection of the lotus flower.

parshvottanasana The Side Angle Stretch; a standing posture.

patella The kneecap.

pavana maktasana Also called Wind Relieving pose, this standing pose brings the knee to the chest, with head extended toward the knee.

pectorals Chest muscles that pull in and rotate the arms.

physical body The lowest of the three bodies, the physical body is the body we see; the other bodies are the astral body and the causal body.

pingala A channel on the right side of the spine through which *prana* moves.

pituitary gland A gland attached to the brain that secretes hormones affecting growth.

PMS An acronym for premenstrual syndrome.

postpartum depression A condition experienced by at least 50 percent of new mothers; characterized by depression, anxiety, drastic mood swings, and spontaneous weeping in the week after childbirth.

prana A form of energy in the universe that animates all physical matter, including the human body; the vital energy of respiration and the soul of the universe.

prana-maya-kosha The vital body and second sheath of existence.

pranayama Breathing exercises designed to help you master control of your breath.

pratyahara Withdrawal of the senses.

premenstrual syndrome A syndrome experienced by some women one to two weeks before the onset of menstruation; symptoms may include irritability, depression, restlessness, back pain, bloating, and swelling.

purvottanasana The Hands to Feet pose; a variation of the Plough; an inversion.

raga Attachment.

Raja Yoga Also known as The Royal Path, this type of yoga emphasizes control of the intellect to attain enlightenment.

rajas The quality of high activity and agitation; a *guna*.

Rig Veda Literally "Knowledge of Praise," the *Rig Veda* consists of 1,028 hymns and is the oldest known reference to yoga and possibly the oldest known text in the world.

roga Sickness.

samadhi The state of meditation in which ego disappears and all becomes one; a state of absolute bliss.

samyama When in a state of *samyama*, the yogi has investigated, concentrated on, meditated upon, and contemplated an object or subject until everything about it is known and understood.

santosha One of the *niyamas*; contentment.

sartorius The muscle that twists the thigh and bends the hip and knee.

sarvangasana The Shoulderstand; an inversion.

sattva The quality of clarity and lightness; a *guna*.

Saturn *chakra* Located just above the anus at the base of the spine, this energy center involves elimination and your sense of smell.

satya One of the *yamas*; truthfulness.

saucha One of the *niyamas*; purity, or inner and outer cleanliness.

scapula The shoulder blade.

sciatic nerve A long nerve that starts in the hip and runs down the leg.

sciatica A painful condition felt in the hip or thigh and down the back of the leg, resulting from inflammation of the sciatic nerve.

sensory nerves The nerves that carry messages from the brain to the body.

setu bandha sarvangasana The Bridge; an inversion.

shat kriyas Purification rituals.

shavasana Also known as Corpse pose, this pose is meant to bring the body and mind into total, conscious relaxation.

shirshasana The Headstand; an inversion.

shodhana Yogic cleansing rituals.

sitali A breathing technique involving rolling the tongue, then inhaling through it like a straw; a cooling technique.

sitar A stringed instrument from India, similar to a mandolin.

sprain An injury to a ligament.

sternum The breastbone, a flat bone to which the ribs are attached.

sthala basti A yoga cleansing ritual for the colon, also called ground colon cleansing, involving the churning of the abdominal muscles.

sthira Steadiness and alertness.

strain An injury to a muscle or its tendon.

sukha Lightness and comfort.

sukhasana Easy pose; a meditative pose.

Suchakra Located in the middle of your brow, this energy center is also known as the third eye, or center of unclouded perception.

surya namaskara Sun Salutation; a *vinyasana*.

sushumna A hollow passageway between *pingala* and *ida* that runs through the spinal cord, and through which *kundalini* can travel once it is awakened.

svadhyaya One of the *niyamas*; the process of inquiring into your own nature, the nature of your beliefs, and the nature of the world's spiritual journey.

svamin A title of respect for a spiritual person who is master of her- or himself rather than others.

svasthya Health.

swami The Anglicized form of *svamin*.

Swami Vivekananda A guru from India who addressed the Parliament of Religions in 1893, and quickly became a popular figure; he was followed by a number of other *swamis* who came to the United States to teach and guide Westerners along the Eastern path of yoga.

tadasana   The Mountain; a standing posture.

tamas   The quality of heaviness and inactivity; a *guna*.

Tantra Yoga   This type of yoga is characterized by certain rituals designed to awaken the *kundalini*.

tapas   One of the *niyamas*; self-discipline.

tendon   Tough, connective tissue attaching muscles to bones.

thoracic cavity   The cavity containing your lungs and heart.

Thousand Petalled Lotus *chakra*   Located at the crown of the skull, this energy center is the core of self-realization, perspective, unity, and enlightenment.

thyroid gland   Located near the trachea, this gland secretes hormones that affect growth.

tibia   The inner and thicker bone of the two bones of the lower leg.

tibialis anterior   Muscles that raise the foot.

trachea   The passageway through which air travels after inhalation.

Transcendental Meditation   Also known as TM, this form of meditation involves the mental repetition of a *mantra*.

trikonasana   The Triangle or Happy pose; a standing posture.

uddiyana bandha   A *bandha* that locks the abdomen.

ujjayi   A breathing exercise that produces sound in the throat with the inhalation; literally, "she who is victorious."

ulna   The larger of the two bones of the forearm.

Upanishads   Scriptures of ancient Hindu philosophy.

urdhvamukha shvanasana   The Upward Facing Dog; a backbend.

ustrasana   The Camel; a backbend.

utkatasana   The Lightning Bolt; a standing posture.

uttanasana   Standing Head to Knee; a forward bend.

uttanatavasana   Leg Lifts.

vajrasana   Kneeling pose; a meditative pose.

vashisthasana   The Arm Balance; a balance posture.

veganism   A form of vegetarianism in which no animal products of any kind are consumed.

vegetarianism   A diet in which no meat is consumed.

Venus *chakra*   Located behind your heart, this energy center is the seat of your compassion.

vidya   Correct understanding.

vijnana-maya-kosha   The intellect sheath and fourth sheath of existence.

vinyasana   A steady flow of connected yoga *asanas* linked with breathwork in a continuous movement; a particularly dynamic form of yoga.

virabhadrasana   The Warrior; a standing posture.

virasana   The Hero; a sitting posture.

vrikshasana   The Tree; a balance posture.

vyadhi   Disease.

yamas   Five abstinences that purify the body and mind, as defined by Patanjali in his *Yoga Sutras*; the *yamas* are *ahimsa*, *satya*, *asteya*, *brahmacharya*, and *aparigraha*.

yoga *mudra*   A forward bend.

Yoga Sutras   The source of Patanjali's Eightfold Path, this collection of succinct aphorisms has largely defined the modern concept of yoga.

yogi   Someone who practices yoga.

yogic   An adjective describing things that are associated with yoga.

yogini   A female yogi.

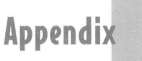

Farther Along the Yoga Path: Suggested Reading

Welcome! Now that you've begun your yoga practice with *The Complete Idiot's Guide to Yoga Illustrated, Third Edition*, no doubt you'll want to read more about the many aspects of yoga, find out how to incorporate yoga into your everyday life, and enhance your yoga practice. Here's a great list of books to help guide you on your yoga path!

Adamson, Eve, and Linda Horning, R.D. *The Complete Idiot's Guide to Fasting*. Indianapolis: Alpha Books, 2002.

Anderson, Sandra, and Rolf Sovik, Psy.D., *Yoga: Mastering the Basics*. Honesdale, PA: The Himalayan Institute Press, 2000.

Balch, James F., and Phyllis A. Balch. *Prescription for Nutritional Healing, 2nd Edition*. Garden City Park, NY: Avery Publishing Group, Inc., 1996.

Ballentine, Rudolph. *Transition to Vegetarianism*. Honesdale, PA: The Himalayan Institute Press, 1999.

Bender Birch, Beryl. *Beyond Power Yoga: 8 Levels of Practice for Body and Soul*. New York: Fireside, 2000.

———. *Power Yoga*. New York: Simon & Schuster, 1995.

Bhagavad Gita (multiple translations available).

Bouanchaud, Bernard. *The Essence of Yoga*. Portland: Rudra Press, 1997.

Bstan-'dzin-rgya-mtsho, Dalai Lama XIV (His Holiness the Dalai Lama). *The Art of Happiness*. New York: Riverhead Books, 1998.

———. *Healing Anger*. Ithaca, New York: Snow Lion Publications, 1997.

Budilovsky, Joan. *Fat-Free Yoga*. Oak Brook, IL: YOYOGA!, 1997.

———. *The Little Yogi Energy Book*. Oak Brook, IL: YOYOGA!, 1997.

———. *Yoga for a New Day*. Oak Brook, IL: YOYOGA!, 1996.

Budilovsky, Joan, and Eve Adamson. *The Complete Idiot's Guide to Massage*. Indianapolis: Alpha Books, 1998.

———. *The Complete Idiot's Guide to Meditation, Second Edition*. Indianapolis: Alpha Books, 2002.

Carper, Jean. *Jean Carper's Total Nutrition Guide*. New York: Bantam Books, 1987.

Chearney, Lee Ann. *Visits Caring for an Aging Parent: Reflections and Advice*. New York: Three Rivers Press, 1998.

Chopra, Deepak. *Ageless Body, Timeless Mind*. New York: Harmony Books, 1993.

Choudhury, Bikram. *Bikram's Beginning Yoga Class*. New York: G.P. Putnam's Sons, 1978.

Christensen, Alice. *The Easy Does It Yoga Trainer's Guide*. Sarasota, FL: American Yoga Association, 1995.

———. *Yoga of the Heart*. New York: Daybreak Books, 1998.

Cloutier, Marissa, M.S., R.D., Deborah S. Romaine, and Eve Adamson. *Beef Busters: Less Beef, Better Health!* Avon, MA: Adams Media Corporation, 2002.

Cloutier, Marissa, M.S., R.D., and Eve Adamson. *The Mediterranean Diet*. New York: HarperTouch, 2001.

Couch, Jean. *The Runner's Yoga Book*. Berkeley, CA: Rodmell Press, 1990.

de Mello, Anthony. *Wellsprings: A Book of Spiritual Exercises*. New York: Doubleday, 1984.

———. *Awareness: The Perils and Opportunities of Reality*. New York: Doubleday, 1992.

———. *Sadhana, A Way to God: Christian Exercises in Eastern Form*. New York: Doubleday, 1984.

Desikachar, T.K.V. *The Heart of Yoga: Developing a Personal Practice*. Rochester, VT: Inner Traditions International, 1995.

Dewey, John. *Experience and Education*. New York: Touchstone Edition, 1997.

Duff, Gail. *Eating Vegetarian: A Step-by-Step Guide*. Great Britain: Element Books Limited, 1999.

Farhi, Donna. *The Breathing Book: Good Health and Vitality Through Essential Breath Work*. New York: Henry Holt and Company, 1996.

Feldman, Gail, Ph.D., and Katherine A. Gleason. *Releasing the Goddess Within*. Indianapolis: Alpha Books, 2002.

Feuerstein, Georg. *The Shambhala Guide to Yoga*. Boston: Shambhala Publications, Inc., 1996.

———. *The Yoga Sutra of Patanjali: A New Translation and Commentary*. Rochester, VT: Inner Traditions, International, 1979.

Feuerstein, Georg, and Stephan Bodian, eds., with the staff of *Yoga Journal*. *Living Yoga: A Comprehensive Guide for Daily Life*. New York: Jeremy P. Tarcher/Perigee Books, 1993.

Flinders, Carol Lee. *At the Root of This Longing: Reconciling a Spiritual Hunger and a Feminist Thirst*. San Francisco: HarperSanFrancisco, 1998.

Francina, Suza. *The New Yoga for People over 50*. Deerfield Beach, FL: Health Communications, Inc., 1997.

Franks, Samskrti, and Judith. *Hatha Yoga Manual Two*. Honesdale, PA: The Himalayan International Institute, 1979.

Gandhi, Mahatma. *All Men Are Brothers.* India: Navajivan Publishing House, 1960.

Gandhi, Mohandask. *Gandhi's Health Guide.* Freedom, CA: The Crossing Press.

Gunther, Bernard. *Energy Ecstasy and Your Seven Vital Chakras.* North Hollywood, CA: Newcastle Publishing, 1983.

Hanh, Thich Nhat. *Peace Is Every Step.* New York: Bantam Books, 1991.

Hanna, Thomas. *Somatics.* Reading, MA: Addison Wesley, 1988.

Harrar, Sari, and Sara Altshul O'Donnell. *The Woman's Book of Healing Herbs.* Emmaus, PA: Rodale Press, Inc., 1999.

Harvey, Andrew. *The Essential Mystics: The Soul's Journey into Truth.* San Francisco: HarperSanFrancisco, 1996.

Hess, Herbert J., and Tucker, Charles O. *Talking About Relationships.* Kendall/Hunt: Dubuque, IA, 1976.

Hewitt, James. *Teach Yourself Yoga.* Lincolnwood (Chicago), IL: NTC Publishing Group, 1993.

Hittleman, Richard. *Yoga for Health: The Total Program.* New York: Ballantine Books, 1983.

Iyengar, B.K.S. *Light on Yoga.* New York: Schocken Books, 1979.

———. *Yoga: The Path to Holistic Health.* New York, DK Publishing, 2001.

Japananda, Swami K. *Yoga, You, Your New Life.* Chicago: The Temple of Kriya Yoga, 1981.

Kabat-Zinn, Jon, Ph.D. *Full Catastrophe Living: Using the Wisdom of Your Body and Mind to Face Stress, Pain, and Illness.* New York: Delta, 1990.

Komitor, Jodi M., and Eve Adamson. *The Complete Idiot's Guide to Yoga with Kids.* Indianapolis: Alpha Books, 2000.

Kraftsow, Gary. *Yoga for Wellness.* New York: Penguin, 1999.

Kriyanada, Goswami. *Extraordinary Spiritual Potential.* Chicago: The Temple of Kriya Yoga, 1988.

———. *The Laws of Karma.* Chicago: The Temple of Kriya Yoga, 1995.

———. *The Spiritual Science of Kriya Yoga.* Chicago: The Temple of Kriya Yoga, 1992.

Kriyananda, Sri (J. Donald Walters). *Yoga Postures for Higher Awareness.* Nevada City, CA: Crystal Clarity, 1967.

Lasater, Judith, Ph.D. *Relax and Renew.* Berkeley, CA: Rodmell Press, 1995.

Lerner, Michael. *Choices in Healing: Integrating the Best of Conventional and Complementary Approaches to Cancer.* Cambridge, MA: MIT Press, 1994.

LeVert, Suzanne, and Gary McClain, Ph.D. *The Complete Idiot's Guide to Breaking Bad Habits, Second Edition.* Indianapolis: Alpha Books, 2001.

Levitt, Atma JoAnne. *The Kripalu Cookbook.* Stockbridge, MA: Berkshire House Publishers, 1995.

Mahabharata (numerous translations available).

Marshall, J. Dan, James T. Sears, and William J. Schubert. *Turning Points in Curriculum: A Contemporary American Memoir.* Upper Saddle River, NJ: Prentice Hall, 2000.

McClain, Gary R., Ph.D., and Eve Adamson. *The Complete Idiot's Guide to Zen Living.* Indianapolis: Alpha Books, 2000.

McHugh, Richard P., SJ., Ph.D. *Mind with a Heart.* India: Sadhana Institute, 1998.

McLaren, Karla. *Rebuilding the Garden.* Columbia, CA: Laughing Tree Press, 1997.

Mehta, Silva, and Shyam Mihra. *Yoga the Iyengar Way.* New York: A.A. Knopf, 1990.

Mishra, Rammurti S., M.D. *Fundamentals of Yoga.* New York: Harmony Books, 1987.

Monro, Robin, R. Nagaranthna, and H. R. Nagendra. *Yoga for Common Ailments.* New York: Fireside, 1990.

Moyers, Bill. *Healing and the Mind.* New York: Doubleday, 1993.

O'Brien, Paddy. *Yoga for Women: Complete Mind and Body Fitness.* London: Thorsons, 1994.

Paley, Vivian Gussin. *The Boy Who Would Be a Helicopter.* London: Harvard University Press, 1990.

Prabhupada, A. C., and Swami Bhaktivedanta. *Bhagavad-Gita as It Is.* Los Angeles: Bhaktivedanta Book Trust, 1968.

Rama, Swami. *Living with the Himalayan Masters.* Honesdale, PA: The Himalayan Institute Press, 1999.

———. *Path of Fire and Light.* Honesdale, PA: The Himalayan Institute Press, 1996.

Ramayana (numerous translations available).

Ravindra, Ravi. *Christ the Yogi.* Rochester, VT: Inner Traditions, 1998.

Rieker, Hans-Ulrich. *The Yoga of Light: Hatha Yoga Pradipika.* Middletown, CA: The Dawn House Press, 1971.

Rig Veda (multiple translations available).

Rush, Anne Kent. *The Modern Book of Yoga.* New York: Dell Publishing, 1996.

Satchidananda, Yogiraj Sri Swami. *Integral Yoga Hatha.* Satchidananda Ashram-Yogaville, VA: Integral Yoga Publications, 1998.

Scaravelli, Vanda. *Awakening the Spine.* New York: HarperCollins, 1991.

Schatz, Mary Pullig, M.D. *Back Care Basics.* Berkeley, CA: Rodnell Press, 1992.

Schiffmann, Erich. *Yoga: The Spirit and Practice of Moving Into Stillness.* New York: Pocket Books, 1996.

Sivananda Yoga Vedanta Center. *Learn Yoga in a Weekend.* New York: Alfred A. Knopf, 1995.

———. *The Sivananda Companion to Yoga.* New York: Simon & Schuster, 1983.

———. *Yoga Mind Body.* New York: DK Publishing, 1996.

Somar, Sonia. *Yoga for the Special Child.* Buckingham, VA: Special Yoga Publications, 1998.

Stewart, Mary, and Kathy Phillips. *Yoga for Children.* London: Webster's International Publishers, 1992.

Takoma, Geo, and Eve Adamson. *The Complete Idiot's Guide to Power Yoga.* Indianapolis: Alpha Books, 1999.

Tigunait, Pandit Rajmani. *Inner Quest: The Path of Spiritual Unfoldment.* Honesdale, PA: Yoga International Books, 1995.

Upanishads (multiple translations available).

Vishnudevananda, Swami. *The Complete Illustrated Book of Yoga.* New York: Bell Publishers, 1960.

Yogananda, Paramahansa. *Autobiography of a Yogi.* Los Angeles: Self-Realization Fellowship, 1946.

———. *Journey to Self-Realization: Discovering the Gifts of the Soul.* Los Angeles: Self-Realization Fellowship, 1997.

Yogi Bhajan, Ph.D. *Kundalini Yoga: The Flow of Eternal Power.* Los Angeles: Time Capsule Books, 1996.

Yukteswar, Swami Sri. *The Holy Science.* Los Angeles: Self-Realization Fellowship, 1949.

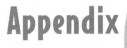

Appendix **C**

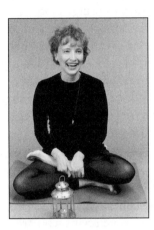

Yo Joan!

The "Yo Joan" column began appearing on Joan's Yoyoga! website in 1996. Letters quickly started coming in from all over the world. Today, Joan writes globally and locally in areas of alternative health care and stress reduction. Go Yo Joan! What's your question? Write to Joan at www.yoyoga.com.

Q: I want to lose weight quickly. Is yoga for me?

Joan: *Yoga* means "union"—union of bodymindspirit. Yoga isn't a weight-loss program. It's a practice and a lifestyle approach that can make us more aware of where we're out of sync and where we're in sync. As you study yoga, you will become more keenly aware of your potential and the beauty that's within you. You'll grow to also see more clearly the beauty that exists within all of life. When you begin to see this, you begin to bring your life into balance.

For example, let's say you're focused on one part of your body that you feel is grossly overweight—let's say it's your stomach. Every time you look at your body in the mirror, your eyes gravitate toward your stomach and you become upset. Yoga helps you see that you are more than your stomach. No matter how grand your stomach is, you are ever so much grander than that!

And so, you begin to learn ways of helping your stomach, rather than hurting it. You begin to see it as part of you and not as a separate part of you. In this process, you begin to learn nonviolence. Soon, you develop an appreciation for your stomach and treat it more kindly by what you ingest and also how you move and hold yourself. Soon, your eyes begin to love your stomach. When you look in the mirror, you begin to see a reflection of health. Your stomach size will change as your view of who you are deepens. This is an example of the study of yoga.

Q: I have a very stressful and busy life. Will the time I take practicing yoga help me?

Joan: Yoga is stress-reducing. Yoga works in harmony with the balance of your body and the balance of nature. We spend much of our life fighting nature, trying to control it. For example, on a physical level, gravity is constantly pulling at us. Yoga says yes to gravity! Yoga plays with it. It befriends it. It helps us understand we can actually move our bodies in various directions and gravity can help in the movements. We don't fight gravity. We say "Welcome! Let's be friends!" So if you're looking for an oasis of peace in a stressful world, the study of yoga helps create a more peaceful environment.

Q: My daughter has Downs syndrome. Will yoga help her?

Joan: Because yoga is a study of balance, we can all benefit from studying yoga no matter what our physical or mental condition. Yoga calms the nerves. It helps us take the time to realize that something as simple as one's breath can have a profound influence on one's life and the lives around us. It's not complicated—although some of the poses might appear that way. It's the limitations of the mind that encourages complicated approaches. Some of us don't need advanced poses to derive the benefits of yoga. The benefits come about from a reordering of priorities. A benefit can be as simple as learning to take a slow breath before making an important decision.

I would encourage not only your daughter to take a yoga class, but for you to as well—or, even better, with her. Although the particular struggles we have in life vary from person to person, we're all here, today, intimately connected in this healing journey we call life. According to yoga, we are all one. *Om.*

Q: Do you have to give up meat to practice yoga?

Joan: Many yogis practice vegetarianism, but not all yogis are vegetarians. Nonviolence (*ahimsa*) is a principle that is studied in yoga. There are various ways to bring *ahimsa* more clearly into one's life. Some find the path of vegetarianism to be one of these ways. There are also many other ways, such as abstaining from negative gossip or negative self-talk. What area of your life can benefit from the further development of nonviolence? Vegetarianism might be one way for you.

Vegetarianism does not give someone a kind heart, yet a kind heart often leads to vegetarianism. This might sound like some kind of Zen riddle, so let me explain further: There are many people who are vegetarians who are not kind. They are vegetarians for various reasons—some can not afford meat, others find it healthier to abstain from eating meat, some don't like the taste of meat, still others don't have access to meat, etc. All these reasons for being vegetarian can involve a kind heart, but they don't necessitate a kind heart. A heart that encompasses a sincere love for sentient creatures of all forms is a heart that breathes nonviolence—and this is, indeed, a kind heart.

Q: Will yoga improve my sex life?

Joan: Yoga creates a stronger, more flexible, and more balanced body. This balance extends into all of life. How can your bodymindspirit prosper? As one becomes richer in the knowledge of the self, one becomes richer in the knowledge of all of life. Yoga can help you improve your life—every beautiful aspect of it, and yes, that includes the sexual part.

Index

More Books and Tapes by Joan Budilovsky

Special Offer for Readers of
The Complete Idiot's Guide to Yoga Illustrated, Third Edition

New– *Yoga with Joan* CD

Joan's ever-popular audio recording is now in a beautiful CD! Fifty minutes of invigorating postures and breathwork. Join Joan to start your day the yoga way. **$11.00**

Additional Tapes and Books

Yoga Audio Cassettes

Breathworks! **$10.00**
Thirty minutes of yoga deep-breathing exercises.

Sun-Salutations! with Joan **$10.00**
A dynamic series of yoga postures with meditation exercises.

Total Relaxation with Shavasana **$10.00**
Shavasana + meditation = BLISS.

Beach Blanket Yoga **$10.00**
Thirty minutes of yoga fun in the sun.

Yoga CD

Body and Soul Meditation **$12.00**
Harp music, Joan's voice, and you.

Yoga Books

The Little Yogi Water Book **$8.00**
Splish, splash, and learn water yoga with Joan.

The Little Yogi Energy Book **$8.00**
Energize yourself with these terrific *chakra* postures.

Yoga for a New Day **$10.00**
Compact yoga lifestyle guides with simple postures.

Yo Joan **$10.00**
Thoughtful responses to your yoga questions from the popular Yoyoga! website.

Massage Audio Cassette

The Art of Massage Made Simple **$11.00**
Joan guides you in giving a one-hour full-body massage.

Foot Massage for Body, Mind, and Sole **$10.00**
Relax your feet. Relax your whole body.

Massage Video

My Swedish Massage with Joan **$19.50**
Spirited and instructional video on many of the massage strokes featured in *The Complete Idiot's Guide to Massage*.

Come visit Joan at her "Yoyoga!" website: www.yoyoga.com
Order form on NEXT PAGE

Yes, send me copies of Joan's wonderful tapes and books.

Special CD Offer
❑ *Yoga with Joan* $11.00

Yoga Audio Cassettes
❑ *Breathworks!* $10.00
❑ *Sun-Salutations! with Joan* $10.00
❑ *Total Relaxation with Shavasana* $10.00
❑ *Beach Blanket Yoga* $10.00

Yoga CD
❑ *Body and Soul Meditation* $12.00

Yoga Books
❑ *The Little Yogi Water Book* $8.00
❑ *The Little Yogi Energy Book* $8.00
❑ *Yoga for a New Day* $10.00
❑ *Yo Joan* $10.00

Massage Audio Cassette
❑ *The Art of Massage Made Simple* $11.00
❑ *Foot Massage for Body, Mind, and Sole* $10.00

Massage Video
❑ *My Swedish Massage with Joan* $19.50

Shipping/handling charges:
Audio/book   Add $2.50 for one or two items; add $.50 for each additional item.
Video   Add $4.50 for first videotape; add $1.00 for each additional videotape.

             _____
             _____
         Subtotal _____
Illinois residents add 6.75% sales tax _____
Outside United States add $5.00 additional shipping and handling _____
TOTAL _____

Payment to be made in U.S. funds. Prices and availability are subject to change without notice.
❑ Check or money order enclosed.
❑ I would like to charge to: ❑ MasterCard   ❑ Visa
     Acct. #: _____
     Exp. Date: _____
     Signature: _____

Send this order form with your check, money order, or charge information to:

Yoyoga, Inc.
PO Box 5013
Oak Brook, IL 60522
Phone: 630-963-1906
Fax: 630-963-4001

Allow four to six weeks for delivery.

Ship to:
Name: _____
Address: _____
City, State, Zip: _____
Telephone: _____